Encyclopedia of Diet Fads

ENCYCLOPEDIA OF DIET FADS

Marjolijn Bijlefeld and Sharon K. Zoumbaris

GREENWOOD PRESS
Westport, Connecticut • London

Library of Congress Cataloging-in-Publication Data

Bijlefeld, Marjolijn, 1960–
    Encyclopedia of diet fads / Marjolijn Bijlefeld and Sharon K. Zoumbaris.
      p. cm.
    Includes bibliographical references and index.
    ISBN 0–313–32223–6 (alk. paper)
    1. Reducing diets—Encyclopedias. 2. Weight loss—Encyclopedias.
I. Zoumbaris, Sharon K., 1955– II. Title.
RM222.2.B535 2002
613.2'5'03—dc21   2002192821

British Library Cataloguing in Publication Data is available.

Library of Congress Catalog Card Number: 2002192821
ISBN: 0–313–32223–6

First published in 2003

Greenwood Press, 88 Post Road West, Westport, CT 06881
An imprint of Greenwood Publishing Group, Inc.
www.greenwood.com

Printed in the United States of America

The paper used in this book complies with the
Permanent Paper Standard issued by the National
Information Standards Organization (Z39.48–1984).

10 9 8 7 6 5 4 3 2 1

Contents

Introduction

What will Americans do to lose weight? Just about anything, it seems. Over the past century, a variety of quick and easy fixes have flooded the market. Many of these products or devices are costly; some are not safe; and some are simply outrageous. Consider a bristle brush to scrub fat away or magic weight loss earrings.

Dietitians and physicians will say that there is only one fundamental combination to help most people lose weight: eat less and exercise more. Through its Dietary Guidelines for Americans, the government recommends an assortment of foods that include vegetables, fruits, grains, fat-free or low-fat milk products, fish, lean meat, poultry, and beans.

This volume introduces a wide variety of weight loss means and methods. Some entries describe a particular diet; some describe a support group or service; and some entries focus on the people who have changed the way Americans eat. It combines advice from nutritionists and physicians, weight loss gurus, and government and private agencies whose role it is to oversee the weight loss industry.

No doubt, there will be disagreements about the effectiveness of a certain diet plan. One person may swear by the high-protein diet while another may swear by a plan that restricts or permits only certain foods. Entries may contain a description of the diet plan and arguments from those who say it is unsafe.

While weight loss may not seem like a topic of debate, there are distinct and seemingly opposing voices. Indeed, the voices of those who advocate a low-carbohydrate diet have gained volume recently. In essence, they say that the emphasis on low-fat diets over the past few decades has not resulted in weight loss for Americans. In fact, just the opposite. More American adults and children are overweight and obese today than just a decade ago. They blame carbohydrates, which cause insulin levels to spike, which in turn make people feel hungrier again sooner. They say that diets rich in high-fat foods and low in carbohydrates will help people lose weight.

Yet that doesn't mean that Americans should immediately forgo the salad and order more fries. The headlines may be more sensational than the truth. Much of mainstream medicine still stands by its emphasis on a balanced diet limiting high-fat and high cholesterol foods.

What is happening with the current debate mirrors what happens so often with weight loss topics: Americans are looking for a quick fix. People want to eat a food or type of food that will make the pounds disappear. Or they want to avoid a food or certain foods that will cause them to put on weight.

There's no doubt that people have lost some weight following specific diet plans. But is it the best way, or even the only way to lose weight? Probably not. For most people, moderation may do the trick. Cut down on sweets, cut down on fats, cut down on carbohydrates. Increase your level of daily physical activity. The result is fewer calories consumed and more calories burned. In the long run, this combination results in long-lasting weight maintenance, not just a quick-fix weight loss.

In all cases, before starting a diet to aggressively lose weight, see a doctor. Too sudden or rapid a weight loss can have severe consequences. And realize, too, that losing weight is just one part of healthy living. Maintaining a good weight and a diet that provides you with enough energy to feel good and be active is a lifelong goal.

Early History of Dieting and Fad Diets

In dieting, as in life, everybody wants a quick answer, a quick meal, and quick success. The elusive promise of quick weight loss is the driving force behind the popularity of best-selling books, powders, liquids, pills, and programs. Each year these new fad diets appear on the scene—everything from high-protein, low-carbohydrate plans to fasting and liquid meals. And Americans—teens included—desperate to lose weight, embrace them enthusiastically. At any given time, 15 percent to 35 percent of Americans are actively dieting. And they have good reason to be concerned about losing weight since the latest findings from the Centers for Disease Control and Prevention's National Health and Nutrition Examination Survey (NHANES) show an estimated 61 percent of U.S. adults are either overweight or obese. Those 1999 survey results also show the number of overweight teenagers 12 to 19 years old increased from 11 percent to 14 percent in the six years studied.

These sobering statistics go a long way toward explaining why the lure of quick, easy weight-loss schemes is so hard to resist. Unfortunately, fad diets aren't healthy and don't work for the long haul. Consider this: 95 percent of all dieters will regain their lost weight in one to five years; 35 percent of "normal dieters" progress to pathological dieting or full-blown eating disorders; Americans spend more than $40 billion on dieting and diet-related products each year.

Not only are diet theories and products nothing new, they date back centuries to a time when people had no scientific understanding of digestion and food assimilation. And while today's consumers make their decisions based on improved research and understanding of how the body works, they still fall victim to fad diets that focus on one true aspect of nutrition, which is then exaggerated to an extreme. For women in particular, the lure of fast, effortless weight loss is strongly tied to the demands of fashion and beauty.

Thinness as a beauty ideal surfaced in the early 1800s with the emerging Victorian woman. This thin, genteel, docile creature replaced the idealized voluptuous women painted in the sixteenth and seventeenth centuries by artists like Rembrandt and Rubens. And as thinness became the defining feature of beauty in the United States, an eighteen-inch waist became the Holy Grail of physical perfection. Unfortunately, this measurement was so out of line with normal body dimensions that to achieve it most women resorted to a practice called tightlacing, a procedure immortalized in Margaret Mitchell's *Gone With the Wind*. This extreme corset tightening eventually caused headaches, fainting spells, and uterine and spinal disorders.

In the 1830s, as literacy increased, technology advanced, and the publishing industry expanded, American women became the target of medical-advice books as well as beauty manuals, all of which encouraged thinness. Still, there were critics like writer Harriet Beecher Stowe who vigorously lamented the increasing problems associated with dieting and the national preoccupation with thinness. Lois Banner in *American Beauty,* quoted Beecher Stowe's opinion of the misuse of dieting by American women. "We in America have got so far out of the way of a womanhood that has any vigor of outline or opulence of physical proportions, that, when we see a woman made as a woman ought to be, she strikes us as a monster. Our willowy girls are afraid of nothing so much as growing stout; and if a young lady begins to round into proportions like the women in Titian's or Gorgione's picture, she is distressed above measure, and begins to make secret inquiries into reducing diet, and to cling desperately to the strongest corset."

A decade earlier the popular English poet, Lord Byron, influenced beauty and diet practices and standards in America as well as in Europe. According to scholars, Byron was known for his tendency to gain weight. By 1822 the poet had starved himself into what biographers call an unnatural thinness. In fact, Banner in *American Beauty* traces the popularity of drinking vinegar to lose weight to Byron, whose favorite weight-loss regimen was to subsist for some days on vinegar and water. But Byron's most lasting contribution to the popularity of fad diets came from his statement that the sight of a woman eating was disgusting. Biographer Leslie A. Marchand attributed this quote to the poet in *Byron: A Portrait.* "A woman," he wrote, "should never be seen eating or drinking, unless it be lobster salad and champagne, the only truly feminine and becoming viands." Following this remark, fashion historians say women in Europe and the United States took up systematic fasting. Indeed, thanks to Byron and other cultural factors, dieting was commonplace by 1900.

Others who influenced society's early love affair with diets included Englishman William Banting, credited with writing the first diet book. Born in 1797, by age forty the 5-foot-5-inch Banting was extremely obese. He consulted doctor after doctor but nothing helped and his growing girth was ruining his life. By age sixty he was unable to stoop and tie his shoes and he walked backwards down the stairs to lessen the stress on his joints. Finally, in 1863 at age sixty-six, he consulted Dr. William Harvey, a surgeon known for his starch- and sugar-free diet treatment for diabetes. Banting immediately lost weight by eating only lean meats and dry toast and eventually went from a high of 202 pounds to a comfortable 156 pounds. Eager to share his success with the world, Banting wrote his diet book, a testimonial titled *A Letter on Corpulence*. Following its publication, *Banting* or *to bant*, meaning to diet, became a household word in England and in America. At his death in 1878 more than 58,000 copies of his diet book had been sold, and a total of twelve editions had been published between 1863 and 1902.

Meanwhile, in America in 1837, talk of diet and health nearly incited a riot in Boston. Sylvester Graham, an evangelical New England preacher and speaker faced an angry mob one evening as he attempted to lecture on food and hygiene reform. Graham was a controversial figure whose Spartan views on diet and drinking had strongly divided the Boston crowd. Critics of Grahamism included the writer Ralph Waldo Emerson, who mocked Graham as "the prophet of bran bread and pumpkins." While Graham was also called the father of all modern diet crazes, he is most widely remembered as the namesake of the graham cracker. His career as a lecturer grew out of his earlier study of human physiology, diet, and nutrition, a choice largely influenced by his 1830 appointment as general agent for the Pennsylvania Temperance Society. During this time Graham developed the "Graham system," as he liked to call it, based on the French vitalist school of medicine. He believed nutrition had moral as well as physical qualities and any desire for food or drink, except for stark hunger and thirst, was depraved. Gluttony was a debilitating expression of an unhealthy urge and Graham was determined to launch an all-out war on debauchery and gluttony.

Graham was one of the first American health reformers to reach a mass audience via lectures. He traveled a circuit through Massachusetts, Rhode Island, Maine, New York, New Jersey, and Pennsylvania. In his talks he recommended a strictly vegetarian diet but did allow for a small daily ration of roasted beef or boiled mutton for those who wanted some meat. He did not believe in cooking vegetables or in warm food in general since he considered heat a stimulant. And he was particularly adamant about the evils of commercially baked white bread, made from highly refined flour. Graham argued that any good wife and mother must feed her family homemade, coarse bread, served stale after twenty-four hours. Long after Graham's death in 1851 his followers, called "Grahamites," whose ranks included John Harvey Kellogg of cornflake fame, would continue to advocate vegetarianism, temperance, and bran bread. Many of the most ardent Grahamites were women who were attracted to his recommendations on diet, health care, and dress reform, which criticized disfiguring corsets and advocated loose, comfortable clothing. And while knowledge about nutrition would not be discovered until the early twentith century, Graham was also ahead of his time in understanding the importance of fiber in the diet. Even though the modern version of graham crackers are a far cry from the coarse, whole-wheat bread Graham championed in his time, he was clearly an early voice in preaching that you are what you eat.

Sylvester Graham died in 1851 but his influence on the American diet was only beginning. Per capita meat consumption began to decline as Americans shed their fears of fresh fruit and vegetables and began to eat more balanced meals. Graham had moved public opinion away from gluttony and poor digestion toward slenderness and eating to produce good health. Although Graham died in the nineteenth century, his way of thinking significantly influenced another man who founded a twentieth-century version of Grahamism. Like Graham, Bernard Adolphus McFadden, born in 1868 near Mill Spring, Missouri, believed there was a specific way to eat and live that would produce ultimate health and longevity. He was a man who practiced what he preached and historians believe his philosophy, known as physical culture, is largely at the root of today's health and fitness consciousness in America.

The core belief of McFadden's philosophy was that people got sick because of poor diet, lack of proper exercise, stale air, lack of sunshine, tobacco, alcohol, and drugs. Like Graham, McFadden believed meat should play a minor part in the diet. He preferred fruits, vegetables, and whole grains and, like Graham, he also thought white bread was the worst food a person could eat. He advocated fasting on a regular basis and believed it was a cure for all ailments. Another important component of his physical culture regime was regular exercise, such as walking, and he encouraged women not to wear corsets or any kind of restrictive clothing. In 1892 Bernard McFadden changed his first name to "Bernarr" and his last name to "Macfadden." His third wife, Mary, wrote in her book titled *Dumbbells and Carrot Strips,* that Macfadden believed the changes would glamorize his name while at the same time making him sound more robust.

Macfadden's ultimate philosophy of health was shaped by his early years as a sickly child. By the time he was eleven, both his parents were dead—his father of alcoholism and his mother of tuberculosis. He finally overcame his poor health when relatives in Illinois took him in. Working on their farm turned him into a strong, healthy teenager. At 5-feet-6-inches tall he was not a big man but he had incredible stamina and energy and developed his 145 pounds into a powerful upper body and a strong chest.

In 1899 Macfadden launched *Physical Culture* magazine with its motto, "Weakness is a Crime: Don't Be a Criminal." It was an immediate success and by the 1930s his publishing empire included *True Story, True Romances, Photoplay,* and the sensational tabloids *Midnight* and the *New York Graphic,* a publication where young Walter Winchell got his start as a writer. At the same time Macfadden also began to organize and promote bodybuilding competitions for men and women. Macfadden was so convinced he was right about health and nutrition that he campaigned to be the country's first Secretary of Health in the cabinet of President Franklin D. Roosevelt. When that failed, he campaigned for the Republican nomination for president in 1936, promoting himself through his publications and funding campaign expenses with money from his business. The results were disastrous: stockholders ousted him from his publishing company, he failed to win the nomination, and he lost a great deal of money.

Macfadden's eventual undoing came from his need to carry his ideas to an extreme. In 1955 he developed a urinary tract blockage. Since he believed fasting was a cure for all ailments, he attempted to treat his final illness by fasting but instead became severely emaciated. By the time he reached a hospital, doctors could do nothing to save him. He died October 12, 1955.

At the same time that American men and women were trimming their waistlines through programs like Macfadden's physical culture, medical doctors were telling patients that obesity was bad for their health. This advice added authority to the new insurance industry ideal height-and-weight charts. Many insurance companies had been charging larger premiums for heavy clients since the 1830s but as more middle-class families bought policies and as medical examinations became mandatory, Americans now looked to these ideal tables as an the most important indicator of their overall health. Self-styled obesity experts quickly followed, and those entrepreneurs helped shape the lucrative diet business with a hastily created array of prescription and patent medicines guaranteed to dissolve and expel unwanted fat.

These early digestive cures included Berledets, made of boric acid, cornstarch, milk, and sugar, and Human Ease, a combination of sodium bicarbonate and lard. Sassafras tea was a chief ingredient in Densmore's Corpulency Cure, while mineral water made up the bulk of Lucile Kimball's powder, along with a little soap and Epsom salt. Arsenic, used for years to stimulate the flow of digestive juices, was turned into an obesity tablet by mixing it with strychnine, caffeine, and phytolacca. Hillel Schwartz describes in *Never Satisfied* how Phytoline, made from phytolacca or pokeberry, a well-known emetic and purgative, was created and marketed as a fat-dissolving preparation. In 1936, another manufactured drug, dinitrophenol, was sold as a weight-loss medicine. Dinitrophenol, a derivative of benzene, was commonly used in the synthesis of different color dyes. At low dosages it would speed up metabolism. Unfortunately, dieters quickly experienced serious side effects: rashes, loss of the sense of taste, and blindness from cataracts. Some who exceeded the recommended dosages of dinitrophenol died from hyperpyremia, a condition where the body literally burns itself up, according to Carl Malmberg in *Diet and Die*. Finally the government in 1938 banned dinitrophenol. The American Medical Association's *Nostrums and Quackery* series, first published in 1912, detailed these and some of the other most blatant examples of the various fake obesity cures.

Early diet books were also growing in popularity, such as Dr. Lulu Hunt Peter's *Diet and Health* or Vance Thompson's *Eat and Grow Thin,* which reached its 112th printing in 1931. The early 1930s also saw the introduction of another new weight loss product, the diet drink. One of the best-known reducing drinks was Dr. Stoll's Diet Aid, sold through beauty parlors in the 1930s. A combination of milk chocolate, starch, and an extract of roasted whole wheat and bran, users mixed it by the teaspoon into a cup of water as a diet substitute for breakfast and lunch. Twenty years later in 1959 doctors at the Rockefeller Institute, studying metabolic changes, mixed together evaporated milk, corn oil, dextrose, and water and created another low-calorie diet drink whose balance of protein, fat, and carbohydrate closely resembled breast milk. Metrecal, a product of the Mead Johnson Company famous for its Pablum baby food, reawakened the public's interest in diet drinks. Today Nestlé, another distributor of infant formulas, markets Metrecal under the brand name Carnation Slender.

Even at the height of the Depression, the diet industry was flourishing, soon to grow by leaps and bounds with the introduction of amphetamines in the late 1930s. First used clinically in the mid-1930s to treat narcolepsy, a rare disorder resulting in an uncontrollable tendency to sleep, amphetamines skyrocketed in use when doctors began prescribing them for appetite suppression and the treatment of depression. At the time, pharmacologists were actually looking for a synthetic substitute for the expensive ephedrine, which had been used to treat asthma. Under the trade names Benzedrine, Methedrine, and Dexedrine, amphetamines, with their clear effect on appetite and weight loss became the new darling of the diet industry. Amphetamines stimulate the central nervous system by increasing heart rates and blood pressure while reducing fatigue. However, people who use amphetamines on a regular basis build up a tolerance to them until dieters need higher doses to achieve the same effects. So widespread use by dieters in the 1930s created related problems of drug dependency and addiction. As early as 1943, the American Medical Association (AMA), publicly opposed the use of amphetamines for the treatment of obesity because of problems of dependence, but doctors continued to recommend them for dieters. Five years later, doctors began recommending Dexedrine as the drug of choice for weight loss and justified it by adding a prescription for barbiturates to calm the amphetamine jitters.

With dieting now a growing national pastime, diet foods became fashionable. For example, in New York, Minneapolis, and five other cities,

Stouffer's restaurants offered special low-calorie lunches and the Pennsylvania Railroad featured a 470-calorie "Streamliner" on its dining car menus. Some 80 percent of U.S. supermarkets added dietetic departments filled with low-calorie foods whose sales totaled some $25 million according to an August 10, 1953, article in *Time*. Postwar Americans began joining dieting groups. Take Off Pounds Sensibly (TOPS) was the first of the group programs and boasted a membership of 30,000 by the late 1950s. Overeaters Anonymous was started in 1960, Weight Watchers in 1961, and the Diet Workshop in 1965.

Calories Don't Count, was the catchy title of a diet book written in 1960 by Dr. Herman Taller, a Rumanian-born physician who practiced obstetrics in Brooklyn. He told people they could eat as many protein and fatty foods as they wanted but he recommended that dieters severely cut back on carbohydrates. His diet also prescribed six capsules a day of safflower oil. While book sales jumped to more than a million copies in less than a year, in 1962 Taller was fined $7,000 for violating the federal Food, Drug and Cosmetic Act, and was sharply criticized by the U.S. Food and Drug Administration (FDA). FDA Commissioner George Larrick, quoted in the July 13, 1962, issue of *Time,* said, "This best-selling book was deliberately created and used to promote these worthless safflower oil capsules for the treatment of obesity, cardiovascular diseases and other serious conditions. One of its main purposes was to promote the sale of a commercial product in which Dr. Taller had a financial interest." Larrick went on to say that there is no easy, simple substitute for weight loss, but added that in the end calories do count.

And so today's consumers find themselves inundated with every kind of diet product and program from Dr. Atkins to The Zone. To lose unwanted pounds, desperate dieters continue to look for magic pills and easy programs from Slim Fast to Nutri/System or Jenny Craig, from herbal capsules, skin patches, or pills to liposuction. Yet, ironically, in most cases the pounds come back once the fad diet ends. And as Americans move into a new century, the dieting public seems ready to embrace a whole new crop of schemes and fads no matter how far-fetched. Yet, the real solution has always been available. Simply eat more fruits, vegetables, and whole grain food, fewer junk and fast foods, and, most important, exercise. Experts recommend at least thirty minutes of vigorous activity five days a week. If you can't find thirty minutes, try two 15-minute intervals, or even three 10-minute intervals.

Additional Reading

Adams, Samuel Hopkins. *The Great American Fraud*. Denver: Nostalgic American Research Foundation, Inc., 1978.

Banner, Lois W. *American Beauty*. New York: Alfred A. Knopf, 1983.

"Benzedrine and Dieting." *Newsweek*, 8 September 1947, 48–49.

"Calories Do Count." *Time,* 13 July 1962: 56–57.

Cambridge World History of Food. New York: Cambridge University Press, 2000.

Malmberg, Carl. *Diet and Die.* New York: Hillman-Curl, Inc., 1935.

Pillsbury, Richard. *No Foreign Food: The American Diet in Time and Place.* Boulder, Colo.: Westview Press, 1998.

Roberts, Paul. "The New Food Anxiety." *Psychology Today,* March–April 1998, 30–40.

Schwartz, Hillel. *Never Satisfied: A Cultural History of Diets, Fantasies and Fat.* New York: Macmillan, 1986.

Aerobic Activity

During aerobic activities, oxygen breaks down carbohydrates and converts them into lasting energy. Aerobic exercise is ideal for burning fat. Examples of good aerobic activities are running, swimming, and aerobics classes, which combine fast-paced stretching, strength, and endurance exercises—all activities that make your

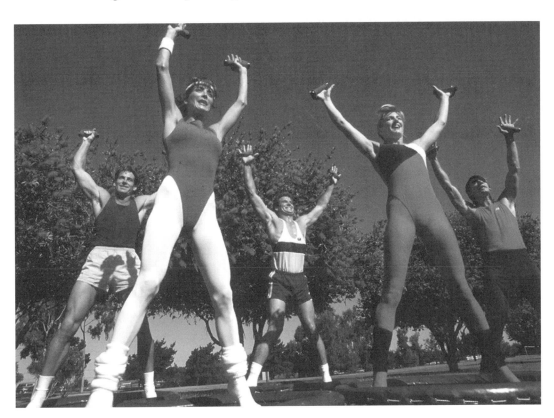

There are plenty of ways to get your heart pumping. Go for a walk, take the stairs, or join a group like this one. (Painet)

muscles use oxygen. Aerobic exercises are repetitive—bicycling, swimming, jogging, brisk walking, basketball, skating, dancing, jumping rope.

What do aerobic exercises do for you? By strengthening your heart, aerobic exercises get fresh blood pumped more rapidly to muscle groups. That helps tone those muscle groups because they can keep moving longer. Aerobic workouts break down carbohydrates, fats, and proteins so they are the ideal workouts for losing fat.

To make the most of aerobic exercises, work out for at least 15 to 30 minutes at your target heart rate. If you can't go that long, break it down in ten-minute intervals, but aim for thirty minutes a day, three or four days a week. Have rest days in between so your body can recover and to prevent injuries. As your body gets stronger, increase the level of intensity or the time of the activity. Do it gradually, though. Don't expect to jog thirty minutes one month and an hour and a half the next. Instead, try covering more ground in that 30 minutes, or extend the slow jog to 40 minutes or so.

Amphetamines

Amphetamines belong to a group of medicines called central nervous system (CNS) stimulants. They act on the CNS—the brain and the spinal cord—increasing heart rate and blood pressure while reducing appetite and fatigue. Dieters have used amphetamines to treat obesity for many years, in both prescription and over-the-counter forms. However, medical use of amphetamines is now restricted primarily to treating narcolepsy, a sleep disorder, and attention-deficit hyperactivity disorder (ADHD). Ritalin is a drug in the amphetamine family most widely recognized for the treatment of

ADHD and hyperactivity. In treating ADHD, these medicines are part of a total program that includes social, educational, and psychological components.

When initially taken, amphetamines produce feelings of well-being, increased competence, and alertness. Their effects are similar to those of cocaine, but their onset is slower and their duration is longer. High doses of amphetamines can cause tremors, sweating, heart palpitations, or anxiety. Exhaustion and depression follow when the drug wears off. In general, chronic abuse produces a psychosis that resembles schizophrenia and is characterized by paranoia, picking at the skin, preoccupation with one's own thoughts, and auditory and visual hallucinations. Violent and erratic behavior is frequently seen among chronic abusers of amphetamines. Amphetamines have a high potential for abuse, since regular use can lead to greater physical tolerance, requiring higher doses to achieve the same effect. This causes psychological dependency, characterized by a craving for the drug and a belief that one cannot function without it. Doctors caution weight-loss patients that without long-term changes in exercise and eating habits, using amphetamines is not a long-term weight-loss solution and is not an appropriate substitute for good nutrition and a healthy lifestyle.

Additional Reading

"Obesity." In *Gale Encyclopedia of Medicine.* Detroit: Gale Group, 2002.

Anaerobic Activity

Anaerobic energy is created by burning carbohydrates, not oxygen. Anaerobic exercises are characterized by maximum bursts of energy, of short duration, to build muscle strength. They include weight lifting and sprinting, for example. Muscle-strengthening activities let you work on specific groups of muscles by using resistance. These exercises can be performed with free weights, weight machines, or even the resistance created by the weight of your own body—push-ups, chin-ups, or sprinting. Before doing a muscle-building routine, make sure you warm up with stretches to prevent painful cramping that can result from lactic acid buildup in muscle tissue. Stretching at the end of the workout is also important.

Anemia

Anemia is a condition in which a deficiency in the size or number of red blood cells or the amount of hemoglobin they contain limits the exchange of oxygen and carbon dioxide between the blood and the tissue cells. It results from a variety of conditions, such as hemorrhage, genetic abnormalities, chronic disease states, or drug toxicity.

During the teenage years, iron requirements are higher than at other times in life. The human body needs iron for energy production: too little iron leaves you tired and at risk for iron-deficiency anemia. Iron is especially important for teenage girls who are menstruating, since iron is essential for the expansion of blood volume. The highest incidence of iron deficiency occurs in adolescent girls.

Iron is a trace mineral found in red meat, liver, fish, green leafy vegetables, enriched bread, and some dried fruits such as prunes, apricots, and raisins. Some people consume most of their iron requirements by eating meats, but the incidence of iron-deficiency anemia in vegetarians is not significantly different from that in omnivores, according to the American Society of Clinical Nutrition. Foods high in iron include spinach, broccoli, raisins, chickpeas, pinto beans, whole grains, and blackstrap molasses. In fact, calorie for calorie, spinach has fourteen times the iron of sirloin steak. However, as with calcium, absorption of iron is also affected by diet, and iron from plant foods is not as easily absorbed as iron from animal foods. For that reason vegetarians and people who need to boost their iron levels should eat foods rich in vitamin C to help increase how much iron the body can absorb. Citrus fruits and juices, tomatoes, and broccoli are all good sources of vitamin C.

Recommended iron intake for young women is 15 milligrams per day; for boys age fifteen to eighteen, it's 12 milligrams per day, decreasing to 10 milligrams per day after age nineteen. The level of iron required for women stays the same until menopause. Blood loss, such as that which occurs during menstrual cycles, is a major cause of iron deficiency, which can be corrected either by eating more foods that are higher in iron content or by taking iron supplements. Coffee, tea, wheat bran, eggs, and soy inhibit iron absorption. Medications such as antacids, for example, can also interfere with iron absorption.

Iron demands also peak for pregnant women. The requirement for iron doubles in the second trimester and triples in the third as blood volume increases and the fetus grows dramatically.

Antioxidants

Many claims have been made about the health benefits of antioxidants. These are substances that counteract the harmful free radicals created by oxidation. Oxidation, for example, can rust cars. Some oxidation in the body is good because it produces energy and kills bacterial invaders. But, in excess, it can damage tissues. Antioxidants are found naturally in many foods, primarily fruits and vegetables. They are also available as supplements, but whether or not they are helpful is still a matter of debate. There are claims that antioxidants in large quantities can help prevent or reduce the effects of a variety of diseases, including cardiovascular disease, diabetes, Alzheimer's, and various forms of cancer. Vitamins with antioxidant properties include vitamins E, C, and A as beta carotene. Some minerals, such as selenium, are also considered to have antioxidant properties. On April 10, 2000, a panel at the Institute of Medicine of the National Academies of Science reported that megadoses of antioxidants haven't yet been proven to be helpful and might in fact be dangerous. According to the press release announcing the findings, "A direct connection between the intake of antioxidants and the prevention of chronic disease has yet to be adequately established," said Norman I. Krinsky, chair of the study's Panel on Dietary Antioxidants and Related Compounds, and a professor of biochemistry, at Tufts University School of Medicine, Boston. "We do know, however, that dietary antioxidants can in some cases prevent or counteract cell damage that stems from exposure to oxidants, which are agents that affect a cell's molecular composition. But much more research is needed to determine whether dietary antioxidants can actually stave off chronic disease."

As such, the panel established the following recommendations for dietary supplementation of antioxidants. It increased recommended intake levels of vitamin C to 75 milligrams per day for women and 90 milligrams per day for men. Smokers, who are more likely to be impacted from the cell-damaging biological processes and deplete more vitamin C, need an additional 35 milligrams per day. The report set the upper intake level for vitamin C, from both food and supplements, at 2,000 milligrams per day for adults, saying intakes above this amount may cause diarrhea. Food sources for vitamin C include citrus fruit, potatoes, strawberries, broccoli, and leafy green vegetables.

Vitamin E recommendations were also increased, and men and women are now advised to consume 15 milligrams of vitamin E from food. Food sources for this vitamin are vegetable oils, nuts, seeds, liver, and leafy green vegetables. Synthetic vitamin E from vitamin supplements should not exceed 1,000 milligrams of alpha-tocopherol per day for adults. Alpha-tocopherol is the only type of vitamin E that human blood can maintain and transfer to cells when needed. People who consume more than this amount place themselves at greater risk of hemorrhagic damage because the nutrient can act as an anticoagulant, according to the report.

The report also recommended that men and women need 55 micrograms of selenium per day. Food sources include seafood, liver, meat, and grains. The upper level of selenium, including natural and supplement sources, should be less than 400 micrograms per day. More could result in selenosis, a toxic reaction that can cause hair loss and nail sloughing.

The report did not set a recommended daily intake or upper intake level for beta carotene and other carotenoids, which are found naturally in dark-green and deep-yellow vegetables. However, it cautioned against high doses, recommending supplementation only for the prevention and control of vitamin A deficiency.

The report stressed that a balanced and varied diet will provide adequate amounts of these vitamins and minerals without requiring supplements. The American Heart Association concurs in a February 1999 Science Advisory, "Antioxidant Consumption and Risk of Coronary Heart Disease: Emphasis on Vitamin C, Vitamin E, and Beta-Carotene," which concluded, "The most prudent and scientifically supportable recommendation for the general population is to consume a balanced diet with emphasis on antioxidant-rich fruits and vegetables and whole grains. This advice, which is consistent with the current dietary guidelines of the American Heart Association, considers the role of the total diet in influencing disease risk. Although diet alone may not provide the levels of vitamin E intake that have been associated with the lowest risk in a few observational studies, the absence of efficacy and safety data from randomized trials precludes the establishment of population-wide recommendations regarding vitamin E supplementation."

Anorexia Nervosa

Anorexia is *not* a diet plan. It is an eating disorder—a pathological fear of weight gain. The National Association of Anorexia and Associated Disorders estimates that more than eight million Americans suffer from full-blown eating disorders—including anorexia nervosa and bulimia nervosa—and 86 percent of them develop the problem before age twenty. Intentional starving often begins around the time of puberty and involves extreme weight loss, defined as at least 15 percent below one's normal body weight. For regularly menstruating adolescent girls and women, skipping three menstrual cycles (except pregnancy) is another medical indicator of a serious problem. Even though someone with anorexia may look

emaciated, she may still be convinced that she's too heavy.

The vast majority of people affected by these eating disorders are adolescent and young adult women. Males and older women can also develop eating disorders, but young women are often most influenced by idealistic—and generally unachievable—standards of beauty. In a survey by the Centers for Disease Control and Prevention, more than one-third of the high-school girls surveyed thought they were overweight. That compares to 15 percent of the boys who answered the same way.

According to the National Institutes of Health, approximately 1 percent of adolescent girls develop anorexia nervosa and

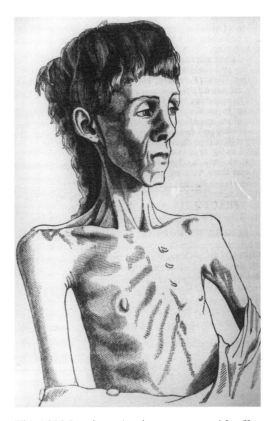

This 1888 London print shows a young girl suffering from anorexia. (National Library of Medicine)

another 2 to 3 percent develop bulimia nervosa. As girls approach adulthood, the numbers increase. Studies indicate that by the time they reach college, somewhere between 4.5 percent and 18 percent of women have a history of bulimia. The National Center for Health Statistics estimates that about 9,000 people admitted to hospitals were diagnosed with bulimia in 1994 and about 8,000 were diagnosed with anorexia. Males account for only 5 to 10 percent of bulimia and anorexia cases. While people of all races develop the disorders, the vast majority of those diagnosed are white.

Both eating disorders are destructive conditions and can lead to serious damage, even death. One in ten cases of anorexia nervosa leads to death from starvation, cardiac arrest, other medical complications, or suicide. About 1,000 women die of anorexia each year, according to the American Anorexia/Bulimia Association. The National Center for Health Statistics noted that anorexia nervosa was the underlying cause of death noted on 101 death certificates in 1994 and was mentioned as one of multiple causes of death on another 2,657 death certificates. In the same year, bulimia was the underlying cause of death on two death certificates and mentioned as one of several causes on sixty-four others. According to the Harvard Center on Eating Disorders, anorexia has the highest mortality rate among eating disorders.

Appetite Suppressants by Prescription

The popularity of prescription appetite suppressants goes up and down like a roller coaster. The drugs work largely by increasing levels of serotonin, which is a brain chemical that controls feelings of fullness. Widespread use of prescription diet pills first began several decades ago with the introduction of amphetamines. In those early days the pills' potential was as great as their abuse by users because they called for increasing doses to be effective. In fact, by the 1970s a crisis of amphetamine abuse had emerged, as people began injecting these drugs intravenously and they were sold on the street as "speed." Doctors responded to the problem by limiting prescriptions, and the drug fell into disfavor as an obesity treatment.

Appetite suppressants made a comeback in the 1990s with the famous combination of drugs, fenfluramine and phentermine. Millions of prescriptions for fen-phen, as it was popularly called, were written before it was pulled from the market in 1997 when the U.S. Food and Drug Administration (FDA) received reports of dangerous side effects; some 30 percent of patients taking the weight-loss pills had developed a fatal form of heart-valve disease. At the same time Redux, or dexfenfluramine, was also withdrawn by the FDA when cases of a rare but fatal type of pulmonary hypertension or lung condition known as PPH developed in those taking the drug for more than three months.

Once again prescription appetite suppression sales slumped. But the market has demonstrated another upturn with the arrival of the diet drugs Meridia and Xenical. These new choices, like the earlier pills, are being marketed for the short-term treatment of obesity, always with the hope that dieters who use the pills to lose weight will learn new ways to eat and to exercise. Meridia and Xenical have shown some progress.

While amphetamines, fen-phen, and Redux all acted to increase serotonin levels in the brain, Meridia keeps two important brain chemicals in balance, serotonin and norepinephrine. Manufacturers of the pills say this helps increase metabolism and also causes a feeling of fullness along with increased energy levels. Problems, since its side effects are similar to fen-phen, are also similar to those of fen-phen. Most are mild and include dry mouth, headache, constipation, and insomnia. Increases in blood pressure and heart rate are also common and, if severe enough, can lead to termination of the drug therapy by a doctor. Most important, there have been no pulmonary hypertension or cardiac-valve side effects reported with this drug, problems that derailed use of fen-phen and Redux.

In contrast to the other prescription appetite suppressants, Xenical ignores brain chemicals and instead interferes with the absorption of fats in the digestive system. The drug works by blocking an enzyme needed to digest fat and prevents about 30 percent of ingested dietary fat from being absorbed by the body. That undigested fat shows up in the stools, and side effects include bloating, flatulence, oily stool diarrhea, and fecal incontinence. And because Xenical can deplete fat-soluble vitamins, doctors say users must take a multivitamin.

Health care professionals say they do not recommend the use of appetite-suppressing drugs to anyone who is not clinically obese, since there are side effects and risks to taking the medications. These medicines are available only with a doctor's prescription and must be used in conjunction with a reduced-calorie diet and increased exercise. And while they are useful during the first few weeks of a weight-loss program, their appetite-reducing effects tend to decrease over time, just as the other, earlier prescription choices did, creating the potential for abuse. Doctors note that many dieters also do not realize that once they stop taking the appetite suppressants, the body may need time to adjust. During this transition period, anyone who experiences extreme tiredness or weakness, mental depression, nausea or vomiting, stomach cramps or pain, or trouble with sleeping or nightmares should contact a physician. When deciding to use an appetite suppressant, health-care professionals suggest weighing the risks of taking the medicine against the good it may do.

See also:

amphetamines; fen-phen; Meridia; Xenical.

Additional Reading

"Obesity." In *Gale Encyclopedia of Medicine*. Detroit: Gale Group, 2002.

Artificial Sweeteners

Sugar has fifteen calories per teaspoon. For anyone trying to lose weight, sugar-sweetened snacks and drinks can present a real problem. Yet few people are willing to give up sweets entirely. As a result, artificial sweeteners that provide the taste of sweetness without the caloric punch, are popular. These sweeteners are hundreds of times sweeter than sugar. In other words, a little goes a long way. There are four kinds of artificial sweeteners on the market: saccharin, aspartame, acesulfame potassium, and sucralose.

Artificial sweeteners are known as non-nutritive sweeteners. They provide no energy, as other caloric foods do. There are also nutritive sweeteners, such as honey, molasses, barley malt, and fructose. Nutritive sweeteners typically have about the same caloric impact as sugar.

Saccharin was first developed in 1879—the result of an accidental spill during research on food preservatives. The sweetener saw huge jumps in popularity during World War I and World War II when sugar was being rationed. Some research starting in the 1960s suggested there was a link between saccharin and cancer. The U.S. Food and Drug Administration (FDA) considered banning it based on animal research that suggested the link to bladder cancer in rats. Indeed, it was banned in Canada in 1977, but it has never been banned in the United States. For twenty-five years, however, products that contain saccharin did carry a warning label that saccharin had caused cancer in lab animals. That label was a requirement of the 1977 Saccharin Study and Labeling Act. In December 2000, a bill passed that essentially gave saccharin a clean bill of health. Saccharin is between 200 and 700 times sweeter than sugar; Sweet and Low is a brand name.

Aspartame was discovered in 1965 and was first approved in 1981 as a tabletop sweetener. Aspartame breaks down as it heats up, so it is not an effective sugar substitute in most baked goods. As of 1996, it had been approved for use in foods and beverages, some snack foods, and products such as syrups and salad dressings. It is about 200 times sweeter than sugar. It is sold in the United States by Ajinomoto USA, Daesang America, the Holland Sweetener Company, and the NutraSweet Company. Equal is also an aspartame sweetener.

According to an article in the *Journal of the American Dietetic Association*, "demand for aspartame in the United States rose from 8.4 million lb in 1986 to 17.5 million lb in 1992, a figure that represents more than 80% of the world demand. Although soft drinks account for more than 70% of aspartame consumption, this sweetener is added to more than 6,000 foods, personal care products, and pharmaceuticals." Overall, the United States consumes about 50 percent of the world demand and leads the world in consumption of high-intensity sweeteners.

The third sweetener, acesulfame potassium, was approved in 1992 for gums and dry foods and its approval was expanded to liquid use in 1998. Pepsi immediately included it in its new Pepsi One drink. It is about 200 times sweeter than sugar, and according to its manufacturer, Nutrinova, it is used in more than 4,000 products.

The fourth sweetener is sucralose and its trade name is Splenda. It's 600 times sweeter than sugar and is the only artificial sweetener actually derived from table sugar. Sucralose cannot be digested; therefore, it adds no calories to food. Before approving sucralose in 1998, the FDA reviewed data from more than 110 studies in humans and animals.

Indeed, the FDA has determined that these four artificial sweeteners are safe for human consumption. However, computer users surfing the Internet can find many claims that artificial sweeteners are linked to the development of cancer, tumors, birth defects, brain damage, and other serious medical conditions. It is the role of the FDA to ensure that food products sold in the United States are safe. Indeed, the FDA banned the sweetener cyclamate in 1969 out of concerns that it could be carcinogenic to some people.

While the FDA and the medical establishment note that the approved sweeteners are generally recognized as safe, physicians and nutritionists recommend moderation in sweet foods. Whether the sugar is nutritive or artificial, sweet foods still make up the top layer in the U.S. Department of Agriculture Food Guide

Pyramid and should be considered as a small part of a balanced diet.

Additional Reading

FDA Talk Paper: "FDA Approves New High-Intensity Sweetener Sucralose." FDA, 1 April 1998.

Henkel, John. "Sugar Substitutes: Americans Opt for Sweetness and Lite." *FDA Consumer* (U.S. Food and Drug Administration) November/December 1999.

"Use of Nutritive and Nonnutritive Sweeteners—Position of the ADA." *Journal of the American Dietetic Association* 98 (1998): 580–87.

www.aspartame.org

www.caloriecontrol.org

www.saccharin.org

www.sucralose.com

Atkins Nutritional Approach

The Atkins Nutritional Approach was developed by the late Dr. Robert C. Atkins and published in his best-selling books, *The Atkins Diet Revolution* (1972) and *Dr. Atkins' New Diet Revolution* (1992). The Atkins Center for Complementary Medicine calls its eating plan a controlled carbohydrate program for weight management and good health. Critics call the diet a high-protein, high-fat, and low-carbohydrate ketogenic diet. The Atkins theory is that excess carbohydrate intake prevents the body from burning fat efficiently. He maintained that drastically reducing the daily intake of carbohydrates will rebalance an individual's metabolism and force the body to burn reserves of stored fat for energy through a condition known as ketosis. Critics counter that a ketogenic diet lacks carbohydrates for fuel, which triggers the body's production of large amounts of ketone bodies, producing ketosis. Symptoms of ketosis include nausea, dehydration, constipation or diarrhea, and bad breath.

The four-step diet begins with a two-week Induction program when dieters may eat liberal amounts of fat and protein while holding carbohydrate intake to just 20 grams per day. Dietary intake recommendations from the U.S. Department of Agriculture (USDA) and the National Institutes of Health allow a daily intake of up to 300 grams of carbohydrates for a healthy adult male eating an average of 2,000 calories a day. During Induction, meals are planned around Atkins's acceptable foods, such as beef, pork, bacon, fish, chicken, eggs, and cheese. Under the Atkins plan, cream is allowed but not skim milk, and sour cream can be eaten but not yogurt. A typical breakfast might include a cheese omelet served with strips of bacon but no orange juice. In later phases, whole fruit, which is a healthy source of fiber, is introduced, but fruit juice is not recommended because it elevates blood sugar.

A typical Induction lunch menu is a Caesar salad with grilled chicken and seltzer water. Dinner might be a shrimp cocktail, clear consommé, followed by roasted salmon, a tossed salad, and a sugar-free gelatin dessert. Snacks during Induction focus on choices such as a slice of cheese, half an avocado, a handful of olives, or vegetables with tahini dip. Depending upon food choices, a typical caloric intake during Induction is between 1,800 and 2,400 calories. It is not necessary to count calories when following the Atkins program, since, according to Atkins representatives, there is ample food to allow dieters to feel satiated and to discourage cheating or overeating. According to the Atkins Center, the original edition of the diet did occasionally imply that individuals could eat unlimited portions of protein and fat. However, a spokesperson stressed that the newest edition of the book clears up this mixed message and anyone following the diet should eat these foods until satisfied but not stuffed.

Atkins also encourages dieters on his plan to take vitamin supplements to correct any nutritional deficiencies they may encounter. In his book he stresses that the early period of the diet is not a lifetime regimen unless the dieter has a particularly stubborn metabolic resistance. Following the Induction period, the pre-maintenance period, known as the Ongoing Weight Loss (OWL) phase, is a time when weight loss is deliberately slowed in an effort to introduce more variety in foods. Now dieters can choose from more vegetables, as well as seeds and nuts, plus low-glycemic fruits such as strawberries and blueberries. According to the Atkins plan, as long as weight loss continues, individuals can gradually increase their carbohydrate intake. The first week they can eat 25 grams of carbohydrates per day; the second week, they move to 30 grams, and so forth until weight loss stalls. Finally at the Maintenance stage dieters are allowed 60 to 90 grams of carbohydrates per day, which might include legumes and whole grains as well as other fruits.

By limiting carbohydrate intake, the Atkins diet eliminates many of the foods and food groups called for in the USDA Food Guide Pyramid. Those include fruits, cereals, breads, grains, starches, dairy products, and starchy vegetables. However, in direct contrast to the Atkins plan, the USDA encourages people to eat sparingly of foods high in fat like butter, oil, meat, poultry, fish, eggs, cheese, and cream and instead suggests that a healthy diet should include five servings of fruits and vegetables each day.

Critics of fad diets that eliminate several foods or food groups say studies show dieters following these plans have the worst failure rates over time. Nutritionists also criticize high-protein, high-fat, low-carbohydrate diets because they suggest the rapid initial weight loss is made primarily of water and lean muscle mass instead of fat. In response to critics, the Atkins Center says Dr. Atkins devoted a new chapter in the most recent edition of *Dr. Atkins' New Diet Revolution* to what they call repeated errors and misconceptions. such as the question of water weight loss. Atkins explained that although early weight loss will be water, he identified research that shows water balance soon returns to normal and weight loss comes from burning body fat for energy.

On another front, the American Heart Association charges that high-protein diets are rich in saturated fat and can accelerate heart disease and dehydration. In rebuttal, the Atkins Center cites a growing body of scientific literature that demonstrates that a controlled carbohydrate-eating plan, if followed correctly, promotes heart health. Atkins representatives point to the Harvard School of Public Health and its Nurses' Study. Those study results suggest that total fat consumed has no relation to heart disease risk; that monounsaturated fats like olive oil lower risk; and that saturated fats are little worse, if at all, than the pasta and other carbohydrates that the Food Guide Pyramid suggests be eaten. According to the Atkins Center, the Nurses' Study research makes the case that consuming less fat and cholesterol actually resulted in more weight gain and higher blood cholesterol.

In his book, Atkins stated that people who follow his plan and then return to eating their prediet amount of carbohydrates will find the pounds returning. The Atkins

Lifetime Maintenance phase begins when dieters reach their goal weight. Then, depending upon age, gender, exercise level, and genetics a person can decide how much carbohydrate to consume, usually from 90 to 120 grams per day. For most people this means occasionally eating modest portions of foods like potatoes, other starchy vegetables, whole-wheat pasta, and whole-grain bread without regaining weight. The Atkins diet is not recommended for lacto-ovo vegetarians, since it would be difficult to find enough nonanimal sources of protein to eat. And vegans cannot follow this diet since a vegan diet is very high in carbohydrates, according to Atkins. Instead, the Atkins Center recommends that vegetarians with a serious weight problem give up vegetarianism, or at least include fish in their diet.

Atkins claimed that his eating plan causes no adverse side effects, yet many health care organizations disagree with his recommendations. Over the years he has been criticized by the American Medical Association (AMA), the American Dietetic Association, the American Society of Bariatric (controlled weight loss) Physicians, and the American Heart Association. Critics also call attention to the fact that the Atkins diet has been in circulation for thirty years, but national obesity rates are continuing to rise at alarming rates. Atkins turned the tables on those critics by charging that Americans who follow the USDA-recommended daily allowances are becoming fatter and fatter. Plus he called the rising incidence of Type 2 diabetes in this country part of the "twin epidemics of diabesity."

See also:

Atkins, Robert C.; Food Guide Pyramid; ketones/ketosis; Ornish, Dean.

Additional Reading

Atkins, Robert C. *Dr. Atkins' Health Revolution: How Complementary Medicine Can Extend Your Life.* New York: Houghton Mifflin Company, 1988.

———. *Dr. Atkins' New Diet Revolution.* New York: Avon Books, 1992.

Brody, Jane E. "Senate Nutrition Panel to Focus on Perils of Being Overweight." *New York Times,* 13 April 1973, 18.

Taubes, Gary. "The Soft Science of Dietary Fat." *Science* 291, no. 5513, 30 March 2001, 2536–45.

Underwood, Anne. "The Battle of Pork Rind Hill: When the Nation's Best-selling Diet Gurus Squared Off in a Raucous Food Fight, One Thing Was Clear: There's No Easy Way to Shed That Ugly Flab. So Get Out the Jogging Shoes." *Newsweek,* 6 March 2000, 50.

Willett, Walter C. *Eat, Drink, and Be Healthy: The Harvard Medical School Guide to Healthy Eating.* New York: Simon and Schuster, 2001.

Atkins, Robert C.

Dr. Robert C. Atkins (b. October 17, 1930, in Columbus, Ohio, d. April 18, 2003) was the founder and executive medical director of the Atkins Center for Complementary Medicine in New York City. The Center was founded in 1976 with the stated philosophy "that the best medicine integrates the safest and most effective therapies from all the healing arts, both traditional and alternative." Dr. Atkins was the author of several best-selling diet books, including *Dr. Atkins' Diet Revolution* (1972), as well as *Dr. Atkins' New Diet Revolution* (1992), and *Dr. Atkins' New Diet Revolution: Revised and Updated* (1999). His last book before his death was *Atkins for life* (2003). He and his wife, Veronica, coauthored *Dr. Atkins' Quick and Easy New Diet Cook-*

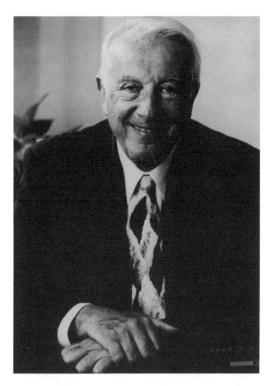

Dr. Robert C. Atkins wrote controversial diet books for more than twenty years, beginning with his first best-seller, *Dr. Atkins' Diet Revolution*. The Atkins eating plan recommends traditional sources of protein, like red meat, eggs, and bacon, and limits carbohydrates. Atkins also encouraged supplements and maintained that his diet could eliminate many health problems. (Atkins Center for Complementary Medicine)

book (1997) and he wrote a guide to using vitamins, minerals, and other supplements, titled *Dr. Atkins' Vita-Nutrient Solution: Nature's Answer to Drugs* (1998).

The Atkins diet is a ketogenic diet, a high-protein, high-fat, and low-carbohydrate plan that causes rapid initial weight loss without limiting calories. However, the Atkins Center refers to its program as the Atkins Nutritional Approach, labeling it a controlled carbohydrate program for weight management and good health. The Center objects to those who classify the diet as high-protein or ketogenic. Cen-

ter spokespeople maintain that when the Atkins program is followed correctly, the amount of protein consumed is no higher than that in the typical American diet. A diet is called a ketogenic diet when the lack of carbohydrates for fuel triggers the body's production of large amounts of ketone bodies, a condition known as ketosis. Symptoms of ketosis include nausea, dehydration, constipation or diarrhea, and bad breath. Atkins Center representatives answer critics by saying a true ketogenic diet is 90 percent fat and 10 percent protein while the first phase of the Atkins program is 60 percent fat, 30 percent protein, and 10 percent carbohydrates. They say the aforementioned symptoms are rare when individuals follow their program correctly.

In *Dr. Atkins' New Diet Revolution*, Atkins encouraged the onset of ketosis, calling it, "one of life's charmed gifts," and a "dieter's best friend." Atkins maintained that, as long as an individual consumes sufficient calories from protein and fat, there is no health risk involved in ketosis. Both the original Atkins diet and the updated version start off with a two-week Induction program designed, according to Atkins, to rebalance an individual's metabolism by causing ketosis. During the first fourteen days, the plan allows dieters to eat liberal amounts of fat and protein, however it restricts carbohydrates to 20 grams per day. That equals about three cups of salad vegetables such as lettuce, cucumbers, and celery.

Dietary intake recommendations from the U.S. Department of Agriculture (USDA) and the National Institutes of Health call for a daily intake of up to 300 grams of carbohydrates for an average, healthy adult male. Atkins argued that the USDA 300-gram recommendation has done nothing to help the growing number of Americans who are becoming fatter and fatter as well as the rising incidence of Type 2 diabetes. Dr. Atkins called these the "twin epidemics of diabesity."

However, this emphasis on an almost carbohydrate-free diet worries critics like the National Cancer Institute, which urges Americans to eat five servings of fruits and vegetables each day to reduce the risk of certain kinds of cancers. The premaintenance phase of the Atkins program gradually adds one to three servings a week of carbohydrate-rich fruits and vegetables. The maintenance phase typically allows for 60 to 90 grams daily of carbohydrate foods.

Atkins began his study of medicine at the University of Michigan where he earned his Bachelor of Arts degree in 1951. He received his medical degree from Cornell University in 1955. Atkins practiced as an internist and cardiologist for some twenty years before he published his first book and best-seller, the *Dr. Atkins' Diet Revolution*. His diet was followed by another very popular high-protein, low-carbohydrate eating plan, *The Complete Scarsdale Medical Diet*, written in 1978 by physician and cardiologist Dr. Herman Tarnower.

Over the years a number of leading medical and health organizations have denounced Atkins's diet, including the American Medical Association, the American Dietetic Association, and the American Heart Association. In 1973 Atkins was called to testify before the Senate Select Committee on Nutrition and Human Needs to answer charges that his diet would compromise the lives of unborn children. Appearing with his attorney, Atkins declared that he stood by everything in his book, including his recommendation that overweight women could follow the diet during pregnancy. During testimony at the hearing, according to an April 13, 1973, *New York Times* article, a New York obstetrician cited extensive research evidence that the kind of diet Atkins recommended would compromise the well-being and possibly the life of an unborn child. Dr. Karlis Adamsons said, "If I were a fetus, I would forbid my mother to go on such a diet." Several other physicians, appearing in front of the Senate committee, said the full impact of such a low-carbohydrate diet may not become apparent until many years later and that obstetricians might not detect damage to a fetus until it was too late.

Although he is better known for his work in weight control, Dr. Atkins also built a reputation as a supporter of what he called natural medicine and nutritional pharmacology, which he advocated as an alternative to pharmaceutical drugs and surgery for many debilitating illnesses. Criticism of Atkins's belief in alternative medicine reached its peak in 1993 when New York Health Commissioner Mark Chassin briefly suspended Atkins's medical license. Calling Atkins's medical practice "an imminent danger to the health of the people of this state," the commissioner's action was in response to how the doctor treated one of his patients who complained of headaches and weakness after injecting herself with ozone. Atkins at the time was a strong advocate of the use of ozone gas to treat cancer and AIDS. Atkins, in an August 1993 *Time* magazine article, called the commissioner's action harassment and said the suspension was a reaction to Atkins's belief in the use of alternative medicine. Atkins's medical license was restored less than a month later.

Critic of Atkins's diet plan also include Dr. Dean Ornish, author of *Eat More, Weigh Less*, who said in a 2000 *Newsweek* interview, "The problem with low-carbohydrate diets is, even if you lose weight, you're mortgaging your health in the process." In answer to critics like Ornish, Atkins Center representatives cite research at Harvard that found that excessive carbohydrate intake has been linked with an increased incidence of heart disease. The Atkins Web site lists other studies as well as anecdotal evidence to further support the program.

See also:

Atkins Nutritional Approach; Scarsdale Diet; ketones/ketosis; Ornish, Dean.

Additional Reading

"Atkins diet." In *Gale Encyclopedia of Medicine,* Detroit: Gale Group, 2001.

Atkins, Robert C. *Dr. Atkins' New Diet Revolution.* New York: Avon Books, 1992.

Atkins, Robert C. *Atkins for Life.* New York: St. Martin's Press, 2003.

Brody, Jane E. "Senate Nutrition Panel to Focus on Perils of Being Overweight." *New York Times,* 13 April 1973, 18.

"Fad Diets: Don't Look for Magic Bullets." *Consumers' Research Magazine,* July 2000, 24–26.

"License Suspended, Dr. Robert Atkins." *Time,* 23 August 1993, 21.

Taubes, Gary. "The Soft Science of Dietary Fat." *Science,* 30 March 2001, 2536–45.

"The Trendy Diet That Sizzles: A Counterintuitive Program Reaches Critical Mass." *Newsweek,* 6 September 1999, 60.

Underwood, Anne. "The Battle of Pork Rind Hill: When the Nation's Best-Selling Diet Gurus Squared Off in a Raucous Food Fight, One Thing Was Clear: There's No Easy Way to Shed That Ugly Flab. So Get Out the Jogging Shoes." *Newsweek,* 6 March 2000, 50–52.

Barnard, Neal

Dr. Neal Barnard, a psychiatrist by training, has made a name for himself as a champion of the critical role diet plays in maintaining good health. He is a

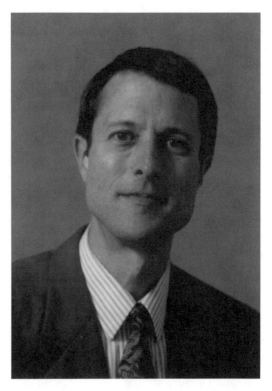

Dr. Neal Barnard, a psychiatrist and author, is a well-known advocate of good nutrition and its role in maintaining good health. He is a strong supporter of vegan and vegetarian diets and founded the Physicians Committee for Responsible Medicine, an organization on the front lines of the national debate on dietary guidelines. (Physicians Committee for Responsible Medicine, PCRM)

strong supporter of vegan and vegetarian diets. He is also known for his work advocating animal-rights issues, including the end of reliance on animals as experimental models for humans. Barnard founded the Physicians Committee for Responsible Medicine (PCRM) in 1985 with the stated mission of promoting preventive medicine through exercise and diet. He has written several books about nutrition and its impact on health. His newest title, *Turn Off the Fat Genes* (2001), looks at new genetic information and the role that genes play in determining body weight.

Like Dr. Dean Ornish, Nathan Pritikin, and Dr. John McDougall, Barnard emphasizes a high-fiber diet filled with whole grains, legumes, vegetables, and fruits. He writes in *Turn Off the Fat Genes* that carbohydrates are not the enemy people think they are; instead, it's the butter, sour cream, oils, and other fats that create overweight people and obesity. Like Ornish and McDougall, Barnard also disagrees with those who support high-protein diets, like Dr. Barry Sears in his Zone diet or Dr. Robert Atkins in his New Diet Revolution program. He says the theory that insulin is not affected by meat because meat has no carbohydrate, is false. According to Barnard, research has shown protein to be a powerful stimulus for insulin release, just as sugar is. He believes a better answer to the problem of insulin resistance is for dieters to choose high-fiber, natural plant foods.

In his latest book Barnard also suggests that five key genes influence a person's appetite and affect the body's tendency to store fat. In *Turn Off the Fat Genes* he discusses how people can manipulate their fat genes by switching to a high-fiber diet rather than a low-calorie eating plan that will eventually lead to bingeing. Barnard makes a strong case for his theory that it's not how much we eat but what we eat that determines our health and weight. The book also features a three-week "gene-control program" and suggested menus and recipes by Jennifer Raymond.

As part of his dietary tips, Barnard divides different foods into those that release sugars slowly and those that release them quickly. He blames the American tendency to overeat on the rapid rise and fall of blood sugar and the signal to eat again that it produces. According to Barnard, the best choices for a slow, steady energy release are beans, vegetables, fruits, and certain grains and grain products like pasta, barley, bulgar, and whole-grain breads. However, refined sugars found in food like white bread, white potatoes, and some sweeteners release their natural sugars more rapidly. He added that weight loss is often seen in people who consume large amounts of raw foods like melons, carrots, and apples, since these foods contain natural sugars but release them only gradually.

Barnard has been recommending a low-fat, high-fiber, vegetarian diet for many years. This opposition to eating meat and dairy is apparent in all of his books, including the earlier titles *Foods that Fight Pain: Revolutionary New Strategies for Maximum Pain Relief* (1998); *Food for Life* (1994); and *Eat Right, Live Longer* (1997). Physical activity is another important part of Barnard's message. He recommends brisk walking for a half hour three times per week as a way to burn calories and to counteract the fat-storage effect of lipoprotein lipase or LPL, which he believes plays a role in whether calories are stored as fat or lost as body heat. Barnard also suggests that exercise can help raise a naturally low metabolism and it can help control eating binges by taking the dieter away from temptation and replacing eating with activity.

Barnard's interest in healthy eating evolved over many years, according to a biography released by the PCRM. Before going to medical school he worked as an autopsy assistant, where he observed heart disease and other deadly effects of an unhealthy diet. Barnard received his medical degree in 1980 from the George Washington University School of Medicine and Health Sciences in Washington, D.C. As president of the PCRM, he currently works to promote preventive medicine and to address controversies in modern medicine as well as ethical issues in research.

See also:

Atkins, Robert C.; McDougall Program; Ornish, Dean; Sears, Barry; The Zone.

Additional Reading

Barnard, Neal, M.D. *Eat Right, Live Longer.* New York: Harmony Books, 1995.
————. *Turn Off the Fat Genes: The Revolutionary Guide to Taking Charge of the Genes that Control Your Weight.* New York: Harmony Books, 2001.
Brandt, Peter. "Dr. Neal Barnard." *Salon.com,* 12 March 2001.
"Eat Right, Live Longer: Using the Natural Power of Foods to Age-Proof Your Body." *Publishers Weekly,* 242, no. 33 (14 August 1995): 80.
Kennedy, Barbara Ferguson. "Turn Off the Fat Genes and Control Your Weight." *Health Science,* 24, no. 3 (Summer 2001): 16.

Beverly Hills Diet

The Beverly Hills Diet by Judy Mazel has been labeled among the most nutritionally outrageous of the fad diets. The original six-week plan, published in 1981, began with ten days of eating only fruit in unlimited amounts. Pineapples, bananas, papayas, mangoes, watermelon, blueberries, strawberries, apples, prunes, raisins, and grapes were all to be eaten in a certain order on specific days. In *The New Beverly Hills Diet* (1996), Mazel said she has fine-tuned the plan following fifteen years of research and experimentation. The book calls this newest diet "a lifestyle eating plan" and says the changes help the plan "meet all standards set by the Senate Committee on Nutrition and Human Needs as recommended for a balanced weekly diet." A key change: the original diet did not include any animal protein until day nineteen, but the new diet allows foods from all food groups, including protein, in the first week.

Mazel tells readers they will see how successfully "the right combination of foods can trigger astonishing weight loss and weight maintenance." Those combinations start with Day 1 when dieters can eat only pineapple, corn on the cob, and the author's favorite LTO Salad—iceberg lettuce, tomatoes, onion, cucumbers, and the Mazel dressing. Minor substitutions can be made, for example, when fruits like watermelon are not in season or readily available. Day 2 allows limitless strawberries, a half-pound of prunes, and baked potatoes. Mazel reminds dieters of the "Waiting Rule"; when going from one fruit to another, dieters must wait one hour, when moving from food group to food group, wait two hours.

Fruit portions are generous, from the half a pound of prunes on Day 2 to five pounds of grapes on Day 3. Nutritionists say five pounds of grapes would equal only 1,350 calories. But nearly all those calories come from sugar; only a small portion would provide any protein or dietary fat. Critics say that eating so little protein means dieters quickly become protein deficient and are likely to lose lean muscle tissue rather than fat. That happens because the human body has no storage organ for protein and when there isn't enough to meet daily needs, the protein in body tissues is broken down to fill in. However, when normal eating patterns return, so do the pounds in the form of increased body fat.

The theory behind the Beverly Hills Diet is simple, according to Mazel. She writes that when food isn't digested properly due to enzyme confusion, unused food turns to fat. Mazel says this confusion develops when proteins, carbohydrates, and fats are mixed together during meals. Calling this Conscious Combining, Mazel explains that the enzymes in each specific fruit along with the combination of foods eaten are critical to the success of her diet. "It isn't what you eat or how much you eat that makes you fat; it is when you eat and what you eat together!" Critics argue that all foods except for plain sugar or fat are a mixture of carbohydrates, protein, and fat and the body produces all the enzymes needed to digest them without complicated food-combining plans. According to Mazel, the principles of Conscious Combining go back thousands of years to China and ancient Persia. This theory also has modern supporters, such as Suzanne Somers. Her Somersizing diet is based on a similar concept of separating fats and proteins from carbohydrates for complete digestion.

Weight loss comes easily on the Beverly Hills Diet, since fruits are very low in calories, but the generous portions of fruit can also cause diarrhea and gas. Even though the diet quickly became a bestseller, critics were also quick to point out concerns with its basic lack of standard nutrition. In a report released in 1981 in the *Journal of the American Medical Association,* doctors called the Beverly Hills Diet "full of medical inaccuracies" and criticized Mazel's claim that undigested food causes weight gain. Doctors disagreed, saying the undigested food is not absorbed as fat but instead passes through the digestive tract to the large intestine where it is broken down by bacteria, forming gases, or eliminated as body waste. In an August 1981 *New York Times* interview, Dr. Philip White, director of the AMA's department of foods and nutrition, said, "There is very little in the book in the way of explanation of nutrition, biology or digestion that is in fact the truth." Health organizations say the real solution to being overweight is solved by eating a nutritionally balanced diet and combining that with increased exercise.

See also:

Somers, Suzanne; Somersizing.

Additional Reading

Brody, Jane E. "Another Entry in the Annals of Fad Diets." *New York Times,* 3 June 1981, C17.
Mazel, Judy. *The New Beverly Hills Diet.* Deerfield Beach, Fla.: Health Communications, Inc., 1996.
McDowell, Edwin. "Behind the Best Sellers." *New York Times,* 23 August 1981, 26.
Rhodes, Maura. "America's Top 6 Fad Diets." *Good Housekeeping,* July 1996, 100–103.

Body for Life

Body for Life: 12 Weeks to Mental and Physical Strength by Bill Phillips and Michael D'Orso, published in 1999 by HarperCollins, tells dieters they can change the shape and the fitness of their body in twelve weeks with reasonably hard work. Pound for pound this is a very specific diet with precise exercise requirements and limited food choices.

The eating plan warns users away from a majority of carbohydrates. Phillips and D'Orso say eating too many carbohydrates over a long period of time can create "insulin resistance." Instead they encourage a diet that features protein, which they suggest can provide stable energy levels and help control appetite. With its focus on protein foods, the Body for Life eating plan shares characteristics with several other diets like The Zone and Dr. Atkins's New Diet Revolution.

Critics of Atkins, The Zone, and other high-protein, low-carbohydrate diets contend that there is no reliable scientific evidence that insulin resistance develops from eating a reasonable amount of carbohydrates such as the serving recommendations in the U.S. Department of Agriculture Food Guide Pyramid.

The diet instructs users to count "portions" of food rather than calories and includes a chart of some eighteen authorized food choices that dieters can mix and match. Another important component in the Body for Life eating plan is the Myoplex drink mix, designed and distributed by Phillips's company, Experimental and Applied Sciences (EAS). The powdered formula contains a "precise blend of nutrients" that Phillips designed to help dieters maintain proper health and recover quickly from strenuous workouts. He writes, "Without the advantage it offers, I don't believe I would have been able to stick with this nutrition method," something critics say is a problem with diets that rely heavily on special foods or shakes. Statistics show that a large percentage of dieters who use prepackaged foods or shakes fail to learn to make healthy food selections or to eat sensible meals and are often at the greatest risk of regaining weight after the program ends.

For each meal, dieters choose one of the eighteen protein options along with something from the carbohydrate column. A vegetable serving is recommended for two of the daily meals. Dieters eat a grand total of six small meals per day, spread out to reduce feelings of hunger and fatigue. The book includes suggestions for six weeks' worth of meals,

which dieters can then repeat again during the twelve-week period. Nutritionists agree that more frequent, small meals and snacks can help dieters maintain a steady energy level and avoid intense feelings of hunger that can trigger unhealthy eating.

The book lists sample menus such as the Wednesday meals that start with a breakfast of one vanilla Myoplex shake made with half a fresh orange and three ice cubes. Midmorning the meal is a portion of cottage cheese along with a portion of fat-free, sugar-free yogurt and two cups of water. Lunch is a skinless chicken breast with freshly squeezed lemon and lime juice plus a plain potato served with fresh carrots and a tall glass of iced tea. Midafternoon calls for another Myoplex shake. Dinner includes a serving each of steak and brown rice. And the final meal that day is a chocolate Myoplex shake blended together with one serving of fat-free, sugar-free hot cocoa mix and three ice cubes.

Phillips and D'Orso then add a strenuous exercise program, something critics consider to be a plus, since many other diets fail to emphasize the importance of physical exercise. *Body for Life* offers a number of success stories along with before and after pictures on the dust jacket in an effort to prove that the program works. What is lacking, critics say, is any mention of long-term weight-loss success or any nutritional studies that support the diet.

Phillips defends his 20-Minute Aerobics Solution and High-Point Technique as a way to create a more metabolically efficient body. He charts a six-day exercise program, with aerobics three times a week and intense weight-training workouts three days a week, on alternate days. What sets this plan apart is the intensity of the sets at the end of each exercise designed to compound the training effect on each muscle group. The same is true for the cardiovascular exercise, which follows a schedule of increasing and decreasing intensity. This up and down, according to Phillips, allows dieters to burn more calories in less time.

He also suggests that dieters can keep metabolism levels from slowing by setting aside one free day each week—free of exercise and diet restrictions. The free day stems from Phillips's theory that eating regularly one day every week tricks the body into holding metabolism levels steady rather than letting them slow down in response to perceived starvation. The weightlifting program is simple; anyone who has spent time in a gym will immediately be comfortable following Phillips's directions. As founder and executive editor of *Muscle Media,* a strength-training magazine, Phillips knows his way around exercise equipment.

With a detailed twelve-week training schedule and daily progress reports, users can easily follow the exercise script and chart their progress in the back of the book. Phillips predicts people can lose up to twenty-five pounds of body fat in the twelve-week program but cautions that losing more than two pounds per week could signal the loss of muscle tissue as well. Critics say that in the short term any diet will cause a weight loss but because of its many restrictions, this diet and other low-carbohydrate, high-protein eating plans are difficult to follow for long periods. The fact remains that carbohydrates help store fluid in the body, so when a dieter restricts carbohydrates the body releases some of those fluids. And when dieters resume eating carbohydrates they can expect a quick weight gain of from 5 to 10 pounds as the lost fluids returns.

See also:

Atkins Nutritional Approach; Food Guide Pyramid; The Zone.

Additional Reading

Phillips, Bill, and Michael D'Orso. *Body for Life: 12 Weeks to Mental and Physical Strength.* New York: HarperCollins, 1999.

Body Mass Index

Researchers developed the Body Mass Index (BMI) to help people gauge a healthy weight range for their age. However, for teens who are still growing, the BMI should be used more as a guideline than to actually determine risk level. Here's how to calculate it:

#1. Multiply your weight in pounds by 704.5.

#2. Multiply your height in inches by your height in inches.*

Divide answer #1 by answer #2.

* If you're 5′5″, your height in inches would be 65 inches.

If your BMI is	your risk level is
19–24	minimal to low
25–26	low to moderate
27–29	moderate to high
30–34	high to very high
35–39	very high to extremely high
40+	extremely high

Using this formula, let's calculate the BMI of two people.

One is 5′4″ and weighs 130 pounds.

#1. $130 \times 704.5 = 91,585$

#2. $64 \times 64 = 4,096$

BMI = 91,585 divided by 4,096 = 22.4

Look at the chart above. That figure is within the range of minimal to low risk.

Now let's look at another person who is 5′9″ and weighs 210 pounds

#1. 210 × 704.5 = 147,945

#2. 69 × 69 = 4,761

BMI = 147,945 divided by 4,761 = 31

That person is in the range of high to very high risk and needs to put some serious effort into losing weight.

Bulimia Nervosa

Bulimia nervosa is an eating disorder characterized by a binge-and-purge eating pattern. Either by forcing herself to vomit, taking laxatives or diuretics, or giving herself enemas, the bulimic is purging to rid herself of the food she ate. There is also a nonpurging form of bulimia, characterized by some other method of keeping the weight off, such as compulsive exercising or fasting.

Binges and purges can range from once or twice a week to several times a day. What is visible to family and friends, however, may only be strident dieting. Symptomatic of the disorder is the excessive amount of food being eaten. Someone with bulimia will eat more food and more frequently than most people. Often, while eating, the person seems to lack control or feels as if he or she can't stop eating. For example, normal food intake for women and teens is between 2,000 and 3,000 calories per day. But bulimic binges are often more than that in a span of less than two hours. Some people with the disorder have reported consuming up to 20,000 calories in binges lasting up to eight hours.

Rapidly purging food, either through abuse of laxatives, enemas, and diuretics, or induced vomiting, upsets the body's balance of chemicals, including sodium and potassium. The result is often fatigue, irregular heartbeat, thinner bones, and seizures. Repeated vomiting can also damage the stomach and esophagus and can erode tooth enamel. It can also result in skin rashes and broken blood vessels in the face.

Bulimia typically begins during adolescence and can continue for years undetected by others. The longer someone with an eating disorder waits to seek help, the more ingrained her eating habits become and the more difficult the recovery.

Cabbage Soup Diet

The Cabbage Soup diet is a quick weight-loss plan that has circulated like a chain letter across the United States for decades via photocopiers, fax machines, and word of mouth. The diet promises a seventeen-pound weight loss in one week and requires followers to adhere to a rigid eating schedule to achieve that goal. Many versions of this anonymously created diet have surfaced over the years. The basic soup recipe has also been attributed to many sources, including Raymond Dietz, a doctor who proposed it to his patients in the 1930s. The soup was published in the 1960s as Dr. Cooper's Super Soup in *The Doctors' Clinic 30 Program,* by J. T. Cooper. In 1975 another version of the soup and eating plan appeared in the *Oriental Seven Day Quick Weight-Off Diet,* by the one-name author Norvell. Both titles were re-released by the publishers in 1996. The diet has also been called "The Skinny," and the "Basic Fat Burning Soup Diet."

The recipe is a simple one and consists of one head of cabbage, six large onions, two green peppers, one 28-ounce can of tomatoes, one bunch of celery, one packet of onion soup mix, and water. The cook is instructed to chop the vegetables, boil all the ingredients rapidly for ten minutes and then simmer. For one week dieters eat all the soup they want plus a specified food, mostly in unlimited amounts. Meals for Day 1 include soup and any fruit except bananas; Day 2 is soup and vegetables, including a baked potato with butter for dinner. Potatoes are off-limits on the other six days. Day 3 is soup, fruits, and vegetables; Day 4 allows up to eight bananas and skim milk plus soup; Day 5 is soup and six tomatoes plus 20 ounces of beef, chicken, or fish; Day 6 is the same and vegetables are not limited to tomatoes; and Day 7 is soup, brown rice, unsweetened fruit juice, and vegetables.

Nutrition experts call the diet an unbalanced, unrealistic plan and say pounds shed are mostly water weight. Critics acknowledge that the soup is filling, but add that eating two bowls of any low-carbohydrate soup will act as an appetite suppressant. Cabbage soup dieters complain of gas, nausea, and fatigue after a few days on this diet but nutritionists say the one-week duration isn't long enough for most people to suffer any serious health problems. But people on this plan can expect to suffer from extreme boredom and a return of lost pounds once they resume their normal eating patterns.

Additional Reading

Cooper, Sharon, and J.T. Cooper. *The Doctor's Clinic 30 Program*. Erie, Pa.: Green Tree Press, 1996.

Norvell. *The Oriental Seven Day Quick Weight-Off Diet*. West Nyack, N.Y.: Parker Publishing Co., 1996.

Rubin, Rita, and Leonard Wiener. "A Bad Diet With Phony Credentials." *U.S. News & World Report*, 24 June 1996, 69.

Weinraub, Judith. "A Closer Look Into the Cabbage Soup Diet." *Washington Post*, 6 March 1996, E5.

Yazigi, Monique P. "The Cabbage-Soup Diet That Came From Nowhere." *New York Times*, 20 March 1996, C3.

Caffeine

Caffeine is a natural substance found in the leaves, seeds, or fruits of over sixty-three plant species worldwide and is part of a group of compounds known as methylxanthines. The most commonly known sources of caffeine are coffee and cocoa beans, cola nuts and tea leaves. Diets high in sodium and caffeine negatively affect calcium levels because calcium is lost through urine.

Calcium

Calcium is a mineral that contributes to strong bones and teeth. It's found naturally in dairy products, green leafy vegetables, and soy products, including tofu. Calcium requirements are highest for adolescents, whose bones are growing rapidly, and pregnant and lactating women. In 1999, the American Academy of Pediatrics revised its policy statement to read that preteens and adolescents, should have 1,200 to 1,500 milligrams per day of calcium. The policy also recommends exercise as an important component in achieving maximal peak bone mass, and stresses that fat-reduced dairy products such as skim milk are just as nutritious for older children.

So how do you get this much calcium? Consuming four to five glasses of low-fat milk per day is one way. Other milk products are also good sources of calcium. Green leafy vegetables, such as kale, collards, beets, and turnip tops are also natural sources of calcium. So are tofu, dried peas and beans, the soft bones of canned fish, and calcium-fortified orange juice. Many people find they can get enough calcium through a healthy diet, but calcium supplements do exist for those who cannot or who are at particularly high risk for osteoporosis. Read the label of a calcium supplement carefully to find the amount of "elemental" calcium. There are different kinds of calcium supplements—including calcium citrate (which is generally the most easily absorbed), calcium carbonate, and calcium phosphate—that include other elements such as vitamin D, which help with absorption.

While more is generally better, too much is not good. Overdoses of calcium can interfere with the absorption of other nutrients, such as zinc and iron.

Bone mass is also affected by how you use your body. Weight-bearing exercise, such as dancing and running, can increase bone mass and strength. Unhealthy activities, such as smoking, alcohol use, and a poor diet contribute to losing bone mass. Diets high in sodium and caffeine negatively affect calcium levels because calcium is lost through urine.

According to the National Institute of Child Health and Human Development (NICHD), supplementing the daily diets of girls, ages 12 to 16, with an extra 350 milligrams of calcium produced a 14 percent increase in bone density. Researchers say this is a striking difference because for every 5 percent increase in bone density, the risk of later bone fracture declines by 40 percent.

Calcium requirements rise again during the second and third trimester of pregnancy—the period during which the fetal skeleton is developing quickly. The general recommendation is that calcium intake be increased by 400 milligrams per day.

Calorad

Calorad is a weight loss product, advertised as a collagen protein supplement. According to the manufacturer, Essentially Yours Industries, dieters who take one tablespoon of Calorad with water just before bed and don't eat or drink anything but water for three hours before taking the supplement, will lose excess fat and toxins naturally and will see an increase in lean body mass.

Collagen hydrolysat, the main ingredient listed on the label, is the scientific name for gelatin. Other ingredients in Calorad include aloe vera, which has a laxative effect when taken orally; glycerin, a sugar alcohol traditionally used as a mild sweetener; and potassium sorbate and methyl paraben, preservatives to keep the collagen from spoiling. Critics like the National Council Against Health Fraud, say the manufacturer's claims that Calorad helps build lean muscle mass and burn more calories during sleep are inaccurate. They suggest that weight loss associated with Calorad may stem from the fact that users do not eat for three hours before bed. In many adults this would amount to a reduced intake of daily calories, resulting in weight loss.

Critics say studies show human muscle tissue does not spontaneously generate with increased protein consumption; instead, muscle mass is increased through various types of resistance training. Calorad packaging and advertising claims users can increase muscle mass without exercise. Critics also cite the lack of peer-reviewed research published to support the scientific claims of the product. The manufacturer points to anecdotal testimonials as proof of Calorad's effectiveness.

Additional Reading

Czarnecki, Joanne, and Shelley Drozd. "Rating the Fat-fighters." *Men's Health,* January 1999, 60.

Calories

A calorie is a measurement of heat needed to raise 1 kilogram of water 1 degree Centigrade. Since food "stokes the furnace" of our bodies, foods have assigned calorie values. The number of calories in a food can be found on the Nutrition Facts label on any packaged food. Realize, however, that these are calories per serving. If the nutrition label claims the package has two servings—and you've eaten it all, you've eaten double the calories that the label says.

Fat and alcohol are high in calories. Foods high in both sugars and fat contain many calories but often are low in vitamins, minerals, or fiber. There are numerous calorie counters readily available—online and often in cookbooks. If you reduce your caloric intake, you'll lose weight. If you increase the amount of calories you consume, you'll gain weight. A pound equals 3,500 calories. So to lose a pound in, say a week, you'll either have to eat 3,500 calories less or burn off 3,500 calories in exercise, or some combination of the two.

It is possible to estimate about how many calories per day you need to eat to maintain your body weight. Once you use the formula below to calculate that number, you can tweak it. If you want to lose weight, cut the calories or increase your level of activity.

Moderately active males should multiply their weight in pounds by 15. For example, if you weigh 170 pounds, you need about 2,500 calories per day. Moderately active females should multiply their weight by 12. A 130-pound female needs about 1,560 calories per day.

However, if you are not regularly active, you'll need to use a different formula because the number of calories needed per day decreases as the level of activity does. In other words, if you burn fewer calories a day, you'll need fewer of them to maintain your weight. Relatively inactive men should multiply their weight by 13 pounds and women in that category should multiply their weigh by 10. So that a 170-pound man who is relatively inactive needs only 2,210 calories and a 130-pound inactive woman needs only 1,300 calories to maintain body weight.

Calories from Fat

Numerous health and government authorities, including the U.S. Surgeon General, the National Academy of Sciences, the American Heart Association, and the American Dietetic Association, recommend reducing dietary fat to 30 percent or less of total calories. However, that doesn't mean you have to give up all high-fat food products. For example, peanut butter with sugar added has 200 calories in a two-tablespoon serving. Of those, 140 calories are from fat—70 percent. Add that peanut butter to two slices of whole wheat bread, which have 120 calories and 20 calories from fat, and the equation is different: now the fat is down to about 48 percent. It's still higher than the recommendation, but by adding a glass of skim milk and an apple, you start to bring it down to a healthy level.

Keep in mind that the information on nutrition labels is based on a 2,000-calorie-per-day diet. So if your average caloric intake is lower, realize that the overall percentage of fat is higher than what's listed on the label. For example, back to the peanut butter with its 16 grams of total fat and 3 grams of saturated fat. The total fat is 25 percent of the daily value and the saturated fat is 15 percent of the daily value—based on a 2,000-calorie diet, which calls for less than 65 grams of total fat and less than 20 grams of saturated fat per day. Now let's say you're inactive and need only 1,300 calories per day to maintain your body weight. You'd need to cut your overall dietary fat intake accordingly.

In general, restoring physical activity to our daily routines is critical. According to surveys conducted in 1977–78 and 1994–96, reported daily caloric intakes increased from 2,239 kcal (calories) to 2,455 kcal in men and from 1,534 kcal to 1,646 kcal in women.

Eating more frequently is encouraged by numerous environmental changes: a greater variety of foods, some with higher caloric content; the growth of the fast-food industry; the increased numbers and marketing of snack foods; and a growing tendency to socialize with food and drink. At the same time, there are fewer opportunities in daily life to burn calories: children watch more television daily; many schools have done away with or cut back on physical education; many neighborhoods lack sidewalks for safe walking; the workplace has become increasingly automated; household chores are assisted by labor-saving machinery; and walking and cycling have been replaced by automobile travel for all but the shortest distances.

Consider this: the American Institute for Cancer Research says Americans' snack-food intake has tripled in the last twenty years. An average American now consumes 16 to 20 pounds of snack food, or 40,000 snack calories, a year.

Calories Burned During Exercise

Exercise burns calories. For example, walking briskly can burn off about 100 calories per mile. Bicycling for half an hour at nearly 10 mph will burn about 195 calories. The specific number is dependent on the person's weight and the intensity of the activity. A variety of interactive exercise counters, available on the Internet, allow you to plug in your weight and age, and change variables such as the length of time and intensity of the activity. For someone working to lose weight, the combination of exercise and a healthy diet works more effectively than either method by itself. Eat less and you'll lose weight. Exercise more and you'll lose weight and tone muscles and build aerobic endurance. Do both and they'll complement each other.

The more you weigh, the more calories you'll burn. The reason is that your heart has to pump harder to get the blood to the different parts of your body. So a 130-pound person doing medium-intensity aerobic dancing for thirty minutes will burn about 174 calories in that time. A 150-pound person will burn about 201 calories in the same amount of time.

The Austin (Texas) Diagnostics Clinic put together this listing of calorie-burning levels of different activities in the Spring 1998 issue of its fitness publication, *Classics Club Quarterly*. Many such listings and online calculators exist to help provide a more precise gauge on how and what you're doing.

Let's say you eat 2,000 calories worth of food. But your physical activity only uses 1,500 of these. The extra calories are stored in your body—as fat. When you exercise, your body uses fuel, which comes from one of two forms: stored carbohydrates called glycogen or stored body fat. Stored body fat is found in fat

CALORIE BURNING ACTIVITIES CHART

Activity	Calories burned in 30 minutes (by weight)				
	100 lb	125 lb	150 lb	175 lb	200lb
Basketball	192	240	288	336	384
Bicycling (10–12 mph)	144	180	216	252	288
Dancing (ballroom, slow)	72	90	108	126	144
Football (flag)	192	240	288	336	384
Golf (using cart)	84	105	126	147	168
Golf (no cart)	120	150	180	210	240
Racquetball	240	300	360	420	480
Running (5 mph)	192	240	288	336	384
Step Aerobics (low intensity)	144	180	216	252	288
Swimming (50 yds/min, freestyle)	192	240	288	336	384
Tennis (singles)	192	240	288	336	384
Walking (2 mph)	72	90	108	126	144
Walking (4 mph)	96	120	144	168	192

cells and is also stored in small droplets in the muscles.

Most activities use both carbohydrates and fat for fuel. Lower intensity workouts, such as walking, use fat as the primary fuel. As the workout intensifies, the fuel reserves come increasingly from carbohydrates. But that doesn't mean that walking burns more fat than running. When the carbohydrate or glycogen source runs low, the body releases fats for fuels. Also, a higher-intensity workout, such as running, continues to burn fat even after the physical activity itself is over. As the body works to restore glycogen, it continues to use fat to do so. And because higher-intensity workouts burn more calories overall, even though the mix of carbohydrates and fats may be different, you're still burning more fat in the workout.

Carbohydrates

Carbohydrates provide energy for the brain, central nervous system, and muscle cells. They are found largely in sugars, fruits, vegetables, and cereals and grains. Meats generally have no carbohydrates. There are simple carbohydrates, such as sugars, and complex carbohydrates, such as breads and pastas, that the body breaks down into sugars. Someone with a 2,000-calorie-per-day diet should limit carbohydrates to 300 grams. Someone with a 2,500-calorie-per-day diet can consume up to 375 grams of carbohydrates. A medium baked potato with skin has 51 grams of carbohydrates. An apple has about 21 grams of carbohydrates, a tablespoon of sugar has 12 grams, and a slice of pie can pack 60 or more grams of carbohydrates.

On the Nutrition Facts label on food products, total carbohydrates are broken down into two categories: fiber and sugar.

All carbohydrates eventually break down into sugars in your body. The difference is that complex carbohydrates do so more gradually, providing energy over a longer period of time. And complex carbohydrates also contain other nutrients whereas simple sugars generally do not. That's particularly true of "empty" calories, such as soft drinks and candy.

Carbohydrate Addict's Diet

The Carbohydrate Addict's diet, was developed by the husband and wife team of Rachael F. Heller and Richard F. Heller, who hold PhDs in psychology and biology, respectively. It is a low-carbohydrate diet based on the theory that as many as 75 percent of people who are overweight have a carbohydrate addiction. On their Web site, such an addiction is defined as having "A compelling hunger, craving, or desire for carbohydrate-rich foods; an escalating, recurring need or drive for starches, snack foods, junk food, or sweets."

The body counteracts carbohydrate consumption by releasing the hormone insulin. The Hellers say that people with carbohydrate addictions have a hormonal imbalance. The body releases too much insulin when they eat carbohydrates. As a result, they feel hungry again sooner as the excess insulin signals their body to take in more food. Insulin also signals the body to store food energy as fat.

That's why carbohydrate addicts, who may be eating low-fat meals, still gain weight. The diet plan outlined in the Carbohydrate Addict's diet consists of two carbohydrate-restricted meals and one "reward meal" in which anything can be eaten up to one hour following a high-protein meal.

The Web site offers a quiz to help determine if you're a "carbohydrate addict." It asks questions about eating habits: do you eat even though you're not really hungry or if you finish a meal and don't feel satisfied? If so, you may be a carbohydrate addict. Is it hard for you to resist snacking at night and is it difficult to stop snacking once you've started? If so, you may also be a carb addict.

The Hellers, who are carbohydrate addicts themselves, say this diet plan has done much to both help them lose weight and maintain weight loss. They followed up on the *Carbohydrate Addict's Diet* with other books, among them, *The Carbohydrate Addict's Program for Success* and *The Carbohydrate Addict's Gram Counter.*

Are Americans eating too many carbohydrates? Carbohydrate consumption has increased by fifty pounds per person per year over the past decade. As people have turned away from high-fat foods, carbohydrates may have become a greater share of most Americans' diets.

An article in the *Journal of the American Dietetic Association* suggested that carbohydrates became the dieter's taboo "because the low-fat diets of the 1980s and 1990s failed consumers who mistakenly believed that consumption of low-fat products was license to eat voraciously while paying no mind to the amount of sugar and energy being consumed. Many people find irresistible the basis of low-carbohydrate diets: eating as much protein as desired—including steaks, eggs, and other fatty foods that they had previously been told by media reports and medical practitioners to shun—and still losing weight, so long as intake of carbohydrates is strictly limited."

Yet many critics of these restrictive carbohydrate plans say severely limiting carbohydrates is not good either. All high-protein, low-carbohydrate plans put the dieter at risk of loss of vitamin B, calcium, and potassium, resulting from lack of carbohydrates in the diet, and risk of coronary heart disease from eating more high-protein foods that are also high in fat.

While a low-carbohydrate diet will help a dieter lose weight initially, critics say the dieter will feel lethargic. Because there are so few carbohydrates to burn as energy, the body begins to burn lean muscle mass for energy. The Physicians Committee for Responsible Medicine rated the Carbohydrate Addict's Program as unsafe.

Additional Reading

Gotthardt, Melissa Meyers. "The New Low-Carb Diet Craze." *Cosmopolitan,* February 2000, 148.

Heller, Rachael F., and Richard F. Heller. *The Carbohydrate Addict's Program for Success.* New York: Plume, 1993.

————. *Carbohydrate Addicted Kids: Help Your Child or Teen Break Free of Junk Food or Sugar Cravings for Life.* New York: HarperCollins, 1998.

————. *The Carbohydrate Addict's Diet: The Lifelong Solution to Yo-Yo Dieting.* New York: New American Library, 1999.

————. *The Carbohydrate Addict's Cookbook.* Hoboken, N.J.: John Wiley & Sons, 2000.

Physicians Committee for Responsible Medicine press release: "Doctors Rate Popular Diet Books." 9 January 2001.

Stein, Joel. "The Low-Carb Diet Craze." *Time,* 1 November 1999, 71–79.

Stein, Karen. "High Protein, Low-Carbohydrate Diets: Do They Work?" *Journal of the American Dietetic Association,* 100, no. 7 (July 2000): 760.

Turner, Richard, and Joan Raymond. "The Trendy Diet That Sizzles: A Counterintuitive Program Reaches Critical Mass." *Newsweek International,* 13 September 1999, 62.

Wilgoren, Jodi. "Low-Carb Diet: Lose the Bun, Not the Burger." *New York Times,* 11 January 2000, D7.

www.carbohydrateaddict.com.

Childhood Obesity

The combination of diets filled with high-fat foods and too little exercise con-tinues to expand obesity rates for American children and teens. The latest findings from the Centers for Disease Control and Prevention's (CDC) National Health and Nutrition Examination Survey (NHANES) show that more children and teens are overweight. This continues the pattern the survey documented over the past two decades when the number of overweight children and teens in the United States nearly doubled.

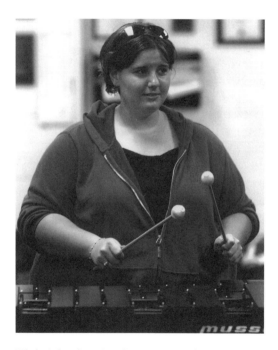

High School senior Courtney Dunham listens to instructions from her section leader during band practice at Milford (Ohio) High School, on September 11, 2002. Despite numerous attempts at dieting to shed weight, Dunham chose obesity surgery at Cincinnati Children's Hospital and as seen in this photo, has lost twenty-nine pounds since the operation. Her goal is to fit into size 16 jeans, twelve sizes smaller than before surgery. The latest government findings show that the number of overweight children and teens in the United States nearly doubled over the past two decades. (AP/Wide World Photos)

Growing along with the obesity rate is the cost of pediatric health care, according to another report released in May 2002 in *Pediatrics,* the journal of the American Academy of Pediatrics. The study, also conducted by the Centers for Disease Control and Prevention (CDC), showed that childhood diabetes doubled during the last two decades, gall bladder disease tripled, and sleep apnea increased fivefold, a substantial increase. Sleep apnea, a disorder in which a sleeping person repeatedly stops breathing for long enough to lower the amount of oxygen in the blood and brain, is more common among overweight children because fat gathers at the back of the neck and can block the airway.

The researchers also found that obesity, in addition to directly contributing to childhood diseases, is turning up more often as a secondary factor in illnesses such as asthma and mental-health disorders. A statement issued by Dr. Jeffrey P. Koplan, director of the CDC, said the figures show a growing epidemic of obesity, which must be addressed so that American children can lead healthier lives. Koplan added that overweight children, like their adult counterparts, would continue to be at increasing risk for cardiovascular diseases, diabetes, and other serious health problems as long as childhood obesity remained a major health problem in the United States.

Parents can exacerbate the problems of overweight children. A press release from the Bassett Healthcare Research Institute in Cooperstown, New York, noted that research found that most parents of overweight children do not think of their children as overweight. Physician and researcher Barbara A. Dennison said, "For example, 68 percent of parents of obese children, those with a BMI above the 95th percentile, reported that their child's weight was 'OK, just right,' and 8 percent even reported their child was 'underweight.' "

The press release also cited research that showed parents can do more harm than good by using dessert as a reward for finishing dinner. "Using foods like desserts as rewards tends to increase the child's preference for those foods, while rewarding a child for finishing dinner may actually encourage overeating," Dennison said.

See also:

obesity; television.

Additional Reading

Bassett Healthcare Research Institute press release. "Bassett Study Reports Early Childhood Obesity Not Recognized By Most Parents." 22 May 2000.

Cholesterol (Blood Types)

Blood cholesterol is divided into three separate classes of lipoproteins: very-low density lipoprotein (VLDL); low-density lipoprotein (LDL), which contains most of the cholesterol found in the blood; and high-density lipoprotein (HDL).

LDL seems to be the culprit in coronary heart disease and is popularly known as bad cholesterol. Too much LDL in the bloodstream can build up within the walls of the arteries and contribute to the formation of plaque, which can ultimately clog the arteries. A blood test can measure cholesterol levels. Ideally, LDL levels should be below 130.

By contrast, HDL is increasingly considered desirable and known as good cholesterol. HDL levels typically range from 40 to 50 milligrams/dL for men and 50 to 60 milligrams/dL for women. Levels below 35 milligrams/dL are abnormally low and pose a risk factor for cardiac problems. Low HDL levels can be caused by cigarette smoking, obesity, and lack of physical activity.

Cholesterol (Dietary)

Dietary cholesterol is found only in animal foods. Abundant in organ meats and egg yolks, cholesterol is also contained in meats and poultry. Vegetable oils and shortenings are cholesterol-free.

Foods high in saturated fat raise blood cholesterol more than other forms of fat. Limiting saturated fats to less than 10 percent of calories should help lower blood cholesterol levels. While polyunsaturated and monounsaturated fats could help lower blood cholesterol levels, the recommendation still holds that total fat should account for no more than 30 percent of daily calorie intake.

Christian Diets

With the 1957 publication of Charlie Shedd's book, *Pray Your Weight Away,* Christian-oriented weight loss programs set their sights on an audience beyond church walls. Today faith-based dieting programs, books, and workouts continue to grow in popularity. Dieting programs such as Gwen Shamblin's Weigh Down workshop are held in thousands of churches across the country. Book titles such as *Slim for Him, More of Jesus, Less of Me,* and *What Would Jesus Eat?* preach the gospel of eating right for God. And Christian exercise videos like Sheri Chamber's *Praise Aerobics* link exercise and spirituality.

Shamblin is among the most visible of a growing list of Christian diet creators. Her approach, grounded in a conservative form of Protestant Christianity, requires no calorie counting or measuring. Instead, she suggests that a person with un-

healthy food cravings may be suffering from a real spiritual hunger. Shamblin advocates eating only when truly hungry and she believes that eating when the body doesn't need food is a sign that an individual needs to get right with God. If overeating is a problem of the soul, she suggests that putting your spiritual life in order will bring weight loss without cutting out foods you love. To illustrate that point she teaches people to stop midway through a candy bar, or eat M&M's one by one, to let their taste buds savor the flavor without feeling guilty. Shamblin organized her first support group in 1986 and now counts over 10,000 Weigh Down workshops with a quarter of a million participants. Shamblin and others find willing followers among the estimated 39 percent of born-again Christians in the United States.

Conservative estimates place the total worth of the American dieting industry at over $30 billion a year and economists say a healthy 5 percent of that is Christian money.

Christian dieting programs, like their secular counterparts, are not created equal. First come the programs that avoid strict rules and focus instead on the spiritual side of eating rather than the calorie counting. At the top of the list in popularity is Shamblin's Weigh Down workshop. But newer titles, like Dr. Don Colbert's *What Would Jesus Eat?: The Ultimate Program for Eating Well, Feeling Great, and Living Longer,* go beyond Shamblin's comfort food choices. Colbert, a family physician, tells dieters to examine and emulate the simple diet of Jesus. Basically he advocates the Mediterranean diet favored by many nutritionists—a diet low in saturated fat, sugar, and red meat and high in whole grains, fruits, and vegetables. Plus he encourages the consumption of fish, the use of olive oil, and a daily exercise regimen.

Colbert received his medical degree from Oral Roberts School of Medicine in Tulsa, Oklahoma. After developing chronic fatigue syndrome as a young doctor, he began looking more closely at the links between physical, spiritual, and mental health. He detailed his experiences in his first book, *What You Don't Know May Be Killing You,* which he wrote after he quit eating processed and fatty foods and took up exercise. He describes his newest plan in *What Would Jesus Eat?* as an "all-natural diet from biblical times," and says those who follow his suggestions can expect good health, fitness, longevity, and spiritual health. In his book Colbert acknowledges the similarities between his diet and other nutrition plans, but writes that his program has a healthy difference. "The low-fat diets, such as the Pritikin and Ornish Diets, also work. People lose weight. However, the low-fat diet doesn't taste as good, and after eating a meal, a person often leaves the table without feeling satisfied. This can lead to binge eating. For all of these diets, an equal and opposite 'binge response' seems to be waiting around the corner." He goes on to suggest that binge eating can be avoided by choosing simpler foods. He writes that such a lifestyle, filled with foods cooked in olive oil, seasoned with herbs and spices, meals of fresh fruits, vegetables, and whole grains leave a person feeling full and nourished. Even less traditional than Colbert's plan is the Hallelujah Diet, founded by George Malkmus. He preaches the benefits of vegetarianism and a raw food diet based on foods found in the Garden of Eden.

Still other Christian dieting programs more closely resemble their secular counterparts and advocate food exchanges, measuring amounts, and counting calories. Carol Showalter's *3D: Diet, Discipline, and Discipleship* is a faith-based twelve-week plan that relies on the American Diabetes Association food exchange lists in a style similar to the Weight Watchers program but unlike Weight Watchers it draws inspiration from the Bible. Founded in 1973 by Showalter, a Presbyterian pastor's wife, this program teaches that Christians can lose weight successfully by meeting in small groups and by leading disciplined lives with disciplined eating and disciplined prayer. The book also emphasizes good nutrition, proper eating habits, sensible weight loss, and a long-term exercise program.

First Place is yet another Christian-based diet program, founded in 1981 in Houston's First Baptist Church. Carole Lewis, national director of the group, said in an article in the September 2000 issue of *Christianity Today* that the group supports a recognized food plan, using food exchanges and the Food Guide Pyramid developed by the U.S. Department of Agriculture (USDA) with the added goal of drawing dieters closer to Christ.

While no formal studies have looked at faith-based weight-loss programs, experts say that adding a spiritual component can be a positive step, since the most successful programs do incorporate a lot of social support. In response to suggestions that there is a link between spiritual hunger and physiological hunger, Shape Up America! even added a "soul food" section to its Web site, featuring a series of tutorials that explore the actual concept of spiritual hunger. Ultimately, nutritionists say any faith-based diet must still be based on healthy eating and regular exercise, not just on the notion that God wants us to be thin.

See also:

Ornish, Dean; Pritikin, Nathan; Shamblin, Gwen; Weigh Down Diet; Weight Watchers.

Additional Reading

Brown, Deneen. "Dieting Faithfully; Proponents of the Weigh Down Diet Turn to God for the Will to Resist Overeating." *Washington Post*, 11 April 2000, Z14.

Colbert, Don, M.D. *What Would Jesus Eat?: The Ultimate Program for Eating Well, Feeling Great, and Living Longer*. Nashville: Thomas Nelson Publishers, 2002.

Showalter, Carol. *3D: Diet, Discipline & Discipleship*. Brewster, Mass.: Paraclet Press, 1973; new, rev. ed. 2002.

Winner, Lauren F. "The Weigh & the Truth." *Christianity Today*, 4 September 2000, 50.

D'Adamo, Peter J.

Peter J. D'Adamo (b. 1956, New York) is a naturopathic physician and researcher who developed the blood type diet, Eat Right 4 Your Type. The diet suggests that one's blood type is the key to healthy eating and living. For example, people with Type O blood are descended from earliest man; a high-protein diet and strenuous physical activities are best suited to them. Type As are descended from a gentler agrarian culture and therefore Type As do best with a vegetarian diet and noncompetitive physical activity.

In D'Adamo's 1996 book, he explained that he is a second-generation naturopathic physician and credited the genesis of blood type diets to his father, James D'Adamo. The Eat Right diet plan has its share of critics who say that categorizing people by their blood type is a flawed basis on which to build a successful diet.

In 1990, D'Adamo was selected Physician of the Year by the American Association of Naturopathic Physicians. He founded *The Journal of Naturopathic Medicine* and works in a private practice in Stamford, Connecticut.

See also:

Eat Right 4 Your Type.

Dehydration

Dehydration occurs when the body loses too much water or the intake of water is too low. Severe diarrhea or vomiting can cause dehydration. Fitness experts suggest drinking a cup of water about half an hour before exercising and immediately after a 20- to 30-minute workout to keep the body adequately hydrated. Don't drink beverages containing alcohol or caffeine, since both promote dehydration.

Dexatrim

Dexatrim is a once-a-day diet pill originally formulated with the controversial appetite suppressant phenylpropanolamine, or PPA. It became a best seller among over-the-counter weight-loss pills following its introduction in 1976. In 2000 company officials pulled Dexatrim from drugstore shelves following a November 2000 public health warning to consumers by the U.S. Food and Drug Administration (FDA), saying PPA was no longer safe for consumption and had been shown to increase the risk of stroke in young women.

The FDA also asked manufacturers of products containing PPA—diet drugs as well as over-the-counter allergy and cold medications—to use another active ingredient in their formulas. Dexatrim, with sales of $200 million in 1999, responded.

Chattem, Inc. withdrew the original formula and released an herbal alternative, Dexatrim Natural. The replacement uses the herb ephedra in place of PPA; an ingredient critics say may be just as dangerous as PPA. Derived from a Chinese herb called mahuang, ephedra/ephedrine is a stimulant used for short-term energy boosts and to increase metabolism and suppress the appetite. Researchers are studying the possibility that the human body may convert ephedra to PPA. Information on the Dexatrim Web site informs consumers that Dexatrim Natural follows the FDA's recommended daily dosage limit of 24 milligrams of ephedrine. In 1997 the FDA called for ephedra labeling to recommend a daily dosage limit after serious complications, including heart attacks, strokes, and several deaths, were linked to the ephedra in some dietary supplements.

In the meantime, Chattem launched another new diet drug, Dexatrim Natural Ephedrine-Free. According to packaging, it contains bitter orange peel, caffeine, and ginger root, plus green tea leaf and guarana, both herbal forms of caffeine. Critics argue that these new formulas share the same side effects as products containing ephedrine, including insomnia, restlessness, nausea, dizziness, irritability, anxiety, high blood pressure, and strokes. Diet pills, both prescription and over-the-counter, when used with increased exercise and behavior modification do play a role in short-term weight loss.

However, health professionals continue to question the long-term effects of these medications and they raise concerns that repeated unsuccessful attempts to diet using pills may lead to eating disorders such as anorexia and bulimia in some teenage users. Even though suppliers of weight-control products like Dexatrim Natural do not target teens and have warning labels on their products, younger teens are turning to over-the-counter weight-control products in growing numbers in response to rising teen obesity levels. According to the FDA, a national survey of high-school students conducted by the National Centers for Disease Control and Prevention found that the most common dieting methods used were skipping meals, taking diet pills, and inducing vomiting after eating.

Diet pills at best offer a temporary solution and at worst may jeopardize health. The safest way for anyone to control his or her weight, according to health professionals, is to eat a healthy diet, using the USDA Food Guide Pyramid as a blueprint, and get enough exercise.

See also:

ephedra/ephedrine; phenylpropanolamine (PPA).

Additional Reading

Berman, Phyllis, and Amy Feldman. "An Extraordinary Peddler." *Forbes,* 9 December 1991, 136–39.

Brink, Susan. *U.S. News & World Report,* 20 November 2000, 74.

"Marketing to Teens a Complex Issue." *Chain Drug Review,* 23, no. 7 (9 April 2001): 29.

www.dexatrim.com.

Diabetes

Diabetes is a disease in which the body can no longer produce or properly use insulin, a hormone required to convert sugars and starches from the food we eat into the energy we need. It is one of the most common chronic illnesses today, affecting an estimated 17 million people in the United States and an estimated 120 million people worldwide. It is affecting an in-

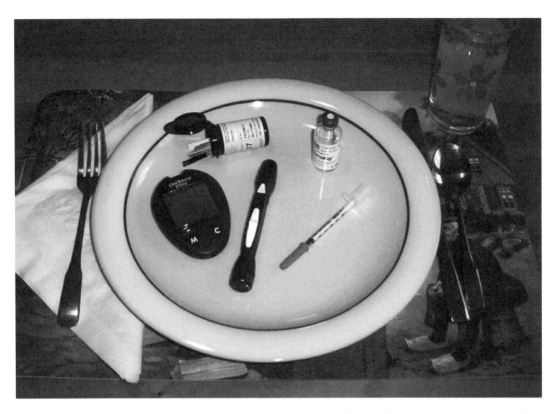

Insulin-dependent diabetics should test their blood sugar several times a day and use the results to adjust their dosage of insulin. The handheld meter requires just one drop of blood to get a glucose level reading. (Courtesy of Marjolijn Bijlefeld)

creasing number of people. The World Health Organization predicts that the total number of people with diabetes worldwide will rise to 300 million by 2025.

There are two major types of diabetes: In Type 1, sometimes called juvenile diabetes or insulin-dependent diabetes, the pancreas no longer produces insulin. Between 5 and 10 percent of people diagnosed with diabetes have Type 1 diabetes. That's between 500,000 and 1 million people in the United States. It usually strikes children or young adults, though it can develop at any age. It occurs when the body's immune system mistakenly attacks the insulin-producing cells in the pancreas. People with Type 1 diabetes must take daily insulin injections to stay alive. While the cause of Type 1 diabetes is unknown, it is likely that heredity plays a role. However, in susceptible individuals, a virus can trigger the disease.

In Type 2 diabetes, the body does produce insulin, but either makes too little or has become resistant to it. More than 90 percent of people with diabetes have Type 2, and it most often strikes older people and those with a history of obesity and inactivity, though increasingly it is appearing in younger people—even children—who are overweight and inactive. Type 2 diabetics can often control their blood sugar levels through weight loss, exercise, and better nutrition, but many also need oral medications and/or insulin.

A third type of diabetes, gestational diabetes, is a temporary condition that occurs during pregnancy, when the body fails to produce the extra insulin needed during some pregnancies. Gestational diabetes requires that the pregnant woman monitor her food and blood-sugar levels carefully. It usually goes away after the pregnancy, but women who have had it are at an increased risk of later developing Type 2 diabetes.

Heredity plays a role in development of Type 1 diabetes. Siblings of people with Type 1 as well as children of parents with Type 1 are at a higher risk of developing the disease. Type 1 most often strikes in puberty, according to researchers, though it can occur at any age. Type 2 diabetes has a hereditary factor as well—people with a family history of Type 2 are more likely to develop the disease themselves. And some racial and ethnic groups have higher rates of diabetes. African Americans and Latinos are nearly twice as likely to develop Type 2 diabetes as the general population.

The warning signs for Type 1 diabetes include frequent urination, excessive thirst, unusual hunger, extreme fatigue, and unexplained weight loss. Victims of Type 2 diabetes can experience the same symptoms, as well as blurred vision, tingling or numbness in the hands or feet, and cuts, bruises, and infections that are slow to heal. Often, though, people with Type 2 diabetes will have no symptoms at all, and the disease won't be discovered until they have developed complications.

Diabetes is the seventh leading cause of death in the United States, and the sixth leading cause of death by disease. Each year, nearly 200,000 people die as a result of diabetes and its long-term complications, which include blindness, kidney disease, heart disease, stroke, nerve disease, and amputations. It is often described as a "silent killer" because in its Type 2 form, it can go undetected for years. It is only when serious and sometimes life-threatening complications develop that many people learn they have the disease. Complications of diabetes—which often take years to develop—stem in many instances from the damage that high blood-sugar levels do to the tiny blood vessels in the body. In instances of kidney failure, for example, damage has been done to the blood vessels inside the kidney that act as filters to remove wastes, chemicals, and excess water from the blood. Poorly controlled diabetes can cause blindness by damaging the tiny blood vessels in the retina.

The most serious short-term complication of Type 1 diabetes is called ketoacidosis. When the body doesn't have enough insulin, it begins to burn fat for energy. Burning fat produces ketones, an acid that can poison the body, leading to coma and even death. Ketoacidosis usually develops slowly—early warning signs include thirst, a dry mouth and frequent urination, and high levels of ketones in the urine. Later, the person may feel nausea, have a fruity odor on the breath, or have difficulty breathing. Ketoacidosis is a serious condition that requires immediate medical attention.

People with diabetes must take a lot of responsibility to make sure their treatment plan works. People with diabetes must balance a variety of factors every day—deciding what to eat and when, or determining how much medication to take and when to take it. Physical activity or illness can also mean adjusting the treatment regimen. The best way to learn that responsibility is to seek advice from a team of health-care professionals.

A primary care physician is a good place to start, but treating diabetes almost always involves specialists in other areas as well. A diabetes care team usually involves an eye doctor, an dietitian, and a certified diabetes educator. If complications arise, a patient might be sent to other specialists.

For people with Type 1 diabetes, insulin is the only option. But there are a wide variety of approaches to insulin therapy. There are more than twenty kinds of insulin available—some act very quickly or peak at different times, and some last all day long. There are also different ways to deliver insulin—syringes, insulin pens, and insulin pumps.

Most people with Type 1 begin by taking two injections of two types of insulin per day. Later they move to taking multiple injections, usually three or four a day, depending on what they're eating or their level of activity. A person with Type 1 diabetes often calculates the amount of carbohydrates she will consume and then injects herself with a number of units of insulin. This formula depends on the individual's reaction to insulin as well as expected activity level.

Injecting insulin before every meal or snack is the most targeted approach to diabetes treatment and allows the greatest flexibility, but some diabetics find it cumbersome. Another approach is to inject a specific amount of insulin in the morning and then eat only those foods that will be covered by that amount of insulin. The second approach is more regimented and doesn't allow for spontaneous snacking.

Another recent innovation in insulin delivery is the insulin pump, a device that looks like a beeper and provides a steady, incremental dose of fast-acting insulin through a tiny tube inserted in the person's abdomen. Insulin pumps are the most expensive approach to diabetes care,

but the device is the closest thing to the normal delivery of insulin that a person with diabetes can achieve. Pumps can be programmed to deliver different amounts of insulin at different times of the day or night, giving the person the ability to fine-tune their treatment regimen.

If you have an insulin-dependent diabetic friend, or if you are insulin-dependent yourself, make sure you discuss this openly with friends. There's the possibility that insulin-dependent diabetics may need help at some point. They may experience an episode of hypoglycemia (low blood sugar) and need help getting a snack or sugared drink. Hypoglycemia occurs when the person has either taken more insulin than needed for the carbohydrates consumed, or is particularly active. The other risk is developing hyperglycemia, or high blood sugar. That happens when the person hasn't taken enough insulin or has eaten more carbohydrates than the insulin can cover. A fast-acting insulin can help counteract these spikes. It's much less intimidating to help a diabetic prepare an insulin injection or provide a sweet snack if you've discussed the symptoms and what to do in advance.

People with Type 2 diabetes have a different set of treatment options. Sometimes, Type 2 diabetes can be controlled through diet and exercise alone. In many cases, though, the body needs help. In people with Type 2, the body doesn't make enough insulin and doesn't use the insulin it does make very well.

Oral medications can help the body reduce blood-sugar levels. There are three classes of drugs for Type 2. The first kind stimulates the body to produce more insulin. The second makes the body more sensitive to the insulin it does have. The third blocks the breakdown of starches and certain sugars, which slows the rise of blood-sugar levels. Sometimes people with Type 2 will take a combination of oral medications, or take pills in combination with insulin. For every person with Type 2, medication combined with improved nutrition and regular exercise is the best treatment.

A key part of self-treatment of diabetes is frequent blood-sugar testing. Pharmacies sell a variety of small blood glucose monitors and test strips that diabetics can (and should) carry with them. The diabetic places a drop of blood on the test strip and within a minute or so has a reading of the blood-sugar levels. The general goal is to achieve blood-sugar levels as close to normal as possible. People without diabetes generally maintain blood-sugar levels between 70 and 120 mg/dl before eating, and less than 180 mg/dl after eating.

People with diabetes can also gauge how well they're controlling their blood sugar by taking a glycated hemoglobin test every three months. The test, done through a doctor's office, measures the presence of excess glucose in the blood over a three- or four-month period and gives a better picture of the effectiveness of the person's diabetes care than a single test on a glucose monitor.

Research has shown that the best way to avoid complications is to keep blood-sugar levels as close to normal as possible. A ten-year study that was completed in 1993 showed the benefits of tight control. The Diabetes Control and Complications Trial (DCCT) followed 1,441 people with Type 1 diabetes for several years. Half of the participants followed a standard diabetes treatment, while the other half followed an intensive-control regimen of multiple injections and frequent blood-sugar testing.

Those who followed the intensive-control regimen had significantly fewer complications. Only half as many developed signs of kidney disease, nerve disease was reduced by two-thirds, and only one-quarter as many developed diabetic eye disease.

Achieving tight control means taking several injections of insulin every day, or using an insulin pump to mimic the release of insulin that occurs in people without diabetes. It also means doing several blood tests a day to gauge how much insulin is needed.

Though the DCCT only followed people with Type 1, researchers believe tight control can have the same effect on people with Type 2. Since most people with Type 2 diabetes do not take insulin, they must take a different approach to tight control. Losing weight is one of the best ways to bring down glucose levels. Regular exercise helps, too, not only to bring down weight but in helping to reduce glucose levels. A recent study of 1,263 men with Type 2 diabetes showed that, over twelve years, the men who did not exercise and stay active were more than twice as likely to die as those who exercised.

Tight control has obvious benefits, but it's not necessarily the right choice for everyone. The DCCT found that people who followed tight control had three times the number of low blood glucose episodes as those using conventional treatment. Plus, people using the tight control approach gained more weight than those on conventional treatment—an average of ten pounds, according to the DCCT.

Those who should avoid tight control include people who already have complications; young children, whose developing brains need glucose; and the elderly, who can suffer strokes or heart attacks from episodes of hypoglycemia.

Additional Reading

American Diabetes Association, www.diabetes.org.

Dietary Fat

Dietary fat is the amount of fat consumed in the foods we eat. Numerous health and government authorities, including the U.S. Surgeon General, the National Academy of Sciences, the American Heart Association, and the American Dietetic Association, recommend reducing dietary fat to 30 percent or less of total calories.

Dietary Guidelines for Americans

In May 2000, the U.S. Department of Agriculture released its revised Dietary Guidelines for Americans. These guidelines are revised every five years, based on new evidence and findings. However, the fundamentals don't change drastically. It's considered more of a refinement. For example, in 1995, the seven dietary guidelines were: eat a variety of foods; balance the foods you eat with physical activity—to maintain or improve your weight; choose a diet with plenty of grain products, vegetables, and fruits; choose a diet low in fat, saturated fat, and cholesterol; choose a diet moderate in sugars; choose a diet moderate in salt and sodium; and if you drink alcoholic beverages, do so in moderation.

The 2000 guidelines are presented as A-B-C or "aim, build, choose" steps. A is to "aim for fitness" with the following two guidelines:

- Aim for a healthy weight.
- Be physically active each day.

B is to "build a healthy base" through the following:

- Let the Food Pyramid guide your food choices.

- Choose a variety of grains daily, especially whole grains.
- Choose a variety of fruits and vegetables daily.
- Keep food safe to eat.

And C is to "choose sensibly" through the following:

- Choose a diet that is low in saturated fat and cholesterol and moderate in total fat.
- Choose beverages and foods that limit your intake of sugars.
- Choose and prepare foods with less salt.
- If you drink alcoholic beverages, do so in moderation.

The most notable changes in the 2000 Dietary Guidelines include greater emphasis on limiting intake of sugar and salt, a focus on a diet that is low in saturated fat and cholesterol, and greater emphasis on physical activity than was evident in the 1995 guidelines.

Dietary Supplement Health and Education Act (DSHEA)

The DSHEA of 1994 was signed into law by President Bill Clinton on October 25, 1994. Congress included several provisions applying strictly to dietary supplements and their ingredients in the DSHEA, hoping to improve the earlier 1958 Food Additive Amendments to the federal Food, Drug and Cosmetic Act (FD&C Act). In findings associated with the DSHEA, Congress stated that there may be a positive link between good dietary practice and good health and there may also be a connection between dietary supplement use, reduced health-care expenses, and disease prevention.

The provisions of DSHEA are designed to ensure that safe and appropriately labeled products remain available to consumers by defining dietary supplements and dietary ingredients; establishing a new framework for assuring their safety; outlining literature guidelines to be displayed where supplements are sold; requiring ingredient and nutrition labeling; providing for use of claims and nutritional support statements; and granting the Food and Drug Administration (FDA) the authority to establish good manufacturing practice (GMP) regulations.

A dietary supplement is now formally defined as a product other than tobacco intended to supplement the diet that bears or contains one or more of the following ingredients: a vitamin, a mineral, an herb or other botanical, an amino acid, a dietary substance used to supplement the diet by increasing the total daily intake, or a concentrate, metabolite, constitute, extract, or combination of these ingredients. A dietary supplement, under the DSHEA is intended for ingestion in pill, capsule, tablet, or liquid form; is not represented for use as a conventional food or as the sole item of a meal or diet; is labeled as a dietary supplement; includes products such as approved drugs, certified antibiotics, or licensed biologics that were marketed as a dietary supplement or food before approval, certification, or license.

The DSHEA also allows the Secretary of Health and Human Services (HHS) to declare that a dietary supplement or dietary ingredient poses an imminent hazard to public health or safety. And the DSHEA restricts manufacturers from statements about the use of a dietary supplement to diagnose, prevent, mitigate, treat, or cure a specific disease.

Under the provisions of the DSHEA, the HHS Secretary may establish an office within the National Institutes of Health to explore the potential role of supplements to improve health care in the United States, to promote scientific study of supplements and their value in preventing chronic diseases, to collect scientific research, and to serve as a scientific adviser to the HHS and the FDA.

Eat Right 4 Your Type

The Eat Right 4 Your Type diet plan suggests that there are four different ideal diets. One for blood type O people, one for blood type A, one for blood type B, and one for blood type AB. Peter J. D'Adamo wrote in the introduction to the 1996 book by the same name, stating that your blood type is the key to understanding much of what your body wants and needs. He breaks down foods into three categories—highly beneficial, neutral, or avoid—for each blood type. His suggestion is that people stop eating the avoid category foods for their blood type. However, people are encouraged to balance their diets by including selections from the neutral categories. Eating only "highly beneficial" foods and eliminating all others will result in too rapid a weight loss and an unhealthy diet, he writes.

He also suggests that some forms of exercise are more beneficial to certain blood types than others. As he writes in the book, "Your blood type plan lets you zero in on the heath and nutrition that corresponds to your exact biological profile."

The Type O diet, for example, should mimic the ancestral high-protein, hunter-gatherer diet, as Type O blood was the earliest in the evolution. Type Os who adopt the Eat Right 4 Your Type diet plan will lose weight because they restrict the amount of grains, breads, legumes, and beans they consume. These foods encourage weight gain in Type Os. Foods that encourage weight loss are seafood, red meat, liver, and some of the leafy green vegetables and kelp. Most meat and fish is either highly beneficial or neutral to Type Os, although bacon, ham, pork, catfish, caviar, and some others should be avoided. Wheat products overall aren't recommended for this blood type; cereals and breads are generally considered neutral at best and the list of grains to avoid is long.

Type Os should exercise vigorously to relieve stress and to lose weight, if needed. Type Os "have the immediate and physical response of our hunter ancestors: stress goes directly to your muscles."

Type A people, however, are the descendants of the "more settled and less warlike farmer ancestors" and therefore, a vegetarian diet suits them best. Type As who cut meat out of their diets will lose weight rapidly "as you eliminate the toxic foods from your diet." That's because Type As store their meat as fat. Most meats should be avoided; seafood can be substituted for red meats. Beans, grains, cereals, breads, vegetables, and fruit are staples of this diet. Stress relief for Type As comes through "quieting techniques" such as yoga and meditation. Competitive sports "will only exhaust your nervous energy, make you tense all over again, and leave your immune system open to illness or disease."

The other two blood types are more difficult to peg. Type Bs, for example, display many of the characteristics of Type Os, but show "a sophisticated refinement in the evolutionary journey, an effort to join together divergent peoples and cultures." Wheats and grains encourage weight gain; green vegetables, meats, eggs, and low-fat dairy products encourage weight loss. In terms of stress reduction and physical activity, Type Bs again show their hybrid past, represented by "both barbarians and agrarians...You're less confrontational than Type Os, but more physically charged than Type As." So physical activities should be a balance between the competitive and the psychic—group hiking, biking, tennis, and aerobics classes are suggested.

Type ABs, which make up only between 2 percent and 5 percent of the population, should take their cues from Type As and Type Bs. Red meats and poultry should be limited; seafood is typically recommended. Tai chi, golf, walking, swimming, hiking, and low-impact aerobics are good for this group, according to the plan.

Eat Right 4 For Your Type provides detailed suggestions for beneficial foods and those to avoid. It further specifies how often certain foods should be eaten, based on the individual's ethnic background. The chapters include menus, beneficial beverages, condiments, and listings of supplements that are best suited for each blood type.

In 2001, D'Adamo followed up with another book, *Live Right 4 Your Type,* suggesting that blood types are not just the key to diet, but the key to each individual's lifestyle. In this volume, D'Adamo lists the characteristics of certain blood types and develops "lifestyle strategies." For example, Type Os are typically impulsive. Therefore, they shouldn't make big decisions when feeling stressed. Methodical eating is recommended—Type Os should sit at the table for each meal and put down the fork and knife between bites. Physical activity is a good outlet for them.

Type As crave consistency in all aspects of their lives. Smaller more frequent meals suit them better. Type Bs also benefit from smaller, more frequent meals. They should seek out ways to connect to their community and find methods to express their nonconformity. Type ABs take their cues from a combination of other blood types—small, frequent meals; a combination of aerobic activity and relaxing techniques; and time alone and time spent with others are all recommended as lifestyle strategies for these people.

The diet has its share of critics. *The Tufts University Health & Nutrition Letter* gave the diet plan an F. Even its fundamental philosophy of tracing blood types back to ancestors is flawed, the review said. "It is a fallacy even to speak of 'original' type Os or 'original' type As because blood types did not originate with humans," explains Stephen Bailey, PhD, a nutritional anthropologist at Tufts. "They came on the biologic scene long before humans did. Furthermore, there is no anthropologic evidence whatsoever that all prehistoric people with a particular blood type ate the same diet."

Additional Reading

D'Adamo, Peter J., with Catherine Whitney. *Eat Right 4 Your Type.* New York: G. P. Putnam's Sons, 1996.

———. *Live Right 4 Your Type.* New York: G. P. Putnam's Sons, 2001.

"Eat Right 4 Your Type" book review. *Tufts University Health & Nutrition Letter,* 15, no. 6 (August 1997): 6.

Williams, Deirdre B., and John J. McMahon. "The Blood Type Diet: Latest Diet Scam," posted on http://www.vegsource.com/articles/blood_hype.htm. Accessed 12 June 2003.

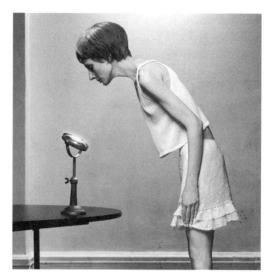

People with eating disorders often have a distorted image of what they look like. (© Dennis Galante/CORBIS)

Eating Disorders

Anorexia nervosa and bulimia nervosa are eating disorders. Food and weight control are the avenues through which the eating disorders are expressed, but eating disorders aren't just about food. People with eating disorders often have issues with self-esteem, stress, fear of becoming overweight, and a feeling of helplessness. What they eat or don't eat becomes a tool of control, either as self-control or even control over others.

Researchers are not precisely sure of what causes eating disorders. They suspect these disorders may stem from a combination of factors—behavioral, genetic, and biochemical. People who develop anorexia often share some similar characteristics: they tend to be obedient, perfectionists, good students, and often excellent athletes. People who develop bulimia and binge eating often eat large amounts of junk food and then feel guilty about it. They eat to relieve stress, but the subsequent guilt increases stress. And the cycle continues.

See also:

anorexia nervosa; bulimia nervosa.

Eicosanoids

Eicosanoids are powerful, hormonelike substances that help control many body processes, including the transfer of oxygen into muscles and the use of fat and carbohydrate as energy sources. Eicosanoids have very diverse effects and are extremely short-lived and hard to study.

In the current culture and its obsession with thinness and weight loss, fats have almost been eliminated from our diet. However, the human body needs small amounts of two types of essential fatty acids that it cannot manufacture. The omega-3s include EPA and DHA. Top sources of omega-3 fats are fish high in oil, like salmon and mackerel. The average American consumes a minuscule one-quarter of a teaspoon of EPA and DHA daily. The second variety of omega-3 fatty acid is alpha-linolenic acid, which comes from plant foods and is then converted to EPA and DHA. Top sources of this fat are flaxseed oil and canola oil. Most average Americans consume less than a third of a teaspoon of alpha-linolenic acid per day.

The second variety of essential fatty acid the body needs is linolenic acid and it is plentiful in modern diets. In fact, today's foods are saturated with it in the form of vegetable oils like corn, soybean, and safflower oils, and it can be found in margarine, mayonnaise, and other processed foods; our current ratio of linolenic acid to the omega-3s is now 10 to 1. Scientists say early diets had a ratio of 1 or 2 to 1, which amounted to a more equal balance between the two essential fats.

What scientists now suspect is that when the linolenic acid predominates, as it does in today, and when omega-3s are in short supply, this affects the kind of eicosanoids our bodies produce as well as the overall health of our cardiovascular and immune systems. Eicosanoids that lack omega-3s tend to provoke inflammation, blood clots, and so forth. This has led to the label of "good" or "bad" eicosanoids.

Researchers are now examining the role of omega-3 fatty acids in our diet and their effects on cell functions. In November 2000, based on the strength of current omega-3 research, the FDA determined that manufacturers could promote evidence that omega-3 supplements may reduce the risk of coronary heart disease.

While research continues, some diet promoters have taken that need for essential fatty acids and turned it to their own advantage by calling for diets higher in protein and lower in carbohydrates than what nutritionists and health experts suggest. For example, in his book *The Zone,* Dr. Barry Sears supports a daily intake of 30 percent fat, 30 percent protein and 40 percent carbohydrates. He says that ratio will cause weight loss while at the same time it will keep eicosanoids in balance. By eating this way, dieters are in what he calls "the Zone." His theory also claims that the traditional carbohydrate-rich American diet dramatically raises the level of insulin in the bloodstream, which in turn influences the production of too many "bad" and not enough "good" eicosanoids.

Even though critics call this an oversimplification of the problem, there is agreement that it is just as unhealthy to eliminate all fat from the diet as it is to eat those fats to excess. So even though not everyone agrees on the numbers, they all agree that a balanced ratio of fats in the diet is essential for normal growth and development and good health.

See also:

Sears, Barry; The Zone.

Additional Reading

Lawrence, Ronald M. "Fat in the Diet: How to Retain the 'Good' Fats and Avoid the 'Bad.'" *Total Health,* 1 March 2001, 50.

McCord, Holly, R.D., and Teresa Yeykal. "The Fat You Need: Can This Forgotten Nutrient Ward Off Illness From Head to Toe?" *Prevention,* 1 January 1997, 100–104.

Ephedra/Ephedrine

Ephedrine is a drug from the plants of the genus ephedra, and is promoted in many herbal diet remedies as a "natural" weight-loss product. Derived from a Chinese herb called mahuang, ephedra is a

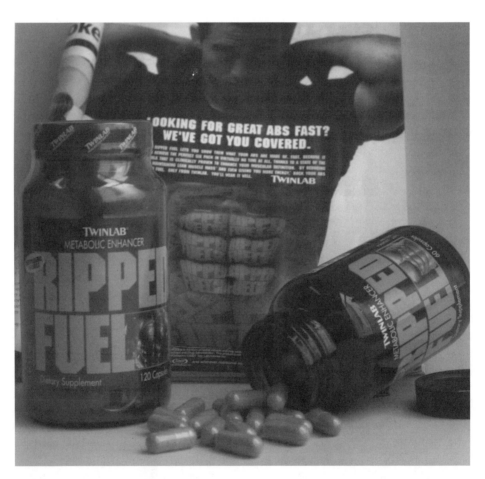

Bottles of Ripped Fuel Metabolic Enhancer, which contains ephedra, are shown in New York on June 18, 2002. Quite a few NFL players, it turns out, were taking ephedra, a stimulant banned by the league in September 2001. Reportedly, a bottle of Ripped Fuel was found in the locker of Minnesota Vikings tackle Korey Stringer after he collapsed and died during a training camp practice in 2001. (AP/Wide World Photos)

stimulant, used for short-term energy boosts to enhance athletic performance and endurance, to help people exercise longer and feel more alert, to increase metabolism, and to dampen or suppress appetite. Ephedra has been an ingredient in several popular diet supplements, including Metabolife, Diet Pet, and Dexatrim, all part of the multibillion-dollar weight-loss industry.

Research published in the December 2000 issue of the *New England Journal of Medicine,* outlined serious complications from dietary supplements containing ephedra, including 10 deaths, 32 heart attacks, 62 cases of cardiac arrhythmia, 91 reports of hypertension, 69 strokes, and 70 seizures. Those figures were compiled between 1993 and 2000. Another possible problem with ephedrine, according to researchers, is the possibility that the human body may convert ephedra to PPA, short for phenylpropanolamine, an ingredient the FDA banned after it was shown to increase the risk of a kind of stroke in young women. Although the FDA has taken no formal action, in 1997 the agency called for ephedra labeling recommending that daily consumption be held to 24 mg. The agency also suggested that users take the supplements no more than seven days in response to studies showing that users who take ephedrine-containing supplements may develop a tolerance to it and must take more of the supplement to achieve the same effect.

The alarm over ephedra use rose after the drug was considered a factor in the death of several high-profile athletes such as Steve Bechler, a twenty-three-year-old minor-league baseball player who collapsed and died while training with the Baltimore Orioles in February 2003. Bechler had been taking a weight-loss supplement containing ephedra at the time of his death. The first statewide ban on ephedra use was signed into law in May 2003 by Illinois Governor Rod Blagojevich after the death of a sixteen-year-old high school football player. The governor has urged other states and the federal government to adopt similar bans.

Health organizations, businesses, and professional athletes have all started to distance themselves from the use of ephedra. Nutritional supplement retailer General Nutrition Centers announced in May 2003 that it would stop selling products containing ephedra. Following Bechler's death, minor-league-baseball officials took steps to stop their players from using supplements with ephedra, a restriction already in place for professional and college football players as well as for NCAA and Olympic athletes. Ephedra was considered a factor in the deaths of college football players Rashidi Wheeler and Devaughn Darling and Minnesota Viking Korey Stringer. One baseball agent quoted in the March 2003 *Sporting News* estimated that 75 percent of ball players use ephedrine.

The American Medical Association continues its efforts to remove ephedra from the market. Following Bechler's death, Health and Human Services Secretary Tommy G. Thompson called for warnings on ephedra labels and for a ban on its use. The American Heart Association has also been vocal in its opposition to supplements containing ephedra.

Researchers also caution that supplements containing ephedrine and caffeine, when used in combination, can produce dangerous side effects similar to those of the banned drug methamphetamine. Those side effects include insomnia, restlessness, euphoria, palpitations or cardiac arrhythmia, high blood pressure, strokes, and seizures. The information, featured in the December 2000 issue of the *New England Journal of Medicine,* prompted critics to call for a halt in the production and sale of dietary supplements containing ephedrine alkaloids, charging they increase the already apparent risk for heart attacks, strokes, seizures, and hypertension. Industry officials, quoted in a 2001 article in *Drug Topics,* maintain the 200 products containing ephedra aimed at U.S. dieters and bodybuilders are not a health risk. However, in response to the continuing controversy, some of those manufacturers are now marketing an ephedra-free version of their product, such as Metabolife and Dexatrim. Nutritionists say the safest way to increase metabolism is to increase physical activity.

See also:

Dexatrim; Metabolife.

Additional Reading

Brink, Susan, "Diet Drugs: What a Pill." *U.S. News & World Report,* 20 November 2000, 74.

The Columbia Encyclopedia. Edition 6. New York: Columbia University Press, 2000.

Conlan, Michael F. "Consumer Groups Want FDA to Ban Dietary Supplements with Ephedra." *Drug Topics* 145, no. 18 (17 September 2001): 18.

Haller, C. A., and N. L. Benowitz. "Adverse Cardiovascular and Central Nervous System Events Associated with Dietary Supplements Containing Ephedra Alkaloids." *New England Journal of Medicine,* 343, no. 25 (December 21, 2000): 1833–38.

Rosenthal, Ken. "No More Delays on Drug Testing." *The Sporting News,* 227, no. 9 (3 March 2003): 50–52.

Smith, Ian K. "The Trouble with Fat-Burner Pills: Be Suspicious of the Dramatic Weight-Loss Claims of These Supplements." *Time,* 27 August 2001, 66.

Exercise

Trying to lose weight without increasing your level of physical activity is like driving a car with no gas in the tank. You may roll forward a little, but you're not really going to get anywhere. Remember that a pound equals 3,500 calories. So to lose a pound in, say a week, you'll either have to eat 3,500 calories less or burn off 3,500 calories in exercise, or some combination of the two. Some combination of the two is easier and healthier in the long run.

Exercise burns calories. While the specific rate at which you burn calories depends on your weight and the intensity with which you perform the activity, here are some examples of calorie-burning activities. Walking briskly can burn off about 100 calories per mile. Bicycling for a half hour at nearly 10 mph will burn about 195 calories. Experts recommend at least 30 minutes of vigorous activity five days a week. If you can't find 30 minutes, try two 15-minute intervals, or even three 10-minute intervals. And realize that what's vigorous for a sedentary person is different from a vigorous workout for an athlete. Work at your own pace.

In 1998, the American College of Sports Medicine (ACSM) created a new Physical Activity Pyramid. It's similar in design to the nutritional pyramid, with the bottom or base, showing the activities that should be performed the most. The pyramid narrows, with less vigorous activity being required less often.

The base of the pyramid, or the bottom level, is "everyday activities," which could include walking, house or yardwork, outdoor play, walking the dog. These bottom-level activities should total

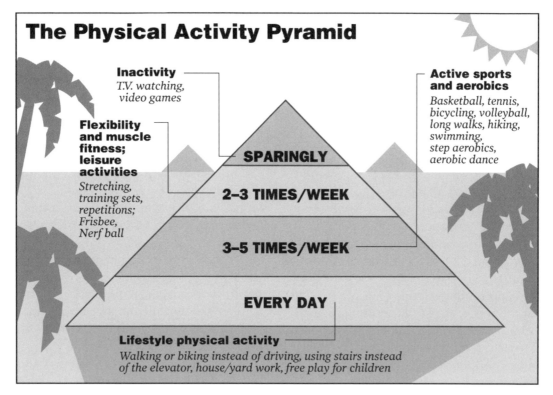

Figure 1 The Physical Activity Pyramid
Source: Courtesy of the U.S. Department of Agriculture, American College of Sports Medicine.

30 minutes done most days of the week. While that satisfies the basic requirement, there's much more people can do to become fit.

The second level of the pyramid is divided between active aerobics and sports and recreation, which should be done at least three times a week. These are more vigorous activities, which involve speeding up the heart rate. These activities could involve aerobic exercises, basketball, tennis, bicycling, soccer, jump roping, and hiking. Because these activities elevate the heart rate, three 20-minute intervals per week have about the same health benefits as the activities done every day.

The third level of the pyramid is divided into flexibility and muscle fitness exercises, which should be done two or three times a week. These activities improve motion and flexibility and include golf, bowling, softball, yardwork. Muscle strength activities include stretching, light weight lifting, push-ups, curl ups, and gymnastics. The ACSM recommends that people exercise each major muscle group three to seven days a week and stretch to the point of mild discomfort, but not pain. For strength, the ACSM recommends doing muscle fitness exercises for each major muscle group two or three days a week with a day of rest in between.

The top level of the pyramid is inactivity. Remember that in the nutritional pyramid, fats and sugars are at this level. Some are required, but they shouldn't be the mainstay of one's diet. Likewise in the activity pyramid, inactivity should be the exception, not the rule. Inactivity should be a small portion of your day—and no more than 30 minutes at a time.

Fat

The reason many people start an exercise program or diet is to lose weight—particularly fat. It's an excellent strategy, and, combined with proper nutrition and diet, it should begin to show results fairly soon. Every human body has some fat in it. A healthy adult male's body should have about 12 to 18 percent fat. Healthy adult females have a slightly higher body fat composition—about 15 to 22 percent fat. Fitness centers often offer body composition tests using calipers or pinchers. People can buy these in fitness and sports stores, too. It's a painless test measuring a fold of skin in several places on your body. Fat lies just below skin level. By measuring a small fold of skin, these calipers can measure how much fat is accumulated. It's a more precise measure of body composition than a simple weigh-in.

However, the bathroom or exercise-room scale is still a good indicator, too. Remember, though, that muscle weighs more than fat. So a person beginning to exercise, turning fat into muscle, may not see as dramatic a weight loss. Don't let that deter you, though. What you'll see and feel is a transformation of your body that will be longer lasting and easier to maintain.

Here's how exercise helps burn fat. Let's say you eat 2,000 calories worth of food. But your physical activity only uses 1,500 of these. The extra calories are stored in your body—as fat. When you exercise, your body uses fuel that comes from one of two forms: stored carbohydrates called glycogen and stored body fat. Stored body fat is found in fat cells

and is also stored in small droplets in the muscles.

Most activities use both carbohydrates and fat for fuel. Lower intensity workouts, such as walking, use fat as the primary fuel. As the workout intensifies, the fuel reserves come increasingly from carbohydrates. But that doesn't mean that walking burns more fat than running. When the carbohydrate or glycogen source runs low, the body releases fats for fuels. Also, a higher intensity workout, such as running, continues to burn fat even after the physical activity itself is over. As the body works to restore glycogen, it continues to use fat to do so. And because higher intensity workouts burn more calories overall, even though the mix of carbohydrates and fats may be different, you're still burning more fat in the workout.

It's not necessary to create a workout regimen that burns the most fat when you're starting out. Create an exercise program that you like and can stick with. As long as you keep using more calories than you consume and start getting those muscle groups active, you will burn fat, strengthen your muscles and your heart, feel better, and lose weight.

Fat Blockers

Imagine a product that lets dieters eat exactly what they want, including cake, pie, candy, and cookies, and still lose weight. Fat blockers, another weapon in the war against obesity, promise "miracles" but deliver health problems.

During the early 1990s, Cal-Ban 3000, a fat blocker, was advertised as an automatic weight-loss solution. Made of guar gum, a soluble fiber used in small amounts as a thickener in sauces, desserts, syrups, and other processed foods, the pills were supposed to decrease appetite and block absorption of fat. Instead, the fiber in Cal-Ban 3000 swelled to four or five times its original size and created havoc for users. The Food and Drug Administration (FDA) received reports of at least seventeen cases of esophageal obstruction among users. According to the FDA, at least ten of those people with obstructions were hospitalized; one reportedly died. Other side effects included stomach obstruction and intestinal blockages, along with nausea and vomiting.

Guar gum is a complex sugar that swells when wet, forms a gel in the stomach, and can create a feeling of fullness. But, unfortunately, in the case of Cal-Ban 3000, the guar gum stuck in the wrong places, in the throat and intestines, forming dangerous obstructions. And critics say that along with the obvious health risks, taking fat blockers does not help those overweight people who eat even when they feel full.

According to the *FDA Consumer,* the FDA had been moving to ban guar gum and some 100 other diet products whose ingredients had not been proven when reports of serious problems with Cal-Ban 3000 prompted them to halt its distribution. Guar gum is still considered safe for use in small amounts in foods like salad dressings, cheese, and ice cream where it acts as a stabilizer, thickener, or binder.

Chitosan is another fat blocker used in weight-loss supplements. Made from the chitin, the outer skeleton of shellfish such as shrimp, lobster, and crabs, chitosan allegedly works as a "fat magnet," according to manufacturers, by binding fats in the stomach and preventing them from being digested and absorbed. The fat is then theoretically excreted via the body's feces.

A study by Judith Stern, a nutrition researcher at the University of California at Davis, showed that chitosan products have no weight-loss value. The results of her study, reported in the May 2001 issue of the *American Journal of Clinical Nutrition,* evaluated subjects taking daily doses of chitosan. Stern measured no change in fecal fat content, debunking the claim that chitosan blocked and then excreted large amounts of dietary fat.

Stern is cofounder of the American Obesity Association and a member of the obesity task force of the National Institute for Diabetes, Digestive and Kidney Diseases. The Napa County, California, district attorney's office partially funded Stern's study and later used the results to bring charges against Enforma, the manufacturer of Fat Trapper Plus, a fat blocker containing chitosan. The company was accused of making false advertising claims and they eventually settled with the government, paying $10 million to the Federal Trade Commission, to be returned to consumers who purchased the product or to the U.S. treasury if that repayment was impractical.

Interest in chitosan as a weight-loss aid grew dramatically in 1997 with the publication of *The Fat Blocker Diet.* Written by Dr. Arnold Fox, the best-seller instructs dieters to eat a healthful diet, exercise, practice positive thinking, and take "something extra, a little lift" of chitosan to help start their weight loss and to keep them going through difficult periods. Fox maintains that chitosan helps dieters avoid any slowing of metabolism, which routinely occurs during low-calorie diets. Instead, Fox suggests that because users do not cut down on calories there is no corresponding message to the body to slow its metabolism. Instead, calorie levels are cut simply because fat is not being digested or absorbed as it was before the dieter took chitosan. Fox tells dieters to follow the U.S. Department of Agriculture Food Guide Pyramid and to eat the recommended daily servings of grains, vegetables, and fruits, and drink at least eight glasses of water per day. He recommends a daily intake of no more than 20 percent of calories from fat, 10 percent from protein, and 70 percent from carbohydrates. In other words, he calls for a basic high-fiber, low-fat eating plan with the addition of daily chitosan supplements. He also goes on to warn against fad diets and provides an eating disorder questionnaire for readers who may show early signs of eating disorders such as anorexia nervosa or bulimia. He recommends they see a physician or registered dietitian before using his diet or taking chitosan.

See also:

anorexia nervosa; Food Guide Pyramid; starch blockers.

Additional Reading

Barrett, Stephen, M.D. "Be Wary of Calorie-Blockers." www.quackwatch.com.
"Better Not Swallow This: Accident Potential of Guar Gum." *Tufts University Diet & Nutrition Letter,* 8, no. 9 (November 1990): 7.
Fox, Arnold, M.D. *The Fat Blocker Diet.* New York: St. Martin's Press, 1997.
"Guar Gum Diet Products Under Investigation." *FDA Consumer,* 24, no. 8 (October 1990): 3–5.
Wallace, Phil. "Study Finds Chitosan Doesn't Block or Trap Fat." *Food Chemical News,* 43, no. 5 (19 March 2001): 11.

Feingold Diet

While most people think of diet plans as a way to lose weight, some diets have different purposes. For example, the Feingold diet program is based on the concept that certain foods can affect behavior—

particularly attention deficit/hyperactivity disorder (ADHD), which affects either 3 to 5 percent of school-aged children or as many as 17 percent of school-aged children, depending on the source. ADHD is commonly treated with stimulants such as Ritalin. In 1974, Dr. Benjamin Feingold wrote the book *Why Your Child is Hyperactive,* espousing what was then called "KP" or the "Kaiser-Permanente" diet—named after the medical center where he practiced and taught. In 1979, Dr. Feingold and his wife wrote *The Feingold Cookbook,* at which time the name Feingold diet began to stick.

The diet program is based on the idea that some people have difficulty tolerating salicylates, natural chemicals made by many plants and chemically related to aspirin. The program also states that other common additives and preservatives can also be difficult to tolerate. This intolerance can show itself in many ways, according to Dr. Feingold and his supporters—including symptoms of attention deficit/hyperactivity disorder (ADHD), and other behavioral or physical problems sometimes associated with ADHD, such as such as bedwetting, asthma, sleep disorders, and frequent ear infections.

Salicylates occur naturally in some fruits such as apples and oranges, and they are synthetic additives to other foods or products. Some people are intolerant of only a few different salicylates; others are intolerant of many different kinds. Therefore, the diet program starts by eliminating most salicylate foods and products at the beginning and reintroducing some slowly as behavior or other symptoms improve. The program also calls for eliminating artificial food dye and flavors, which are petroleum-based additives, and petroleum-based preservatives, such as BHA, BHT, and TBHQ. Eliminating foods and products with these additives will generally show results in one to four weeks, according to the Web site. Younger children typically respond more quickly.

The Feingold program offers participants a food list, a shopping guide with acceptable name brand products. On the Feingold Association Web site it explains that the level of salicylates in foods cannot simply be determined by looking at the Nutrition Facts label or the product contents. For example, Eggo Homestyle Waffles are not acceptable, but Eggo Buttermilk Waffles are, the site says. Sugar isn't restricted, but corn syrup, which is more processed and chemical-laden, is. In fact, the Web site notes that some children who overdo their consumption of candy and seem pumped up on sugar may instead be reacting to the corn syrup, a common ingredient in some candy.

While the Web site offers information about the program and many research links, it doesn't provide someone with the details needed to get started on the program. For that, U.S. members pay $77 for a Foodlist and Shopping Guide and regular updates about new product tests and research. There's also a 393-page companion book, *Why Can't My Child Behave?*

While the Feingold Web site is filled with testimonials from harried parents who say they've been able to take their children off other medication, or have seen marked improvement in behavior and demeanor since starting the diet, there are critics who say the underlying premise that food additives are the root cause of these problems has not been adequately determined.

On the "pro-Feingold" side are the nonprofit Center for Science in the Public Interest, which issued a 32-page report in 1999 titled, "Diet, ADHD, and Behav-

ior." The report cites seventeen controlled studies that found that diet can adversely affect behavior. It also cites six studies that did not detect any change in behavior when a child's diet was changed. In the report, Dr. Marvin Boris, a pediatrician and author of a 1994 study, found that diet affected the behavior of two-thirds of his subjects. "It makes a lot more sense to try modifying a child's diet before treating him or her with a stimulant drug. Health organizations and professionals should recognize that avoiding certain foods and additives can greatly benefit some troubled children."

Among criticism of the program are those studies that show no behavioral changes based on diet. The opposition is summarized in an article by Stephen Barrett, MD, "The Feingold Diet: Dubious Benefits, Subtle Risks." Dr. Barrett writes that "Because the Feingold diet does no physical harm, it might appear to be helpful in some instances. However, the potential benefits should be weighed against the potential harm of (1) teaching children that their behavior and school performance are related to what they eat rather than what they feel, (2) undermining their self esteem by implanting notions that they are unhealthy and fragile, (3) creating situations in which their eating behavior or fear of chemicals are regarded as peculiar by other children, and (4) depriving them of the opportunity to receive appropriate professional help."

A fact sheet from the Web site of Children and Adults with Attention Deficit/ Hyperactivity Disorder lists the Feingold diet as a controversial treatment for ADHD. It says, "Over the years, proponents of the Feingold Diet have made many dramatic claims. They state that the diet—which promotes the elimination of most additives from food—will improve most (if not all) children's learning and attention problems. In the past 15 years, dozens of well-controlled studies published in peer-reviewed journals have consistently failed to find support for the Feingold Diet. While a few studies have reported some limited success with this approach, at best this suggests that there may be a very small group of children who are responsive to additive-free diets. At this time, it has not been shown that dietary intervention offers significant help to children with learning and attention problems."

The good news for parents of children or young adults diagnosed with ADHD is that research into this condition is continuing and seems to be taking a more holistic approach than purely pharmaceutical approach.

Additional Reading

Rowe, K. S., and K. J. Rowe. "Synthetic Food Coloring and Behavior: A Dose Response Effect in a Double-Blind, Placebo-Controlled, Repeated-Measures Study." *Journal of Pediatrics,* 125 (1994): 691–98.
———. "Diagnosis and Treatment of Attention Deficit Hyperactivity Disorder." NIH Consensus Statement Online, 16, no. 2 (16–18 November 1998): 1–37.
Williams, J. I., D. M. Cram, F. T. Tausig, and E. Webster. "Relative Effects of Drugs and Diet on Hyperactive Behaviors: An Experimental Study." *Pediatrics,* 61, no. 6 (1978): 811.

Fen-phen

Fen-phen, a popular combination of the diet drugs fenfluramine and phentermine, sounded almost too good to be true when dieters first discovered the powerful duo. And the pills were a huge success right up until their dangerous side effects prompted the U.S. Food and Drug Administration (FDA) to call for their removal in 1997. While the drugs were supposed to be prescribed for seriously obese patients, doctors wrote millions of prescriptions for women who only wanted to lose a few pounds. Unfortunately, many of those women lost more than weight. Some suffered permanent heart damage while others died from a rare lung disease.

In fact, from 1995 until September 1997, before fenfluramine and dexfenfluramine were taken off the market, an estimated 14 million prescriptions were written for them. FDA statistics also show that up to a total of 4.7 million people were eventually exposed to these deadly diet drugs. Finally, on September 15, 1997, the FDA announced that some 30 percent of patients taking the weight-loss pills had developed a fatal form of heart-valve disease. Manufacturers immediately pulled the drugs from the shelves.

Although fenfluramine was regularly combined with phentermine, another diet drug, to produce the popular fen-phen combination, it was the "fen" that was eventually singled out as the problem. No one taking phentermine alone developed any signs of the disease. Dexfenfluramine, sold under the brand name Redux, was the other deadly diet pill identified by the FDA. It had entered the market in 1996 when manufacturers refined fenfluramine into just its serotonin-stimulating portion, and removed the part that caused extreme drowsiness in users. The diet pills were developed to increase the amount of serotonin, a neurotransmitter released by the brain. This would then suppress a dieter's appetite.

Phentermine was first introduced to dieters in 1959 but was not immediately popular because of its side effects, which included inability to sleep, jitteriness, and constipation. Fenfluramine appeared on the market, approved for short-term obesity treatment, in 1973. Although fenfluramine helped some dieters, its side effects of extreme drowsiness and diarrhea held its popularity in check. But their use rose dramatically in 1992 when the results of a government-funded study published in the journal *Clinical Pharmacology & Therapeutics,* showed that the two diet drugs given in combination cancelled each other's unappealing side effects. Best of all the fen-phen combination doubled the weight loss of study participants when added to a diet and exercise program.

Meanwhile, in 1996, dexfenfluramine received FDA approval for use in obese patients for one year or less. The pills had already been taken by European dieters for about a year with no unmanageable side effects. Redux, like the earlier fen-phen combination was hailed as a revolutionary breakthrough in weight management and doctors wrote tens of thousands of prescriptions for the medications every week.

Until the reports of heart-valve disease surfaced, the only serious side effect of fenfluramine or Redux had been a rare but fatal type of pulmonary hypertension or lung condition known as PPH, that occurred in those taking the drugs for more than three months. In PPH the arteries taking blood from the heart to the lungs thicken, creating high blood pressure in the lungs. Diseases like emphysema or chronic bronchitis typically cause this. But now PPH was showing up in dieters who had no previous history of lung disease but who were taking Redux or fenfluramine. Still, at the time any risk involved with taking the drugs seemed small compared with the serious health problems caused by obesity. And even after the risks of taking fen-phen and Redux were known, patients were willing to continue using the drugs because of the success

they experienced. At the time there were few comparable diet drugs on the market. Since then manufacturers have developed other obesity drugs like Meridia and Xenical. Meridia, or sibutramine, works on neurotransmitters in the brain and makes you feel full sooner. It is intended for people who are at least 25 percent overweight and studies show it can increase blood pressure. Xenical, on the other hand, works by preventing the body from absorbing up to 30 percent of ingested fat but side effects include loose, fatty stools and an urgency to urinate.

Initial concerns about fen-phen's safety came from doctors who detected new heart-valve damage in patients with previously diagnosed heart disease who were also taking the diet drugs. Soon, researchers started finding fen-phen users with no previous heart disease were developing leaky heart valves. As evidence about the severity of the problem grew, the FDA issued new warnings. More and more cases of the rare valve disease were being reported. These reports and a Mayo Clinic study about the valvular disease were described in the August 28, 1997, *New England Journal of Medicine.* A few of the patients with newly diagnosed heart-valve abnormalities were so ill they required valve-replacement surgery. Two weeks before the Mayo Clinic study results were released Jenny Craig Weight Loss Centres stopped staff doctors from prescribing dexfenfluramine (Redux) over concerns about the drug's side effects.

In calling for voluntary withdrawal of the diet drugs, Michael A. Friedman, the FDA's Lead Deputy Commissioner, said the data indicated that "fenfluramine and the chemically closely related dexfenfluramine, present an unacceptable risk to patients who take them." The FDA recommended that patients stop taking the pills and contact their doctors to be tested for heart and lung disease and to discuss treatment. The Department of Health and Human Services also announced its own list of recommendations for patients who had taken the drugs.

In 2000, the largest wrongful death award in the history of Massachusetts was given to the family of a woman whose death was linked to fen-phen. Although the settlement figure was not disclosed, until this time the highest award in the state was $7 million. The settlement also asked for a substantial portion of the damages to fund a foundation, set up by the patient's family, to study and treat primary pulmonary hypertension (PPH). Although the woman only took fen-phen for eleven days, she developed the incurable and fatal PPH, a side effect strongly linked to fenfluramine.

More recent studies show that some 30 percent of those who took dexfenfluramine alone or took fenfluramine in the fen-phen combination developed heart-valve disease, and the longer dieters used the drugs the more likely they were to become sick. Sadly, researchers have also found that the majority of those who lost weight with Redux or fen-phen gained it back once the drugs were no longer available.

See also:

Jenny Craig; Meridia; Xenical.

Additional Reading

Cowley, Geoffrey, and Karen Springen. "After Fen-Phen." *Newsweek*, 29 September 1997, 46–49.

"Fen-Phen Maker AHP Settles Lawsuits." *Claims*, March 2000, 18.

Levine, Hallie. "Fen-phen Killed My Wife." *Cosmopolitan*, December 1997, 196–200.

Rover, Elena. "Rethinking Diet Pills." *Ladies Home Journal*, March 1997, 60.

Stapleton, Stephanie. "Diet Drugs: Problems and Prospects." *American Medical News*, 9 November 1998, 31.

Ukens, Carol. "Fat's in the Fire: Obesity Drugs Pose Weighty Problems for Pharmacists." *Drug Topics*, 141, no. 7 (7 April 1997): 54–56.

Welch, Christine B. "The Miracle That Wasn't: Fen-Phen and Redux." *Diabetes Forecast*, 51, no. 4 (April 1998): 40–46.

Ferguson, Sarah, Duchess of York

Sarah Ferguson (b. October 15, 1959, in London, also known as Sarah Mountbatten-Windsor York and Sarah, Duchess of York) became the Duchess of York through her marriage to Britain's Prince Andrew in July 1986. The couple had two daughters, Princess Beatrice and Princess Eugenie, before divorcing in 1996. The Duchess had a difficult relationship with the British press. At first, she was hailed as a breath of fresh air but soon afterward she was scrutinized and criticized—often about her weight.

Sarah Ferguson's candor about her own struggles with her weight and her personal insecurities have made her an approachable and sympathetic person. As spokesperson for Weight Watchers International, she has coauthored several books with Weight Watchers professionals on weight loss and weight management. On the Weight Watchers Web site, the 2001 release of *Reinventing Yourself With the Duchess of York* was accompanied by this statement from Sarah Ferguson: "Weight Watchers practically saved me by opening my eyes to the unhealthy feelings and behaviors that were behind my eating problems and many of the troubles in other parts of my life," the Duchess says. "It was the weight loss process itself that gave me the opportunity to change my life on many levels," she adds. "My reinvention started at my very core and worked its way outwards."

She's appeared on the lecture circuit and television shows. For example, she and Rosie O'Donnell spoke about their earlier attempts at weight loss. Ferguson mentioned a variety of techniques—from a meat and oranges diet to diet pills to fighting the urge to use food as a comfort

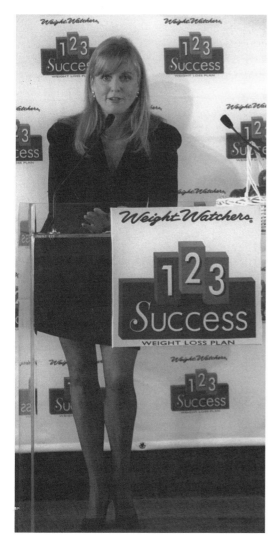

Sarah Ferguson, the Duchess of York, makes a statement during a news conference marking her return as spokesperson for Weight Watchers on October 6, 1997, in New York. (AP/Wide World Photos)

during emotionally difficult periods. Her signature line, "Start with your mind and your bottom will follow," expresses her belief that one of the biggest hurdles in weight loss is in overcoming one's perceptions of oneself.

Additional Reading

Ferguson, Sarah. *Dining With the Duchess: Making Everyday Meals A Special Occasion.* New York: Fireside, 1999.

———. *Win the Weight Game: Successful Strategies for Living Well.* New York: Simon and Schuster, 2000.

Ferguson, Sarah, editor. *Reinventing Yourself With the Duchess of York: Inspiring Stories and Strategies.* New York: Simon and Schuster, 2001.

Ferguson, Sarah, with Jeff Coplon. *My Story.* New York: Simon and Schuster, 1996.

Ferguson, Sarah, with Weight Watchers. *Energy Breakthrough: Jump-Start Your Weight Loss and Feel Great.* New York: Simon and Schuster, 2002.

O'Donnell, Rosie. "When Sarah Met Rosie." *Rosie Magazine,* online at: http://www.rosiemagazine.com/people/archive_2001_08_cover_1.html. Accessed 12 June 2003. www.weightwatchers.com

Five a Day

Five a Day for Better Health is the healthy eating program spearheaded by the National Cancer Institute (NCI). The goal is to encourage Americans to eat at least five servings of fruits and vegetables per day. The effort includes government and private industry sources, including the U.S. Department of Agriculture and the Centers for Disease Control and Prevention. The actual recommendation is that women should eat at least seven and men should eat at least nine servings of fruits and vegetables each day. They add, however, that it's relatively easy to do. For example, the sliced onion on a sandwich counts or a healthy salad with a variety of greens and sliced vegetables would count as several servings in one.

In 2002, the NCI added the concept that these fruits and vegetables should cover the range of color with its "Savor the Spectrum" campaign.

By selecting fruits and vegetables from different color groups, people can get a wider range of phytochemicals—disease-fighting substances found in foods. Specifically, here are the benefits available in different colors of the spectrum.

Blue and purple fruits and vegetables have either anthocyanins or phenolics. Anthocyanins are antioxidants that help control high blood pressure and protect against diabetes-related circulatory problems. Anthocyanins and phenolics help reduce the risk of cancer, heart disease, and Alzheimer's disease, and they may even slow down the aging process. The best sources of anthocyanins are blackberries, blueberries, elderberries, purple grapes, and black currants. The best sources of phenolics are prunes, plums, raisins, and eggplant.

Green fruits and vegetables provide two more important phytochemicals—lutein and indoles. Lutein is an antioxidant that has been connected with better eye health. Lutein helps reduce the risk of forming cataracts and macular degeneration, both of which can cause vision loss in older people. The best sources of lutein can be found in green leafy vegetables such as turnip, collard, and mustard greens; kale; romaine lettuce; green peas; kiwi fruit; spinach; broccoli; and honeydew melon. Cruciferous vegetables—broccoli, cauliflower, cabbage, and brussels sprouts—are excellent sources of indoles, phytochemicals that are linked to a lower risk of breast cancer and prostate cancer. One study showed a 42-percent reduction in the risk of prostate cancer for men who ate cruciferous vegetables at least three times a week. Other sources of indoles are rutabaga, watercress, kale, arugula, turnips, cabbage, bok choy, and Swiss chard.

Deep orange and bright yellow fruits and vegetables contain two other phytochemicals: beta carotene and bioflavanoids. Beta carotene, the antioxidant that has been linked to a reduction in cancer risk and heart disease, also boosts the body's immune system and helps maintain eye health. Excellent sources of beta carotene are mangoes, sweet potatoes, cantaloupe, peaches, carrots, apricots, butternut squash, and pumpkin. Bioflavanoids work together with vitamin C to improve overall health and heart health, reduce the risk of cancer, strengthen bones and teeth, and contribute to more rapid wound healing. Best sources of bioflavanoids are oranges, tangerines, peaches, pears, yellow pepper, grapefruit, clementines, nectarines, pineapple, lemons, apricots, papaya, and yellow raisins.

Red fruits and vegetables—from deep red to bright pink—contain lycopene and anthocyanins. Lycopene has been linked to a reduced cancer risk. Good sources of lycopene are watermelons, pink grapefruits, fresh tomatoes and tomato-based products, such as spaghetti sauce, tomato paste, and tomato juice. Red fruits and vegetables that are good sources of anthocyanins include red raspberries, sweet cherries, strawberries, cranberries, beets, red apples, red cabbage, red onion, kidney beans, and red beans.

Even white vegetables—onions and garlic—contain an important phytochemical called allicin. Allicin has been linked to lowered cholesterol and blood pressure as well as providing a boost to the body's infection-fighting ability. All vegetables in the onion family, including chives, scallions, and leeks, contain allicin.

See also:

Dietary Guidelines for Americans; Food Guide Pyramid.

Additional Reading

Ambrose, Jeanne. "Take 5 at the Very Least." *Better Homes and Gardens,* June 2002, 282.
Sugarman, Carole. "Eat Your Purples: Color Coding Is the Latest Approach to a Healthful Diet." *Washington Post,* 13 June 2001, F1.
www.5aday.gov

Food and Drug Administration (FDA)

The Food and Drug Administration (FDA) is that part of the U.S. Department of Health and Human Services charged with regulating a variety of prod-

ucts, from food ingredients to drugs and new medical devices. According to its Web site, www.fda.gov, "Stated most simply, FDA's mission is to promote and protect the public health by helping safe and effective products reach the market in a timely way, and monitoring products for continued safety after they are in use. Our work is a blending of law and science aimed at protecting consumers."

The FDA reviews new food products, such as artificial sweeteners, before they can be produced for sale. It also reviews and limits the health claims products and foods can make on their labeling.

Food Guide Pyramid

The Food Guide Pyramid is a visual reminder of a balanced and varied diet, developed by the U.S. Department of Agriculture. The foods at the bottom of the

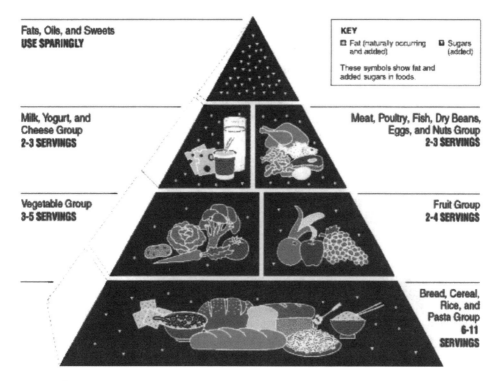

Figure 2 Food Guide Pyramid. (U.S. Department of Agriculture)

pyramid—breads and cereals, for example—should make up the bulk of your diet. The foods at the top—fats, oils, and sweets—should be eaten sparingly.

What's a Serving?

In some cases, the amount of a serving seems intuitive, but the following list shows the amount of a serving. Notice, for example, that a serving of bread is one slice. So a sandwich provides two servings from that category.

GRAIN PRODUCTS GROUP (BREAD, CEREAL, RICE, AND PASTA)

- 1 slice of bread
- 1 ounce of ready-to-eat cereal
- 1/2 cup of cooked cereal, rice, or pasta

VEGETABLE GROUP

- 1 cup of raw, green leafy vegetables
- 1/2 cup of other vegetables—cooked or chopped raw
- 3/4 cup of vegetable juice

FRUIT GROUP

- 1 medium apple, banana, orange
- 1/2 cup of chopped, cooked, or canned fruit
- 3/4 cup of fruit juice

MILK GROUP (MILK, YOGURT, AND CHEESE)

- 1 cup of milk or yogurt
- 1–1/2 ounces of natural cheese
- 2 ounces of processed cheese

MEAT AND BEANS GROUP (MEAT, POULTRY, FISH, DRY BEANS, EGGS, AND NUTS)

- 2–3 ounces of cooked lean meat, poultry, or fish
- 1/2 cup of cooked dry beans or 1 egg counts as 1 ounce of lean meat. Two tablespoons of peanut butter or 1/3 cup of nuts count as 1 ounce of meat.

The food pyramid provides a good guide for getting a varied diet. Now let's get down to the particulars. There are other measurements that are important in eating healthy foods. These include the number of calories, and the amount of carbohydrates, fiber, cholesterol, sodium, and vitamins and minerals found in food.

While meats are included in the USDA Food Guide Pyramid, vegetarians can aim for the same variety and balance in their diets.

See also:

vegetarian diet.

Glycemic Index

The glycemic index is a measurement of how much foods cause blood sugar to rise in two or three hours after consuming them. Consuming carbohydrates causes the body to produce the hormone insulin. The glycemic index is one way to measure the amount of insulin that might be produced as a result of eating foods. This measurement is important for insulin-dependent diabetics who must inject sufficient insulin to cover a meal. It has also become of interest to advocates of a high-protein, low-carbohydrate diet who argue that excess insulin production can lead to other health problems.

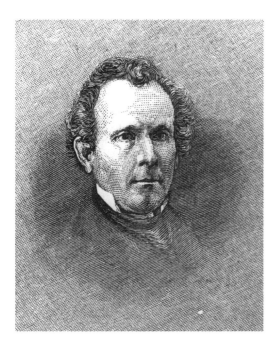

Sylvester Graham was an American preacher in the 1800s who believed that a high-fiber, natural food diet would cure diseases including cholera, alcoholism, and a variety of digestive ills known as dyspepsia. He is most famous as the namesake of the graham cracker, which in his day was hard bread make of coarse flour and bran. (Library of Congress)

Even so, the glycemic index reveals nothing about a food's nutritive value. For example, Skittles and whole wheat bread both have a relatively high glycemic index of around 70. (Glucose has a glycemic index of 100.) Yet that does not make them of equal value in any regard other than the accompanying rise in blood sugar.

Graham, Sylvester

Sylvester Graham (b. July 4, 1794, in West Suffield, Connecticut; d. September 11, 1851, in Northampton, Massachusetts) is considered one of America's first food faddists. Graham believed that a high-fiber, natural-food diet would remedy cholera, alcoholism, premature aging, violence, sexual abuses, and digestive ills. His early followers included the Kellogg brothers, who were famous for their religious colony and health sanitarium at Battle Creek, Michigan. Graham's fanaticism and zeal for natural food attracted early followers, like the Kelloggs; they became known as "Grahamites."

Like many other health reformers, Graham had an early history of bad health. He was the youngest of seventeen children born to Massachusetts minister John Graham who died when Sylvester was just two years old. According to records, Graham's mother was "in a deranged state of mind" after her husband's death so the court appointed a guardian for Sylvester and two older siblings. His health and education suffered as he was passed from relative to relative, finally settling years later in Newark, New Jersey, where he was eventually reunited with his mother and an older brother. It was at this time that he also began to prepare for the ministry. He studied at Amherst Academy but was expelled after one quarter. He then studied privately with a minister and was ordained in 1826, the year he married the woman who had previously nursed him through a nervous breakdown.

While Graham was interested in saving souls, he also lectured on the evils of alcohol for the Pennsylvania Society for Discouraging the Use of Ardent Spirits. This temperance group worked to moderate the per capita consumption of alcohol, but Graham from the first advocated total abstinence. Soon he was also talking about diet and sex as well as alcohol. During this time he studied human physiology and diet. The cholera epidemic of 1832, the first of three cholera epidemics in the

United States during the nineteenth century, gave Graham a renewed platform when he suggested that greasy, spicy meat, combined with "excessive lewdness," caused the cholera outbreak.

But his most famous advice was that thick, coarse bread, baked at home and eaten daily, should be the mainstay of every diet. He believed his bread, made from the whole of the wheat and coarsely ground, known as "dyspepsia or temperance bread," was best when eaten a day old. It was the early version of today's graham cracker and he was convinced of its healing powers. Graham also recommended hard mattresses, open bedroom windows, cold baths, and a raw-food, vegetarian diet as best because it was closest to nature. Even though he realized that people were devoted to white bakery bread, he continued to condemn it as a horrible food choice. Graham's book, *Treatise on Bread*, sold for $4 a dozen and described the breadmaking process as the province of the loving wife and mother. Because he accused bakers of adulterating their products with additives, he was criticized by many, including well-known author Ralph Waldo Emerson, who publicly ridiculed Graham's diet.

The dietary world of the 1830s was filled with disease and bad health caused by consumption, chronic indigestion, and dyspepsia, a blanket term for constipation, stomachaches, headaches, and foul breath. Americans ate meat at every meal—some 180 pounds yearly per person—and foods were soaked in grease or gravy and washed down with whiskey. Long before the discovery of nutrition, fiber, vitamins, minerals, and cholesterol, Graham insisted that diet and health were directly connected. He believed that eating meat, particularly pork, led to sexual excess. Sexual excess then led to increased consumption of more rich foods and unhealthy meat, which, according to Graham, predisposed an individual to disease.

After the cholera epidemics subsided, Graham continued to lecture to mass audiences, traveling through Massachusetts, New York, New Jersey, Pennsylvania, Rhode Island, and Maine. Graham's talks were controversial; he continued to criticize the nation's diet, hygiene, and sexual practices. But it was this obsession with masturbation, what he called the "solitary vice," that eventually alienated many would-be sympathizers. In 1837, as his popularity faded, he moved to Northampton, Massachusetts, with his wife Sarah and their two children. He died there on September 11, 1851, at the age of fifty-seven.

In America, talk of "Grahamism" would continue for many years as followers like abolitionists William Lloyd Garrison, Horace Greeley, and Henry Stanton remained firm believers in his health ideals. Ellen Harmon White, spiritual leader and founder of the Seventh-day Adventist Church and founder of Battle Creek, Michigan's Western Health Reform Institute, also continued to recommend Graham's ideas and diet following his death. Slowly but surely the American medical and scientific communities would one day come to accept Graham's theory that diet and health were interrelated. Although he was ahead of his time, Graham's belief that eating too much salt, meat, and fat can cause health problems is now accepted nutritional wisdom.

Additional Reading

Armstrong, David, and Elizabeth Metzger Armstrong. *The Great American Medicine Show: Being an Illustrated History of Hucksters, Healers, Health Evangelists, and Heroes From Plymouth Rock to the Present*. New York: Prentice Hall, 1991.

DiBacco, Thomas V. "Behind the Graham Cracker, a Health Food Tale: One Man's Battle to Make Americans Think About Nutrition." *Washington Post*, 25 July 1989, 3.

Dictionary of American Biography. Farmington Hills, Mich.: Gale Group, 2001.

Encyclopedia of World Biography, 2d ed. Farmington, Mich.: Gale Group, 1998.

Farmer, Jean. "The Rev. Sylvester (Graham Cracker) Graham: America's Early Fiber Crusader." *Saturday Evening Post*, March 1985, 32–37.

Gordon, John Steele. "Sawdust Pudding." *American Heritage*, July–August 1996, 16–18.

Nissenbaum, Stephen. *Sex, Diet and Debility in Jacksonian America: Sylvester Graham and Health Reform*. Chicago: Dorsey Press, 1988.

Ghrelin

Ghrelin is a new and promising discovery in the fight against obesity. Pronounced GRELL-in, this growth hormone has an effect on whether a person is hungry, raising hopes for a breakthrough in the treatment of obesity. And in a country where obesity is an epidemic, understanding how ghrelin works could lead to effective weight-loss drugs or drugs to promote weight gain in anorexics and cancer patients. Research published in the May 23, 2002, issue of the *New England Journal of Medicine*, suggests that ghrelin may turn out to be one reason people feel hungry and why it's so hard for dieters to keep weight off.

Scientists know that part of the brain's hypothalamus controls food intake, but until recent years the only chemical substances known to turn it on have been found in the brain. New research now shows ghrelin's receptors are in the brain, but its primary site of production is in the stomach. This research suggests that the stomach pumps ghrelin into the bloodstream and the hormone then travels to the pituitary, a vastly different mechanism from other peptides that affect appetite. Those are made in the brain, do not travel into the bloodstream, and only work when injected directly into the appropriate brain regions.

Ghrelin, a peptide consisting of twenty-eight amino acids, was first identified by Kenji Kangawa of the National Cardiovascular Center Research Institute in Osaka, Japan. The name uses the root "ghre," which means "growth" in Hindi and related languages, and the name's initial letters also refer to ghrelin's role as a growth hormone–releasing factor. Following its identification in 1999, doctors have started looking at ghrelin in the treatment of obesity as well as in wasting syndromes stemming from AIDS, cancer, heart disease, and a variety of other illnesses. Although the hormone's role in the body is not yet fully understood, recent studies show that people suffering from wasting illnesses actually manufacture more ghrelin than normal. But, surprisingly, the highest blood concentrations of ghrelin recorded are in people suffering from anorexia nervosa. Apparently while anorexics are starving themselves to death, blood analysis indicates large amounts of ghrelin are released as normal body mechanisms continually signal the need for food.

Another interesting aspect of the report found that after a group of thirteen obese people dieted and lost some 17 percent of their body weight, their ghrelin levels were significantly higher throughout the day then before the weight loss when ghrelin levels would rise before meals but fall afterwards. Scientists suggest this increase in ghrelin in people who have lost weight dieting may reflect the body's attempt to regain lost pounds, a mechanism that originally evolved to defend against starvation during humankind's early history when food supplies fluctuated erratically. Today in developed nations like the United States with an abundance of high-calorie foods, this early survival advantage may now contribute to obesity.

On the other hand, low ghrelin levels were noted in people who underwent gastric-bypass surgery. They experienced a drop in their ghrelin levels but did not appear to suffer any side effects. In fact, according to the study, people who undergo this surgery describe a generalized disinterest in food with a noticeable drop in ghrelin production. Researchers say that following bypass surgery stomach cells that produce ghrelin are no longer exposed to food and ghrelin production may no longer be stimulated. During gastric-bypass surgery, surgeons sew much of the stomach shut, leaving room for a dieter to eat only a small amount of food.

Still, researchers are warning against overenthusiasm about ghrelin's prospects. They say similar hopes were raised years ago for leptin, a hormone that acts as an appetite suppressant. Yet after years of research, no useful medication was developed because researchers found patients quickly developed a tolerance to leptin. Nonetheless, the discovery of ghrelin is a major advance in the understanding of what controls appetite, and this leaves researchers hungry to learn more.

See also:

anorexia nervosa

Additional Reading

Cummings, David E., D. S. Weigle, R. S. Frayo, P. A. Breen, M. K. Ma, E. P. Dellinger, and J. Q. Purnell. "Plasma Ghrelin Levels after Diet-Induced Weight Loss or Gastric Bypass Surgery." *New England*

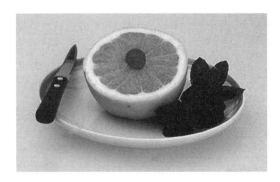

This grapefruit on a plate is part of a diet, popular since the 1930s, which calls for few vegetables, limited protein, and that all-important serving of grapefruit or grapefruit juice with every meal. Dieters hope the grapefruit will act as a special catalyst for fat burning, a false claim, according to scientists. (Painet)

Journal of Medicine, 346, no. 21 (23 May 2002): 1623–30.

Fischman, Josh. "A Hungry Hormone." *U.S. News & World Report,* 3 June 2002, 53.

Flier, J. S., and E. Maratos-Flier. "The Stomach Speaks—Ghrelin and Weight Regulation." *New England Journal of Medicine,* 346, no. 21 (23 May 2002): 1662–63.

Lemonick, Michael D. "Lean and Hungrier: Is a Recently Discovered Hormone the Reason Why Folks Who Lose Weight Can't Keep It Off?" *Time,* 3 June 2002, 54.

Pinkney, Jonathan, and Gareth Williams. "Ghrelin Gets Hungry." *Lancet* 359, no. 9315 (20 April 2002): 1360.

Travis, John. "The Hunger Hormone? An Appetite Stimulant Produced by the Stomach May Lead to Treatments for Obesity and Wasting Syndromes." *Science News,* 161, no. 7 (16 February 2002): 107–109.

Grapefruit Diet

A favorite with generations of dieters, the grapefruit diet has been around since at least the 1930s. This word-of-mouth plan calls for eating a few select vegetables, limited protein, plus the all-important serving of grapefruit or grapefruit juice with every meal. Over the years countless dieters have been encouraged to believe that grapefruit contains a special fat-burning enzyme. Dozens of variations of the grapefruit diet exist, but they all contain that one special ingredient—grapefruit.

Typically the diet lasts two or three weeks. Breakfast consists of half a grapefruit and black coffee. In several variations, breakfast also includes protein foods like bacon and eggs but no carbohydrates. Lunch is half a grapefruit plus an egg, cucumber, dry melba toast, and plain tea or coffee. Again, some variations suggest meat with this meal. Dinner calls for the obligatory grapefruit eaten with half a head of lettuce, a tomato, two eggs, and coffee or tea.

Some variations on the grapefruit diet theme call for dinners that include meat or fish, cooked any way from broiled to fried, baked, or grilled. Every version of this diet is low in carbohydrates and cutting out carbohydrates generally means a big reduction in daily calorie consumption; often less than 800 calories consumed per day. Anyone eating so few calories per day will lose weight no matter what foods they eat. So, on the one hand, nutritionists praise the grapefruit as an excellent food choice, saying it has no fat, is low in sodium, is packed with vitamin C, is high in water and fiber, and the pink variety has beta carotene.

But those same nutritionists laugh at the suggestion that grapefruit or its juice act as a special catalyst for fat burning. Experts say the fat-burning properties of grapefruit are just part of the cultural diet mythology. Scientists add that there are no magical properties in grapefruit or any other citrus fruits to help it burn extraordinary amounts of calories. They suggest that dieters eat grapefruit but they should do it for the right reasons, because it is a healthy food choice.

Healthy People 2010

Healthy People 2010, a federal initiative organized by the U.S. Department of Health and Human Services, considers obesity and overweight to be one of the leading ten health indicators—a measure by which the health of communities and Americans overall can be assessed. The leading health indicators focus on physical activity, overweight and obesity, tobacco use, substance abuse, responsible sexual behavior, mental health, injury and violence, environmental quality, immunization, and access to health care.

Healthy People goals are regularly updated and reviewed and new goals for 2010 were introduced in January 2000. The target for the Healthy People 2010 program is that 85 percent of adolescents in grades 9 to 12 get 20 minutes of vigorous physical activity three times or more per week. That's an increase from the 65 percent level in 1999. Physical inactivity levels rise much higher for adults. In 1997, only 15 percent of adults engaged in the recommended amount of physical activity and 40 percent did none at all. The target for Healthy People 2010 is to get 30 percent of adults engaging in the recommended amount of physical activity. Specifically, Healthy People 2010 sets out to "increase the proportion of adolescents who engage in vigorous physical activity that promotes cardiorespiratory fitness 3 or more days per week for 20 or more minutes per occasion," and "increase the proportion of adults who engage regularly, preferably daily, in moderate physical activity for at least 30 minutes per day."

The reasons are straightforward. The Healthy People 2010 report states that,

"Regular physical activity decreases the risk of death from heart disease, lowers the risk of developing diabetes, and is associated with a decreased risk of colon cancer. Regular physical activity helps prevent high blood pressure and helps reduce blood pressure in persons with elevated levels. Regular physical activity also: increases muscle and bone strength; increases lean muscle and helps decrease body fat; aids in weight control and is a key part of any weight loss effort; enhances psychological well-being and may even reduce the risk of developing depression; appears to reduce symptoms of depression and anxiety and to improve mood."

The initiative specifies those groups of people with low rates of physical activity. Women are generally less active than men at all ages, states the report. African Americans and Hispanics are generally less physically active than whites; adults in northeastern and southern U.S. states tend to be less active than adults in north-central and western states; and people with lower incomes and less education tend to be less active than those with higher education and incomes.

Reducing the rates of overweight and obese people is another primary goal of Healthy People 2010. Total costs related to obesity, calculated by direct medical costs and lost productivity, totaled an estimated $99 billion in 1995. During 1988 to 1994, 11 percent of children and adolescents (6- to 19-year-olds) were overweight or obese. Twenty-three percent of adults were considered obese. The target rates for 2010 are to get those obesity rates down to 5 percent for children and adolescents and down to 15 percent for adults. Obesity for adults is defined as having a body mass index (BMI) of 30 or

more. Overweight is defined as having a BMI of 25 to 30. To calculate BMI:

1. Multiply your weight in pounds by 704.5

2. Multiply your height in inches by your height in inches*

Divide answer to 1 by answer to 2

* If you're 5'5", your height in inches would be 65 inches.

If your BMI is   your risk level is

If your BMI is	your risk level is
19–24	minimal to low
25–26	low to moderate
27–29	moderate to high
30–34	high to very high
35–39	very high to extremely high
40+	extremely high

Being overweight or obese raises the risk of chronic illnesses, from high blood pressure, high cholesterol, Type 2 diabetes, heart disease and stroke, gallbladder disease, arthritis, respiratory problems, and certain types of cancer. As the Healthy People 2010 report points out, "Obese individuals also may suffer from social stigmatization, discrimination, and lowered self-esteem."

The report notes, "More than half of adults in the United States are estimated to be overweight or obese. The proportion of adolescents from poor households who are overweight or obese is twice that of adolescents from middle- and high-income households. Obesity is especially prevalent among women with lower incomes and is more common among African American and Mexican American women than among white women. Among African Americans, the proportion of women who are obese is 80 percent higher than the proportion of men who are obese. This gender difference also is seen among Mexican American women and men, but the percentage of white, non-Hispanic women and men who are obese is about the same."

The entire Healthy People 2010 report, plus periodic updates, can be found online at www.healthypeople.gov.

Herbal Diet Teas

Herbal teas for dieters contain senna, aloe, buckthorn, and other plant-derived laxatives that, when consumed in excessive amounts, can cause diarrhea, vomiting, nausea, stomach cramps, chronic constipation, and, in severe cases, death. By 1997 the Food and Drug Administration (FDA) had received a number of "adverse event" reports about dieter's teas, including information on the deaths of four young women where the teas may have been a contributing factor. Those four deaths involved women with a history of the eating disorders anorexia nervosa and bulimia.

Based on that information, the FDA now advises consumers to carefully follow package directions when using dieter's teas or any other dietary supplements containing senna, aloe, or other laxatives. The agency also encourages anyone experiencing persistent diarrhea, abdominal cramps, or other bowel problems to see a doctor. Although the agency has not required manufacturers to place a warning on the products' label, detailing the potential side effects, some manufacturers are voluntarily doing so.

Herbal diet teas are often purchased in health food stores or through mail-order catalogs. Their popularity comes from the mistaken consumer belief that increased bowel movements would prevent absorption of calories, would stop weight gain, and would even encourage weight loss. However, a special report from the FDA's Food Advisory Committee concluded that studies show using laxatives to cause diarrhea does not work and does not reduce the body's absorption of calories in any significant way.

With words like "dieter's," "diet," "trim," or "slim" in their names, it is easy to understand how consumers would expect weight loss from drinking the teas. Plus, package labeling often promotes the tea as a natural bowel cleanser and may include information about other weight-loss practices. Unfortunately, nutritionists suspect the diet teas are also very attractive to people with anorexia or bulimia because they act quickly and can be extremely effective as a laxative.

FDA reports show three types of problems most often associated with dieter's teas. Short-term problems like stomach cramps, nausea, vomiting, and diarrhea are most likely to occur in a first-time user who drinks more than the recommended amount. More serious chronic problems include ongoing diarrhea, pain, and constipation due to laxative dependency. In one report to the FDA a person who admitted using herbal products with laxatives for decades eventually required surgery to remove their colon when it stopped functioning. People who develop chronic problems have often used these products for years.

Finally, the FDA lists severe side effects such as fainting, dehydration, and electrolyte disorders, which bring with them low blood potassium, a condition that can cause paralysis, irregular heartbeat, and, in some cases, death. Severe problems with

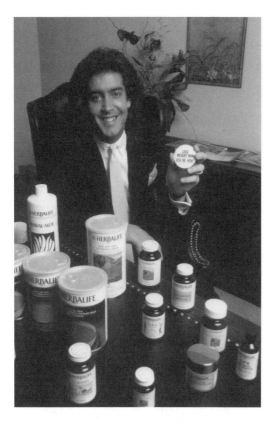

Mark Hughes, founder of Herbalife, poses in 1985 with some of the products from his million-dollar weight-loss business. Hughes, 44, was found dead in his mansion in 2000. He died after accidentally mixing alcohol and other prescription drugs. He began his business in 1980 after watching his mother's struggle with fad diets. Herbalife product advertisements led to federal scrutiny and fines in the 1980s. (© Nation Bill/CORBIS Sygma)

these products may develop when consumers drastically reduce their food intake or when they are already in poor nutritional health because they have an eating disorder.

So while a cup of herbal tea may feel soothing to the soul, people drinking dieter's teas must be careful to follow directions. Otherwise it can be dangerous to their health.

See also:

anorexia nervosa; bulimia nervosa; Food and Drug Administration (FDA).

Additional Reading

Bender, Michele. "Are Herbal Weight-Loss Teas Safe for Me to Drink?" *Cosmopolitan,* January 2001, 89.
Danitz, Tiffany, Karen Riley, and Michael Rust. "Read the Leaves Before Drinking: Health Risks of Herbal Teas." *Insight on the News,* 20 May 1996, 42.
Fraser, Laura. "The Dangers of Natural Diet Aids." *Glamour,* March 1996, 62–65.

Herbalife

Herbalife, a company started in 1980 by a nineteen-year-old high school dropout, Mark Hughes, whose mother died from a diet pill overdose, has been as controversial as it has been successful. The company slogan, "Lose weight now/Ask me how," became a familiar sight on buttons in the early 1980s, but by 1985 regulators from the Food and Drug Administration (FDA) were asking different questions concerning some of the ingredients in the Herbalife products. That same year the California Attorney General's office investigated Herbalife, alleging that the company supported some of its products with false medical claims and that the multilevel marketing operation could be an "illegal pyramid scheme." The company settled with the state of California for $850,000, without admitting fault.

Herbalife uses a multilevel sales approach, in which independent distributors handle all the pills, powders, juices, and other products. To earn money, distributors must sell Herbalife to retail customers, but they also take a percentage of the sales from other distributors they recruit to sell the product. Those recruits, in turn, recruit others. Sales from the diet shakes and vitamin supplements reached $427 million by 1985. Today Herbalife does business in forty-nine countries and has yearly sales of about $880 million.

Right from the start Hughes, the consummate salesman, insisted that his products would help people lose weight—from 10 to 29 pounds per month. And he told distributors and customers that Herbalife could cure a wide variety of ailments, from asthma to baldness or venereal disease, all while boosting energy levels. The original diet, known as the Slim and Trim Plan, included a variety of Herbalife pills and powders along with one 1,000-calorie meal per day, supplemented with two low-calorie skim milk shakes that contained the company's own protein powder. The daily assortment of herbal vitamins and minerals included vitamin B^6, lecithin, senna leaves, kelp, chickweed, and dandelion.

However, back in 1982 trouble first began for the company when the FDA received numerous reports of adverse reactions to Herbalife products. Those reactions ranged from constipation, diarrhea, and nausea to headaches and allergic reactions. The government maintained that Herbalife products contained powerful laxatives and diuretics. The FDA then sent Herbalife a "Notice of Adverse Findings," in which it stated that one of the company's products contained the ingredients mandrake and pokeroot, both considered unsafe by the FDA for food use. Mandrake, used at one time as a suicide drug by American Indians, and pokeroot were voluntarily removed from Herbalife formulas.

Besides side effects, questions were raised about unknown ingredients and about how the products were tested and determined fit for human consumption. Hughes said in an article in *People* that he tests products on himself. For years Hughes also refused to have Herbalife products analyzed by medical experts outside the company and insisted that product nutrition was sound. He suggested that a study of those products was unnecessary, since Herbalife helped more people lose weight than any other institution in the world.

Hughes, the forty-four-year-old founder of Herbalife, was found dead in his Malibu beachfront mansion in 2000. He died after accidentally mixing alcohol and the antidepressant and sleeping aid Doxepin. Today, Herbalife continues to offer a wide range of products for weight loss as well as for skin and hair care and cosmetics. In April 2002, two venture-capital firms acquired the company for approximately $685 million.

Additional Reading

Carey, John. "Selling Herbalife's Way." *Newsweek*, 8 April 1985, 89.

Carlson, P. "Despite Critics and Lawsuits, Herbalife Has Made Mark Hughes Wealthy If Not Healthy." *People*, 29 April 1985, 78–80.

Contemporary Newsmakers 1985. Detroit: Gale Research, 1985.

"Herbalife Founder Dies." *Los Angeles Business Journal*, 22, no. 22 (29 May 2000): 49.

Rakoff, David. "Death Be Not a Punch Line: Vitamin King Takes Pill and Dies." *New York Times Magazine*, 7 January 2001, 3.

High-Protein Diets

High-protein diets, although extremely popular with Americans, have not been proven effective for long-term weight loss. Like other fad diets, nutritionists say these diets pose potential health threats for people who follow them for more than a short period of time. Critics point to popular diets such as the Atkins, Zone, Protein Power, and Sugar Busters! diets as examples of high-protein eating plans.

The diets emphasize foods high in saturated fat, like meat and eggs, and limit high-carbohydrate foods such as cereals, grains, fruits, and vegetables. Concerns from groups like the American Heart Association (AHA) center on the fact that most Americans already eat more protein than their bodies need. Too much protein is not healthy when it comes to the human body. If too much is eaten, the excess is converted to fat and waste. Plus, breaking down that excess strains the kidneys and liver and can increase the risk of osteoporosis. And, according to the AHA and other health organizations, eating too much protein can also increase the possibility of coronary heart disease, diabetes, stroke, and several types of cancer.

According to the U.S. Department of Agriculture (USDA), the average American consumes about 90 grams of protein daily, significantly more than the 50 grams per day average the USDA recommends for healthy adults. The AHA guidelines, similar to the USDA recommendations, urge most adults to consume less than 30 percent of their total daily calories from fat and less than 10 percent of that from saturated fat. Most high-protein diets cannot meet these goals based on their suggested food choices.

The theory behind high-protein diets is that our bodies inefficiently burn carbohydrates, turning too many into fat. By eating fewer carbohydrates foods, these diets suggest that someone will reduce fat production and lose weight. But scientists say carbohydrates are the body's most efficient fuel and, when they are lacking, muscle gets burned for food or worse, ketosis develops. Ketosis is a toxic condition that occurs when ketones are released into the bloodstream. It can be triggered by starvation or untreated diabetes and it brings with it nausea, dehydration, constipation, or diarrhea. Prolonged ketosis may lead to kidney disease, gallstones, and even, in severe situations, cardiac complications. There is considerable disagreement among health organizations and high-protein diet advocates about the benefits and risks of ketosis resulting from high-protein eating programs.

High-protein diets can also fail to provide essential vitamins, minerals, fiber, and other nutritional elements that come from fruits, vegetables, whole grains, and non-fat dairy products because they severely limit these food groups. Many programs, such as the Atkins diet, do recommend vitamin supplements for participants. Health groups like the AHA criticize high-protein diets, saying they work for the same reason all diets work; they limit calories. Fewer calories from any source, whether it's protein, fat, or carbohydrates, will cause weight loss.

In 2001 the AHA issued a strong recommendation against high-protein weight-loss programs, including the Atkins Diet, Protein Power, The Zone, and Sugar Busters!, citing a lack of credible scientific evidence of long-term weight loss for these programs and the possibility of increased risk for those dieters with diabetes and heart disease. The report noted that high-protein weight-loss programs are "especially risky for patients with diabetes," because they can speed the progression of kidney disease even if followed for a short time. Like the U.S. Dietary Guidelines, the AHA's newest guidelines recommend a diet low in fat and high in fruits, vegetables, whole grains, and low-fat dairy products.

See also:

Atkins Nutritional Approach; Carbohydrate Addict's diet; ketones/ketosis; Sugar Busters!; The Zone.

Additional Reading

Albertson, Ellen. "Walking the Protein Tightrope." *Better Homes and Gardens,* April 1999, 118.

Norris, Eileen. "High-Protein Diets: Where's the Beef?" *Harvard Health Letter,* 22, no. 3 (January 1997): 1–4.

Squires, Sally. "Heart Association Skewers Atkins Diet; High Protein Plans Called Unproven, Risky." *Washington Post,* 9 October 2001, F1.

Human Chorionic Gonadotropin (HCG)

Human chorionic gonadotropin (HCG) is a hormone produced during pregnancy. HCG levels are used to determine if a woman is pregnant. Home pregnancy kits can easily measure those levels. During the early 1970s, HCG was a popular component of a low-calorie weight-loss plan. But in 1974 the Food and Drug Administration (FDA) issued a statement that expressed growing concern about the continued use of HCG in weight-loss clinics around the country, saying there was no evidence that the drug was effective in treating obesity. Clinics that offered HCG as part of a weight-loss plan often coupled it with a 500-calorie diet. Diets that low in calories will cause weight loss no matter what foods are eaten or supplements taken.

The FDA also announced that the drug HCG must bear a label saying it is worthless for weight loss. The report stressed that although no injuries had been noted among patients taking the hormone, any active drug can have unexpected adverse reactions. The FDA later issued an alert on the dangers of contaminated HCG reportedly being used by athletes and bodybuilders to counter the effects of steroids.

Doctors legitimately prescribe HCG to treat cases of undescended testicles in men or infertility in women.

Additional Reading

Ballin, J. C. and P. L. White. "Fallacy and Hazard: Human Chorionic Gonadotropin Diet and Weight Reduction." *Journal of the American Medical Association* 230, no. 5 (4 November 1974): 693.

"Disclaimer Ordered on Drug Used in Antifat Clinics." *New York Times,* 15 December 1974, 55.

Prince, Rayma. "FDA Issues Alert on Phony, Contaminated HCG." *Drug Topics* 132, no. 1 (1988): 40.

Insulin

Insulin is a hormone required to convert sugars and starches from the food we eat into the energy we need. Diabetes is a condition in which the body no longer or inadequately produces insulin. People with Type 1, or insulin-dependent, diabetes, must take daily insulin injections—often multiple injections—to stay alive. People with Type 2 diabetes use a variety of controls, including diet, exercise, oral medications, and, sometimes, injections of insulin

Not until 1920 did a Canadian doctor, Frederick Banting, first conceive of the idea of insulin. The first patient treated with insulin was a fourteen-year-old Canadian boy. Oral medications weren't available until the 1950s. Today, there are more than twenty kinds of insulin available—some act very quickly or peak at different times, and some last all day long. There are also different ways to deliver insulin—syringes, insulin pens, and insulin pumps.

Researchers are also making progress in solving the riddle of diabetes. Research

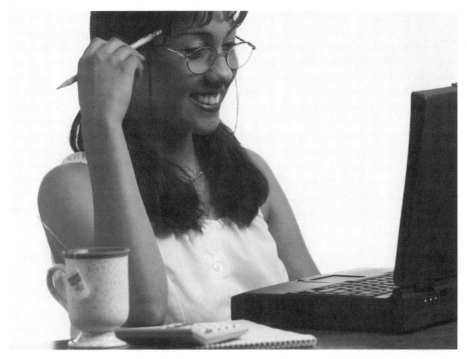

Using a Web-based diet plan can provide support, quick calculations, and an electronic log of your diet plan. (Painet)

into prevention of Type 1 diabetes is under way, as are efforts to transplant insulin-producing cells into the bodies of Type 1 diabetics. Other researchers, meanwhile, are finding new ways to help people who have the condition to control it.

See also:

diabetes.

Internet Dieting

Dieters looking for support and the Internet seem to have been made for each other with the Internet's anytime, anywhere availability. Several Internet-based diet plans have become popular and most of the existing diet plans have enhanced Web sites, featuring, at a minimum, extensive FAQs. Some, such as Weight Watchers, Jenny Craig, and Richard Simmons offer some level of interaction between weight-loss consultants and the dieter.

eDiets is the largest subscription-based, online diet, reporting that it had more than 1.2 million members in mid-2003. The program generates customized diet programs based on individual members' goals, food preferences, and lifestyles. It also sends out e-mail newsletters. The Web site notes, "eDiets does not market a line of food or supplements and weight loss drugs are NOT part of the program. eDieters lose an average of 2 pounds per week—every week—while learning how to enjoy and maintain a healthy lifestyle once their goal weight is reached."

Cyberdiets.com, on the other hand, is a clearinghouse of diet plan information on the Web.

What Internet diet plans offer, of course, is 24/7 access. If you forget what

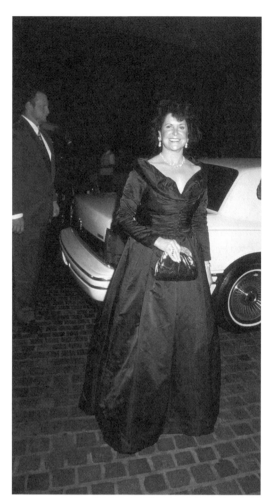

Jenny Craig, cofounder of the weight-loss company that bears her name. (© PACHA/CORBIS)

your meal plan is, you can log on and find out. Snow or icy roads won't prevent you from participating in online meetings or support chat rooms.

Additional Reading

Stroup, Katherine. "Desktop Dieting: Is the Internet the Answer to Losing Those Extra Pounds?" *Newsweek*, 20 May 2002, 70
www.cyberdiets.com
www.ediets.com
www.jennycraig.com
www.richardsimmons.com
www.weightwatchers.com

Jenny Craig

Jenny Craig, Inc., is a weight-loss program combining personalized support with a variety of prepackaged meals. At Jenny Craig In-Centre programs, a dieter meets weekly with a consultant, reviews the past week, plans the menu for the upcoming week, and generally receives support.

Jenny Craig's programs include additional support on exercise, and manuals with strategies for losing weight and maintaining weight loss. The company also offers foods, which the Web site says are "specifically chosen for slow, steady weight loss, with calories levels ranging from 1200 to 2300 calories per day."

Jenny Craig also has some online support, such as an online weight tracker, and the Web site contains motivating success stories.

Jenny Craig was founded in 1983, by Jenny and Sid Craig. They opened their first Jenny Craig Centre in Australia when she was 50 and he was 51. Jenny Craig became interested in weight control after she gained forty-five pounds during a pregnancy. Her biography on the Web site notes that Craig's mother had been overweight after having children and died of an obesity-related stroke at age forty-nine. "In an effort to avoid a similar situation, Jenny joined a local gym and shed her excess pounds using a two-pronged approach of healthy eating and exercise." That combination of nutrition, physical activity, and lifestyle changes are the underpinnings of the Jenny Craig program. With her husband, marketing specialist Sid Craig, the couple grew Jenny Craig, Inc., from that one center to one of the largest weight-loss programs.

In May 2002, Jenny Craig, Inc. was acquired by a private investor group. Sid and Jenny Craig are part of that investor group.

Additional Reading

Thompson, Stephanie. "Two Ad Pitches for Weight Loss Gain More Heft; Weight Watchers and Jenny Craig Stress Personalized Diet Programs." *Advertising Age*, 4 December 2000, 3.
www.jennycraig.com

Ketones/Ketosis

Ketones or ketone bodies are created by the liver when it converts fats into chemicals for the body to use as fuel. Ketosis is an abnormal increase of ketone bodies in the bloodstream, triggered by starvation or by a low- to no-carbohydrate diet. During digestion the liver converts carbohydrates into the simple sugar glucose, an important fuel for most body functions. Proteins replace themselves as needed and any excess protein also becomes glucose.

Ketosis occurs when there is a shortage of carbohydrates for fuel, which triggers the production of large amounts of ketone bodies to compensate for the lack of glucose. Problems develop because the tissue in the brain and in the muscles used for rapid movement cannot use ketone bodies as efficiently as they use glucose for fuel. A low-carbohydrate diet forces the brain to use ketones for its fuel. This change in fuel slows thinking and reaction times. The brain's need for carbohydrates is one of the reasons the USDA Food Guide Pyramid recommends 6 to 11 servings per day of the carbohydrate food group, which includes bread, cereal, rice, and pasta.

The symptoms of ketosis include unpleasant or bad breath odor, nausea, dehydration, constipation, and diarrhea. Severe and prolonged ketosis may lead to kidney disease, gallstones, gout, or cardiac complications. Advocates of high-protein, low-carbohydrate diets, such as the Scarsdale Medical Diet and the Atkins Nutritional Approach, acknowledge that dieters following their eating programs will experience ketosis. However, they claim the condition can enhance the effectiveness of a low-carbohydrate diet.

According to the U.S. Department of Agriculture, a number of factors contribute to weight loss for people following a low-carbohydrate diet. They include water weight loss, decreased appetite, the unpleasant symptoms of ketosis along with the elimination of carbohydrates as a food group, which creates a corresponding decrease in calorie consumption. Doctors have successfully prescribed ketogenic diets for people afflicted with epilepsy. Those ketogenic diets slow down all brain functions, making it less likely the brain will react to the triggers that set off an epileptic episode.

See also:

Atkins Nutritional Approach; Food Guide Pyramid; Scarsdale diet.

Additional Reading

"Fad Diets." *The Nurse Practitioner* 25, no. 10 (October 2000): 1s18.
Merriam-Webster's Medical Dictionary. Springfield, Mass.: Merriam-Webster, Inc., 1995.
Tarnower, Herman, MD, and Samm Sinclair Baker. *The Complete Scarsdale Medical Diet.* New York: Rawson, Wade Publishers, Inc., 1978.

Life Choice Diet

The Life Choice diet by Dr. Dean Ornish is a low-fat, vegetarian eating plan that focuses on beans, fruits, vegetables, and whole grains, and recommends that dieters consume only 10 percent of their calories from fat. Ornish, director of the

Preventive Medicine Research Institute in Sausalito, California, also encourages regular exercise, stress-management techniques, and group support as key components in his plan. Ornish wrote his best-selling book, *Dr. Dean Ornish's Program for Reversing Heart Disease: The Only System Scientifically Proven to Reverse Heart Disease without Drugs or Surgery,* in 1990. The system was developed from Ornish's study data, which showed that program participants who followed his plan had a reduction in overall heart blockages after a relatively short time. The data also showed that his heart patients lost an average of 22 pounds, even though they had not been trying to lose weight during the treatment period.

Ornish published the Life Choice diet in 1993, geared toward people without significant heart disease who wanted to lose weight and improve their health. The book, *Eat More, Weigh Less: Dr. Dean Ornish's Life Choice Program for Losing Weight Safely While Eating Abundantly,* immediately sold half a million copies. According to the author, the Life Choice diet is based on the type of food a person eats rather than the amount of food. This, he said, creates a sense of abundance rather than deprivation. The diet book also echoes the Ornish heart treatment plan by outlining a diet made up primarily of fruits, vegetables, grains, and beans with only 10 percent of calories from mostly polyunsaturated fat. In the book, Ornish explains that the human body needs about 4 to 6 percent of its calories as fat to synthesize essential fatty acids. The Life Choice diet's 10 percent fat goal is less than what is routinely recommended. In fact, a typical 2,000-calorie-a-day diet that follows the Dietary Guidelines for Americans and the American Heart Association's guidelines of less than 30 percent of calories from fat per day, means eating up to 67 grams of fat daily. By contrast, the Life Choice diet, with only 10 percent fat, means participants eat a mere 22 fat grams a day.

The Life Choice diet's simple guidelines are not a list of do's and don'ts. Rather, Ornish suggests a spectrum of foods grouped from most beneficial to least beneficial, based mainly on fat and cholesterol content. Group 1 foods, those that are most beneficial, include whole grains from barley to couscous, oats, brown rice, and soybeans, to name just a few. Good for you vegetables range from A to Z: asparagus and artichokes, kale, leeks, potatoes, squash, turnips, and zucchini. Legumes, like azuki beans, black beans, lentils, all kinds of soy products, plus tempeh and tofu, are also Group 1 choices. And Ornish encourages dieters to eat a wide variety of fruits, including apples, berries, dates, figs, and all kinds of melons.

Next, in Group 2, are foods that should be eaten in moderation: nonfat dairy products such as skim milk, nonfat yogurt, and egg whites, plus nonfat or very low-fat commercially available products, including whole-grain breakfast cereals, nonfat mayonnaise and salad dressings, and fat-free crackers. Ornish also names a variety of Pritikin products, developed by Nathan Pritikin and the Pritikin Longevity Center, in this category. Group 3 foods to be eaten sparingly are things like oils, low-fat dairy products, fish, maple syrup, and honey. Group 4 foods, to be avoided when possible, include poultry, all shellfish, and refined sugar products. Group 5 foods, products which are not considered healthful, range from all beef and pork products to fried chicken, coconut oil, egg yolks, cream, whole milk foods, salt, and alcohol, plus any commercially available product with more than 2 grams of fat per serving.

A typical day on the Ornish diet would feature a breakfast menu with buckwheat pancakes, nonfat yogurt, sliced bananas, kiwi, and fresh strawberries, plus orange juice. Lunch might be tomato and lentil soup, a zucchini salad, and a pear. A dinner entrée might be sweet and sour vegetables with tofu, broccoli, and teriyaki sauce; brown rice pilaf; a green salad with no-fat dressing; and fruit.

While recognizing that these foods sound strange and unfamiliar to many people, Ornish recommends them as part of what he calls comprehensive changes rather than only moderate changes. According to Ornish, big or comprehensive changes disrupt old routines, which in turn makes change easier. For example, if people who usually eat 8 ounces of steak reduce that to just 4 ounces, they feel cheated. They may ultimately find it easier not to eat any steak at all, to eat something totally different. While Ornish acknowledges that big change is stressful at first, in the long run he maintains that it is easier when people abandon their old habits and then form new ones.

Ornish also suggests in his book that conventional dieting doesn't work when the diet tells people what *not* to do and what *not* to eat. He contrasts his approach, saying it allows dieters to make informed and intelligent choices from the options, selections, and preferences he outlines. With a spectrum of choices, he writes, "Each person will see they have the authority to decide what is right for them." He also criticizes some weight loss regimes, which might do more harm than good, especially high-protein diets like the Atkins diet that recommends increasing consumption of meats and eggs while reducing carbohydrates and fiber. Health organizations, including the American Heart Association, warn dieters not to eat excessive animal protein with its accompanying saturated fat, saying studies show that it leads to overweight, heart disease, and other illnesses.

See also:

Atkins Nutritional Approach; Dietary Guidelines for Americans; Ornish, Dean; Pritikin, Nathan.

Additional Reading

Brink, Susan. "The Low-Fat Life." *U.S. News & World Report*, 12 July 1999, 56.

Condor, Bob. "Lifestyle Changes Can Go Right to the Heart." *Chicago Tribune*, 13 February 2000, 3.

Cowley, Geoffrey. "Healer of Hearts." *Newsweek*, 16 March 1998, 50–57.

Gavalas, Elaine. "The Great Diet Debate." *Better Nutrition*, May 2000, 32–36.

Lindley, Sarah. "Heart Smart: Natural Remedies for a Healthy Heart." *Vegetarian Times*, May 1997, 58–66.

Ornish, Dean. *Eat More, Weigh Less: Dr. Dean Ornish's Life Choice Program for Losing Weight Safely While Eating Abundantly.* New York: HarperCollins, 1993.

Thomson, Bill. "The Second Act of Dean Ornish." *Natural Health*, November–December 1998, 112–19.

Liposuction

Liposuction is a surgical procedure to remove pockets of fat from your body. A narrow tube is inserted into a fat layer beneath the skin, and the fat cells are broken up and suctioned out. Typically, liposuction is used to sculpt the abdomen, hips, buttocks, thighs, knees, upper arms, chin, cheeks, and neck. Cost of the surgery ranges from about $2,000 to as high as $14,000.

Liposuction is the most common cosmetic surgery in the country according to

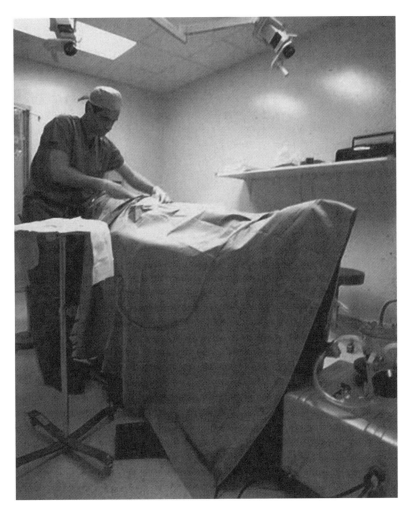

A patient in a Chicago hospital undergoes liposuction surgery in 2001. Liposuction is just one procedure in the rapidly growing list of surgical options developed to treat obesity. (Painet)

the American Society of Aesthetic Plastic Surgeons. In 2002, there were 372,831 surgeries performed, an apparent decrease from the number performed the year before, which estimated that there were about 385,390 liposuction procedures performed.

Recent advances in liposuction, such as ultrasound-assisted lipoplasty (UAL), have made the procedure less rough and the recovery a little easier. However, despite its popularity, the decision to have surgery shouldn't be taken lightly.

Liposuction has distinct risks—including death. There were ninety-five deaths associated with liposuction between 1994 and 1998. The *Philadelphia Inquirer* and other Knight/Ridder newspapers printed an article detailing the death of an eighteen-year-old who died following surgery, apparently from a fat clot that got loose during surgery and traveled through her bloodstream to her lungs. The mother told the newspaper, "We never would have let her do it if we knew she could have died. It wasn't supposed to be a big deal."

In an April 2001 issue of *Teen People,* another mother described the agony and shock at the death of her twenty-three-year-old daughter following liposuction. The family received a $500,000 settlement in a malpractice lawsuit against the doctor, who had reportedly damaged a vein in the young woman's leg. The resulting blood clot traveled to her lungs and she died during a seizure the following day. "Our lawyer thought we should have gotten a much higher sum, but we didn't care. More than anything, we just wanted the public to know what had happened to our daughter," the mother wrote.

Liposuction does not remove cellulite. Nor can a physician guarantee results. Sometimes, the area where the fat was removed may look dimply, a "cottage cheese" effect. Excess skin may stay loose and sag. Fat deposits may develop in new places, and if you gain more than 10 pounds after surgery, the fat may come back to haunt the same area, as well.

The American Society of Plastic Surgeons, which offers a Web-based clearinghouse at www.plasticsurgery.org, suggests that the best candidates "are normal-weight people with firm, elastic skin who have pockets of excess fat in certain areas. You should be physically healthy, psychologically stable and realistic in your expectations. Your age is not a major consideration; however, older patients may have diminished skin elasticity and may not achieve the same results as a younger patient with tighter skin." The site notes that the risks increase for people with medical problems, especially heart or lung disease or poor blood circulation.

The surgeons' site details the different kinds of liposuction procedures, and prospective patients should discuss the options and their expectations with their physician. It also suggests getting help at home for a day or two following surgery. Liposuction can be performed in a office-based center, an outpatient surgery center, or a hospital. Smaller procedures can be done in the first two; the hospital is a more appropriate setting if more fat is to be removed or if other procedures are being done at the same time. How long the surgery takes depends on how much fat is being removed and how many areas are being sculpted. According to www.plastic-surgery.org, following surgery, "You may still experience some pain, burning, swelling, bleeding and temporary numbness." Most people can return to work within a few days and begin to feel better in the next week or so. A noticeable difference in the way you look occurs about four to six weeks after surgery when the swelling has gone down, but it can take about three months for the full effect to emerge.

Additional Reading

"Boom (and Busts) for Plastic Surgeons." *U.S. News & World Report*, 25 June 2001, 10.

Diclementi, Deborah. "Pressure to be Perfect: Since 1996, the Number of Teens Having Plastic Surgery Has Nearly Doubled. Is That a Healthy Choice—or a Dangerous Trend?" *Teen People*, 1 April 2001, 200.

Fitzgerald, Susan, and Marian Uhlman. "A Popular Surgery, a Young Life Lost." *Philadelphia Inquirer*, 5 August 2001, A1.

Gerhart, Ann. "Nipped in the Bud: More and More Young Women Choose Surgical 'Perfection.'" *Washington Post*, 23 June 1999, C1.

Henig, Robin Marantz. "The High Cost of Thinness." *New York Times Magazine*, 28 February 1988, 41.

"Liposuction Rated As Most Popular Procedure for Second Year." *Women's Health Weekly*, 28 February 2002, 11.

Patrick, Stephanie. "Doctors Pioneer Gentler Liposuction." *Dallas Business Journal*, 24, no. 49 (20 July 2001): 3.

www.plasticsurgery.org

Liquid Protein Diets

Liquid protein diets are not a new concept. Protein formula products, both liquid and powdered, were popular as long ago as the 1930s. But this form of fad dieting almost completely disappeared during its most sensational period in the late 1970s, when at least fifty-eight deaths were linked to the use of liquid protein diets. At that time an investigation by the Food and Drug Administration (FDA) and the federal Centers for Disease Control (CDC) revealed a number of deaths from what they called irreversible abnormal heart rhythms. Those who died had used the liquid protein diets for several months and had lost large amounts of weight. Although publicity concerning the deaths and a warning issued by the FDA almost wiped out the market, by changing ingredients, names, and advertising, liquid diet drinks are once again a moneymaker for the $3 billion-a-year weight-loss industry.

Many of those fifty-eight deaths occurred during the diet's two-week period known as refeeding, when dieters stopped eating the liquid protein and started eating conventional foods. Doctors suspect the deaths occurred when large increases in food intake produced changes in metabolic rates and electrolyte balance, which in turn caused the fatal arrhythmias. The women who died were in their mid-20s to mid-30s; most had been on the liquid protein diets for months and had started eating small amounts of solid food again. In studying those deaths, a Harvard Medical School doctor said in a 1978 *New York Times* interview that he believed the patients had been dangerously depleted of essential nutrients, such as potassium and other minerals. This loss of important minerals, in his opinion, contributed to the heart damage seen in the victims.

There are two basic categories of liquid protein diets: the draconian regimes mentioned above, also known as very-low-calorie diets, now modified to be administered under medical supervision; and the over-the-counter cans or powders designed to replace a meal or two per day. Those over-the-counter liquid replacement meals date back to the early 1930s when Dr. Stoll's Diet Aid, the Natural Reducing Food, was sold to women through beauty parlors. Dr. Stoll's was the most famous reducing drink of its day. Directions called for dieters to combine a cup of water with a teaspoon of the protein powder made from milk chocolate, starch, and an extract of roasted whole wheat and bran. Although there were no statistics on the success or failure of Dr. Stoll's Diet Aid, this product was the first in a growing list of popular over-the-counter liquid diet drinks.

In 1959 Metrecal became a household name thanks to the doctors at the Rockefeller Institute. They developed their diet drink to resemble breast milk by including a precise balance of protein, fat, and carbohydrate. That new formula made Metrecal a commercial success. During the 1970s hospitals began offering medically supervised liquid protein plans like Optifast to obese patients. Following the supervised diets came over-the-counter choices with names like Prolinn, Gro-Lean, and Cherrmino. These liquid protein products began innocently enough through the work of Harvard Medical School professor George Cahill, Jr., and his colleague, Dr. George Blackburn. The two were among others studying the problem of malnutrition and the detrimental effects of fasting among postoperative patients. Their solution was to feed people small amounts of pure protein following surgery. Their successful strategy caught the attention of osteopath

Dr. Robert Linn. In 1976 Linn took the idea of liquid protein replacement as the main focus of his own diet program and he explained it all in his best-selling diet book, *The Last Chance Diet.* The book sold more than 2 million copies and laid out his simple plan: take in just enough protein to keep the body going without breaking down lean muscle tissue. For a time dieters could live off their own fat and lose as much as 10 pounds per week. And it was easy, just drink 6 to 8 ounces of liquid protein daily, either straight or mixed with diet soda, and drink plenty of water.

Blackburn's harsh response to Linn's protein diet was quoted in a 1977 *Newsweek* article. He called the Linn diet program "amateurish and totally without credence." Blackburn maintained that insufficient research had been done on the effectiveness of this type of diet, especially problems with long-term maintenance and the need for specific vitamins and minerals. In his book Linn did urge dieters to consult a doctor who could then prescribe the needed supplemental vitamins and minerals. But because the product was sold over the counter, users rarely saw a doctor before starting on the diet. As a result, many suffered from a lack of potassium, a deficiency known to lead to kidney damage or potentially fatal abnormal heart rhythms or arrhythmias.

A study released in 1977 by the FDA noted that three well-known brands of liquid protein contained protein of "extremely poor" quality. Some of the early liquid protein diets were made from ground-up livestock bones and ears. Linn's first liquid diet, Prolinn, contained beef hide. He later switched his main ingredient to pigskin and named it EMF, or Enzymatic Modular Food. Linn admitted there were problems with his early formula; diarrhea was one of the main side effects.

Health groups like the American Dietetic Association say current liquid protein products contain more and better protein, some carbohydrates, and more vitamins and minerals than their 1970 counterparts. Today's liquid diets are still designed to replace solid food entirely for weeks at a time, but now they are handled through hospitals or doctors' offices so that health professionals can check blood pressure, heart function, urine content, and potassium and electrolyte levels. Another common problem with very-low-calorie diets is that dieters risk losing valuable lean muscle if they take weight off too quickly. That problem can be avoided by limiting participants to only those patients who are truly obese, weighing in at over 20 to 30 percent of their ideal weight. Nutrition education and behavior modification training with a psychological component is also part of current very-low-calorie diet programs.

Since 1984 the FDA has required that all very-low-calorie protein diets, meaning diets that provide fewer than 400 calories a day, carry a warning that they can cause serious illness and need to be followed under medical supervision. The initial warning that followed the fifty-eight deaths in 1978 affected nearly all liquid protein products. But newer regulations only require warnings on protein products that provide more than half of a person's calories and are promoted for use in losing weight or as a food supplement. So diet drinks like Slim-Fast protein powder, introduced in 1978, have been able to escape the need for the FDA warning label by recommending that users also eat one sensible meal each day. That way the drinks do not fall into the very-low-calorie range. For example, three Slim-Fast shakes a day provide 660 calories; a snack and sensible dinner add to that for a total of 1,200 or so calories per day. Famous

Slim-Fast users include former New York City mayor Ed Koch, baseball manager Tommy Lasorda, and singer Mel Tormé.

When celebrities lose large amounts of weight, it adds glamour along with an aura of success to the liquid diet programs, but success is far from guaranteed once the pounds are gone. Unfortunately, clinical studies now show that as many as 90 percent of the people who lose 25 pounds or more on any diet gain them back within

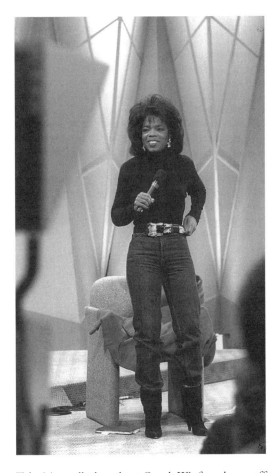

Television talk show host Oprah Winfrey shows off her new figure to her audience in Chicago on November 16, 1988. Winfrey credited her 67-pound weight loss to a liquid diet and exercise. Her goal was to fit into a size 10 pair of blue jeans for the first time on her syndicated TV show. (AP/Wide World Photos)

two years. Medically supervised plans like Optifast have claimed for years that about two-thirds of the patients who complete their programs keep the majority of pounds off for at least eighteen months. Still, health agencies like the American Dietetic Association continue to caution consumers about the risks of liquid protein diets, especially their poor long-term results. And doctors say evidence shows that a high percentage of patients treated by liquid protein diets alone regain weight almost as quickly as they lose it. This is caused by the body's metabolic rate. When dieters lose a lot of lean body mass, their resting metabolic rate slows, and a lowered metabolism makes it that much more difficult to keep off pounds without the help of a daily exercise program—a vital part of any long-term weight loss plan.

For example, in 1988 celebrity Oprah Winfrey lost 67 pounds using the Optifast liquid protein diet. But after one year the star was 17 pounds heavier and went on to regain most of the lost weight. It wasn't until several years later that Winfrey incorporated daily exercise into her weight loss effort. Following her use of Optifast, she vowed she would never again reveal her weight or go on a diet. Oprah's televised Optifast weight loss in 1988 created an initial national frenzy, along with a huge growth in the liquid diet industry, that saw profits of $200 million that year alone. Few Americans had tried liquid diets since the tragic deaths of the 1970s but Winfrey's success gave the industry a needed boost. After the actress regained the pounds, liquid diet drinks came under sharp review by the Federal Trade Commission (FTC). And in 1991 the FTC charged Optifast, Medifast, and Ultrafast with deceptive advertising. The three reached a settlement with the FTC after the companies agreed to stop using what the FTC alleged were deceptive claims about the long-term results and the safety of liquid diets.

Today, liquid diet drinks continue to have the support of some medical professionals who call the programs a successful alternative to high-risk gastric-bypass surgery for very obese patients. While the gastric-bypass surgery reduces the stomach's capacity for food, limiting the amount of food an individual can eat, liquid protein diets take away all food decisions. These rigidly structured programs begin with a fasting period of three months or more, when patients eat only the protein shakes and take in from 400 to 800 calories a day. After patients lose anywhere from 3 to 10 pounds a week and reach their target weight, they begin to reintroduce solid foods, lean meats, salads, or vegetables. Last is the maintenance stage when dieters make their own food choices, a difficult phase according to patients, many of whom haven't learned to eat well-balanced, nutritious meals. Yet doctors say liquid meal replacement is a good option for people who have problems with portion control as long as solid food choices include lots of fruits and vegetables and complex carbohydrates to provide plenty of fiber and phytochemicals. And while the specialists recognize that the risks of liquid diets include heart irregularities and sudden death, they believe medically supervised liquid protein plans can work for people who desperately need to lose weight but have failed for years on other diets.

See also:

Slim-Fast.

Additional Reading

Beck, Melinda. "The Losing Formula: Liquid Diets Take Pounds Off Fast. But a Quick Fix Can Be Risky and Doesn't Ensure Long-Term Success." *Newsweek,* 30 April 1990, 52–58.

Cowley, Susan Cheever, and Patricia J. Seth. "No-Food Diet: Liquid-Protein Regimen." *Newsweek,* 11 July 1977, 74.

Deveny, Kathleen. "Liquid diet plans are staging a comeback." *Wall Street Journal,* 7 September 1993, B5.

Langway, Lynn. "Feasting on Fat." *Newsweek,* 5 December 1977, 83.

Larkin, Howard. "Liquid Diets Suffer Another Blow to Their Image." *American Medical News* 34, no. 42 (11 November 1991): 22.

Mitgang, Lee. "Liquid Protein Dies a Natural Death." *New York Times,* 15 October 1978, 64.

Rhodes, Maura. "America's Top 6 Fad Diets." *Good Housekeeping,* July 1996, 100–103.

Sachs, Andrea. "Drinking Yourself Skinny: Liquid Diets Are Back in Vogue, But Are They Safe?" *Time,* 19 December 1988, 68.

Schmeck, Harold, Jr. "FDA Still Seeking Specific Health Hazard in Liquid Protein Products." *New York Times,* 16 May 1978, 16.

Silberner, Joanne, Pamela Sherrid, and Francesca Lunzer Kritz. "The Real Skinny on Liquid Diets." *U.S. News & World Report,* 28 October 1991, 90.

"Three Liquid Diet Marketers Told to Alter Ad Claims." *New York Times,* 17 October 1991, D2.

Wadden, Thomas A., Theodore B. Van Itallie, and George L. Blackburn. "Responsible and Irresponsible Use of Very-Low-Calorie Diets in the Treatment of Obesity." *Journal of the American Medical Association,* 263, no. 1 (5 January 1990): 83–86.

Macrobiotics

Macrobiotics is a diet considered by followers to be a spiritual and social philosophy of living and eating. Macrobiotic principles stem from the ancient Asian philosophy of yin and yang. Its name comes from the Greek words *macro,* meaning "great," and *bios* meaning "life."

The basic diet, developed by Japanese philosopher George Ohsawa, calls for followers to eat whole foods native to one's environment and to gradually stop eating refined and processed foods.

The diet attempts to balance the intake of yin and yang foods to establish a harmony in the body, which will produce good health. Yin foods include vegetables, grains, beans, and seaweed. Animals and animal products are labeled as yang and include salt, fish, and fowl. Macrobiotic followers aim for a balance of five parts yin to one part yang in their diet. So a macrobiotic eating plan would include 50 to 60 percent of calories from whole grains, including brown rice, barley, millet, oats, corn, rye, wheat, and buckwheat. Fresh vegetables would be 25 to 30 percent of the diet and soybean products, such as tofu and tempeh, along with seaweed might make up 5 to 10 percent of foods eaten. Preparation of the food is an important aspect of macrobiotics. Followers believe vegetables should be lightly steamed, boiled, or sautéed in vegetable oil. Rice must be pressure-cooked, and gas is the only acceptable cooking fuel. Wood utensils are allowed, while plastic ones are to be avoided. Pots should be made of glass, ceramic, or stainless steel. Electric stoves as well as copper, aluminum, and Teflon pots, should be avoided.

During the 1960s the diet was known as "the brown rice diet," and was identified largely with hippies, dropouts, and the drug culture. In 1971 the American Medical Association condemned macrobiotics, labeling it "a major public health problem" that posed a serious hazard to the health of individuals. While the diet is hardly conventional, over the years it has gained support. Recent studies show the diet can decrease the risks for heart disease and some forms of cancer, according to Harvard nutritionist Dr. Frederick Stare. Stare equated macrobiotics to a typical vegetarian diet even as early as 1978 in a *New York Times* interview. Despite some benefits, serious problems can occur with strict interpretations of this diet. Those following it can become deficient in protein, vitamin B^{12}, vitamin D, calcium, iron, and riboflavin. Experts say adding eggs and dairy products or other forms of supplementation to a macrobiotic diet can alleviate those problems.

Additional Reading

Kastner, M. *Alternative Healing: The Complete A to Z Guide to Over 160 Different Alternative Therapies.* La Mesa, Calif.: Halcyon Publishing, 1993.

Sifton, D. W. *The PDR Family Guide to Natural Medicines and Healing Therapies.* New York: Three Rivers Press, 1999.

Wells, Patricia. "Macrobiotics: A Principle, Not a Diet." *New York Times,* 19 July 1978, C1–9.

Woodham, A., and D. Peters. *Encyclopedia of Healing Therapies,* 1st edition. New York: Dorling Kindersley, 1997.

McDougall Program

The McDougall Program, developed by Dr. John McDougall, is a low-fat, starch-based, vegetarian diet designed to promote weight loss along with other lasting health benefits. With a focus on education, the McDougall plan emphasizes nutrition, exercise, and disease prevention. And, according to its founder, successful participants can do everything from lowering their blood pressure, cholesterol, and blood sugar to rebalancing their hormones and reducing their risk of future health problems. Under his close supervision, McDougall says patients have been able to safely reduce or discontinue

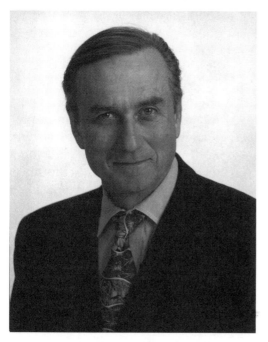

Dr. John McDougall developed the McDougall Program in the Napa Valley area of California. His regimen is based on a low-fat vegan diet that comprises 80 percent complex carbohydrates, is low in calories, and contains no cholesterol. McDougall is an internist and author who has written a number of books to support his belief in better health through vegetarian cuisine. (The McDougall Wellness Center)

their medications for such illnesses as high blood pressure, diabetes, arthritis, and stomach pain, and to avoid what he calls unnecessary surgeries.

McDougall personally cares for all participants during the ten-day, live-in program, which features a complete medical evaluation and health assessment. The personalized program of diet and exercise includes a low-fat, vegan diet made up of 80 percent complex carbohydrates along with activities like walking and swimming. And, according to McDougall, most overweight people who follow his plan lose 6 to 15 pounds of fat a month while eating as much as they want of approved complex-carbohydrate foods. His weight-loss program is also available through his best-selling books, *The McDougall Plan* (1983), *The McDougall Program: 12 Days to Dynamic Health* (1990), and *The McDougall Program for Maximum Weight Loss* (1994).

The cornerstone of the McDougall program is a diet of starchy plant foods from beans and corn to pastas, potatoes, and rice. This approved list of carbohydrate foods also includes unfamiliar grains like quinoa, bulgar, and triticale wheat; exotic fruits such as kiwi, kumquat, mango, papaya, quince, and guava; and unique vegetables like kohlrabi, jicama, aduki beans, arugula, Swiss chard, and turban squash. Typical breakfast menus might be oatmeal, seven-grain cereal, cold breakfast cereals that meet low-fat requirements, whole wheat or oil-free bagels with fruit spread, plus fresh fruit or fruit juices and herbal teas. Lunches range from pita bread stuffed with beans and vegetables, baked potato salad, pasta salad, to various soups made with beans, legumes, or grains.

Dinner selections include bean burrito casserole, Cajun rice with tossed green salad, gingered vegetable soup with seasoned potatoes, a simple pasta with meatless marinara sauce or pasta primavera with cauliflower. Dessert recipes in McDougall's book center around fruit and range from frozen fruit sorbet to easy fruit pudding or something he calls quick apple pie. Beverages consist mainly of water, herbal or iced teas, or fruit juices, and he recommends against caffeine-laden drinks like coffee or soda.

McDougall developed his diet program in response to research, which he believed proved American health problems were due in large part to our typical high-fat, animal-based diet. He said he also experienced firsthand the connection between diet and health during his early years as a doctor at a Hawaiian sugarcane plantation. In his book, McDougall wrote that he treated several generations of workers and their families, from immigrant grandparents to American, third-generation children. He discovered that the older workers were often the healthiest, living on a traditional diet of rice and vegetables, foods low in cholesterol and high in fiber. Each generation that followed became more Americanized, eating richer foods like meats, eggs, dairy products, and processed foods. According to McDougall, those children and grandchildren suffered more chronic diseases like obesity, heart disease, hypertension, and diabetes than their elders.

A graduate of Michigan State University's College of Human Medicine, McDougall performed his internship at Queen's Medical Center in Honolulu, Hawaii, and his medical residency at the University of Hawaii. But he said it was during his time as a plantation physician that he began to show an interest in the connection between diet and health. Years later McDougall and his wife, Mary, left Hawaii and returned to the mainland, where he founded the McDougall Program. First located at St. Helena Hospital in California's Napa Valley, the live-in health program is now housed at the McDougall Health Center in Santa Rosa, California. To support the importance of daily exercise, the McDougall Santa Rosa facility offers an on-site athletic club, education center, tennis courts, and a swimming pool. Supervised outings for exercise are part of the program's educational component as dieters change their lifestyles under Dr. McDougall's medical attention. While at the center, participants can also take vegetarian cooking classes or learn to master grocery shopping or din-

ing out as a vegetarian. Mary McDougall has worked closely with the program over the years, creating recipes to help participants enjoy low-fat meals. She published her own cookbook, *The New McDougall Cookbook* in 1993.

McDougall's other books include *McDougall Medicine: A Challenging Second Opinion* (1985); *The McDougall Health Supporting Cookbooks* (1985); *The McDougall Program for a Healthy Heart* (1996); and *The McDougall Program for Women: What Every Woman Needs to Know to be Healthy for Life* (1999).

For heart disease patients, McDougall's program eliminates all animal foods, even nonfat dairy products. He also limits high-fat plant foods like coconut, avocado, tofu, and nuts, and suggests that the health benefits of dietary oils, even olive oil, do not outweigh the problems they cause. McDougall's program for heart patients is similar to the low-fat, vegetarian eating plan developed by Dr. Dean Ornish. The Ornish program known as the Life Choice diet, focuses on beans, fruits, vegetables, and whole grains, and recommends that dieters get only 10 percent of their calories from fat. Studies by Ornish have shown that his diet can reverse heart disease, lower harmful LDL cholesterol, and promote weight loss. Ornish has published his studies in the *Journal of the American Medical Association,* the *Lancet,* and other major medical periodicals. Critics of both the Ornish and McDougall programs claim the low-fat requirements produce unpalatable food choices. When paired with a strict vegetarian diet, critics say both eating plans are too difficult for most people to follow.

In 2000, McDougall joined other diet doctors Robert Atkins, Barry Sears, and Dean Ornish for the USDA-sponsored Great Nutrition Debate. Agriculture Secretary Dan Glickman said the USDA sponsored the debate to sort out what the Secretary called conflicting information and claims about weight loss and diet. During the panel discussion, McDougall had harsh words for popular high-protein diets, which he said are often based on gimmicks or the mistaken belief that eating large amounts of protein foods will magically prompt weight loss.

In the McDougall newsletter, titled "The Great Debate: High Vs Low Protein Diets," McDougall also criticized the popularity of high-protein diets like The Zone and the Atkins New Diet Revolution. He said those programs are popular only because they cause a quick drop in weight. He suggested that dieters see this rapid weight loss only because stored carbohydrates contain a large amount of water, meaning anyone who switches to a low-carbohydrate diet will release these stores and experience a large initial water-weight loss. But he cautioned that if a diet is low enough in carbohydrates, like the Atkins diet, the body then goes into a condition called ketosis that dulls the appetite and causes nausea and other unpleasant and, in some cases, dangerous side effects.

McDougall said the end result of what he called "the make yourself sick diets," is only a short-term weight loss. But because Americans are desperate to lose weight, he said diets based on protein foods, like beef roasts, hams, butter-drenched lobsters, or crispy bacon, appeal to those who don't want to give up the foods they love—an example of wanting to have their steak and eat it too. McDougall joins other health organizations, including the American Dietetic Association, the American Heart Association, and the American Cancer Society, in recommending that Americans change from a diet full of animal products and saturated fat to a vegetarian diet of nutrient-rich and heart-healthy plant foods.

See also:

Atkins Nutritional Approach; Barnard, Neal; Life Choice diet; Ornish, Dean; Sears, Barry.

Additional Reading

Errico-Cox, Lisa A. "The McDougall Program for Women: What Every Woman Needs to Know to Be Healthy for Life." *Library Journal*, 124, no 1 (January 1999): 141.

Gavalas, Elaine. "The Great Diet Debate." *Better Nutrition*, May 2000, 32.

Lindley, Sarah. "Heart Smart: Natural Remedies for a Healthy Heart." *Vegetarian Times*, May 1997, 58–64.

McDougall, John. *The McDougall Plan*. New York: New Century Publishing, 1983.

———. *The McDougall Program: 12 Days to Dynamic Health*. New York: Dutton/Penguin Books, 1990.

———. *The McDougall Program for Maximum Weight Loss*. New York: Dutton/Penguin Books, 1994.

Wiley, Carol. "Dear Diary...: a Week of Weight Loss at the McDougall Program." *Vegetarian Times*, May 1990, 48–55.

Malnutrition

Malnutrition results from an improper diet. In its extreme, malnutrition can lead to starvation. Poverty is the leading cause of malnutrition, but people in wealthy and developed countries may suffer from malnutrition and undernourishment as well. People who are malnourished are generally weak and lethargic.

Specific deficiencies in a diet result in particular problems: anemia is the most common in developed countries. Anemia results from an iron deficiency. Other dietary problems are less common: night blindness can be a result of a vitamin A deficiency; rickets can be due to a lack of vitamin D or adequate sunlight; and scurvy can result from too little vitamin C in the diet.

According to the *Miller-Keane Medical Dictionary,* "Ignorance of the basic principles of nutrition is probably almost as great a cause of undernourishment as poverty. Misplaced faith in vitamin pills as a substitute for food, for example, can cause undernourishment if carried to extremes. So can overreliance on excessively processed foods."

People who severely cut back their food intake, who eat a very limited diet, or who take megadoses of vitamins to offset the reduction in food could be susceptible to malnutrition. Most commonly, however, malnutrition is a problem in countries where famine and poverty are continuing problems.

Meridia

Meridia (sibutramine hydrochloride) is a prescription drug for weight loss that acts upon the central nervous system by regulating the brain's appetite-control center. It keeps two important brain chemicals in balance, which helps to increase metabolism. It also causes a feeling of fullness and increases energy levels. Meridia is often compared with the diet drug phentermine, part of the fen-phen combination of fenfluramine and phentermine. Although there are differences in how they affect the brain, both Meridia and phentermine affect brain chemistry to give a feeling of fullness. Specifically, Meridia inhibits the reuptake of the neurotransmitters norepinephrine and serotonin while phentermine prevents the reuptake of serotonin at the same time it stimulates its release.

In 1997 the Food and Drug Administration asked manufacturers of fenfluramine and dexfenfluramine to remove them from the market after some users suffered permanent heart-valve damage and others died from a rare lung complication. Dieters taking just phentermine did not develop the heart-valve problems; those problems only occurred when phentermine was used in combination with fenfluramine.

Meridia is taken once a day and is prescribed as part of a nutritious diet and daily exercise program. As a prescription appetite suppressant, it is intended for people who are at least 25 percent overweight. Common side effects include dry mouth, constipation, and insomnia. Studies show it may also increase pulse and blood pressure in some people and those taking the drug who suffer from hypertension are advised to have their blood pressure regularly monitored by their physician. The FDA at first denied approval of Meridia based on concerns about its side effects.

However, Meridia won FDA approval in late 1997 and in early 1998 was distributed nationwide by its manufacturer, Knoll Pharmaceuticals. In its first year of distribution, Meridia saw total U.S. sales of $125 million, but those numbers dropped the following year to $102 million with the introduction of competitor Xenical. That diet medication works by blocking an enzyme needed to digest fat, which prevents about 30 percent of ingested dietary fat from being absorbed by the body. Side effects associated with Xenical include bloating, flatulence, diarrhea, and incontinence.

See also:

fen-phen; Xenical.

Additional Reading

Czarnecki, Joanne, and Shelley Drozd. "Rating the Fat-Fighters." *Men's Health,* January 1999, 60.

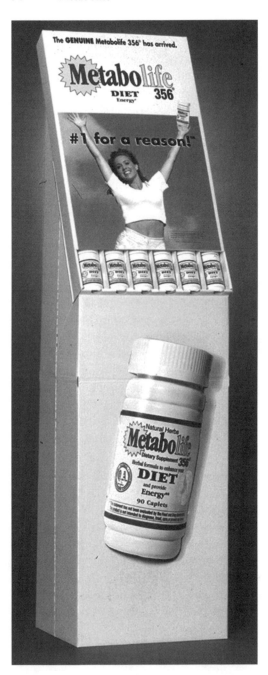

Metabolife is one of America's best-selling weight loss products. Founder Michael J. Ellis developed the herbal blend to enhance his father's energy level during cancer treatments. The formula contains the controversial herb ephedra, an ingredient FDA officials sought to limit in 1997. Metabolife and other manufacturers now market ephedra-free products. (National Archives)

Gleick, Elizabeth. "Available from a Doctor Near You." *Time International*, 25 October 1999, 65.

Shute, Nancy. "FDA Approves New Diet Drug." *U.S. News & World Report*, 8 December 1997, 38.

"Sibutramine Could Sustain Weight Loss, But Question of Safety Remains." *Obesity, Fitness & Wellness Week*, 13 January 2001, 2.

Wilhelm, Carolyn. "Growing the Market for Anti-Obesity Drugs." *Chemical Market Reporter*, 257, no. 20 (15 May 2000): 23.

Metabolife

Metabolife 356 is one of the best-selling herbal dietary supplements in America and the brainchild of San Diego businessman and former police officer Michael J. Ellis. In 2001 the ephedra-based Metabolife line of products accounted for 36 percent of diet pill sales in U.S. drugstores, according to a statement from Eric Larsen, vice president of sales at Metabolife International Inc., reported in the February 2002 issue of *Chain Drug Review*. But the controversy over ephedra-based products is growing along with sales. In November 2002 Metabolife International, Inc., was ordered by a federal court to pay over $4 million to four plantiffs in the first product liability case involving Metabolife 356 to go to trial. Attorneys for the company planned to appeal the decision.

Metabolife 356 was born, according to the company's Web site, metabolife.com, when Ellis developed an herbal blend to boost his ailing father's energy level. Company lore states that the formula was so successful that Joseph Ellis made his son promise to market the herbal combination so that others could reap its benefits.

The Metabolife packaging advertises its ability to raise a dieter's metabolism, cause more energetic feelings, and reduce appetite, reactions that critics attribute to the pill's controversial ingredient, ephedra. Dieters are directed to take the pills, to eat sensible meals, and to increase activity levels. Their success is measured in pounds lost, and the company Web site is filled with testimonials from satisfied customers whose weight loss ranges from 30 to over 100 pounds.

The popular Metabolife 356 is one of a shrinking number of diet supplements on the market made with ephedra, derived from the Chinese herb mahuang. Ephedra is chemically identical to ephedrine, a synthetic compound used in asthma medicine. They are amphetamine-like compounds, powerful stimulants that act on the central nervous system and the heart. They can cause rapid or irregular heartbeats, hypertension, strokes, and seizures, along with psychological side effects such as depression, nervousness, and insomnia.

Because the ephedrine in Metabolife 356 comes from the ephedra plant, Ellis can market Metabolife products as a dietary supplement rather than as a drug, thanks to the Dietary Supplement Health and Education Act of 1994. Under that act, supplements do not carry the same tough restrictions as drugs, which need Food and Drug Administration (FDA) approval for safety and efficacy before they can be sold to consumers. The 1994 law shifted the burden of proving a dietary supplement unsafe onto the regulators rather than the manufacturers.

Since early 1990, the FDA has issued numerous warnings to consumers of diet products and supplements containing ephedra, ephedrine, or mahuang. In 1997 the FDA called for strict new limits on consumption, restricting ephedra amounts to 24 mg per day. The FDA rule also forbids using ephedra or ephedrine products for more than a week or mixing them with other stimulants such as caffeine. According to the FDA, products containing ephedrine extracts have caused hundreds of illnesses, including heart attacks, seizures, strokes, and deaths.

The U.S. Drug Enforcement Administration (DEA) followed on the heels of the FDA ruling and called for tighter controls on ephedra's synthetic counterpart, ephedrine, amid concerns it was being diverted to make methamphetamine. "Meth," or methamphetamine, is a street drug known as speed or crank and is chemically very similar to ephedrine. DEA officials say new, tougher regulations are necessary to keep ephedrine out of the hands of illegal drug manufacturers.

Court documents show that Metabolife founder Ellis was convicted in 1990 on charges linking him to an illegal meth lab. His arrest and conviction were detailed in a 1999 *Washington Post* article. The story states that, following his conviction and while on probation, Ellis launched his first ephedra-based product. Called Fosslip, it contained eighteen vitamins, minerals, and herbal extracts, including caffeine and ephedra. It was designed for weight lifters but sales were disappointing. In 1995 Ellis renamed the formula Metabolife 356 and marketed it strictly as a weight-loss aid. The *Washington Post* reported that sales for the company grew from less than $2 million in 1996 to $600 million in 1998.

During an interview with *Newsweek* in 1999, Ellis conceded that ephedra can be dangerous, but he insisted that his product was safe when used as directed. Ellis and Metabolife International continue to strongly oppose any new government regulations aimed at ephedra; the company, along with other manufacturers, formed the Dietary Supplement Safety and Science Coalition to argue against FDA regulations limiting ephedra use.

Government concerns over ephedra have not slowed development of supplements containing other Chinese herbs, according to the April 2000 issue of *Environmental Nutrition,* which reported that Metabolife International plans to introduce a line of products based on simple versions of complex Chinese formulas. Called Chinac, these supplements are expected to address stress and tension, immune health, menstrual health, joint health, and digestive health. Metabolife claims the formulas are being designed in collaboration with leading Chinese experts. Critics worry about the effects of any new herbs and say there is little research available on these compounds. In addition, what little research has been published has not appeared in English.

Metabolife International also launched a new dietary supplement, 2-ounce Diet & Energy Bars, in December of 2000. The bars were recalled less than six months later when it was discovered that they contained extremely high amounts of vitamin A. Overdoses of vitamin A can cause liver damage, bone and cartilage abnormalities, increased pressure in the brain, and birth defects. Company officials voluntarily recalled the oatmeal-raisin, peanut, chocolate, and lemon bars when their quality assurance audit uncovered the problem. The bars contained over 32,000 International Units of the vitamin; the U.S. Department of Agriculture–recommended daily allowance of vitamin A is 5,000 IU. Metabolife officials said no illnesses have been associated with the bars.

See also:

Dietary Supplement Health and Education Act (DSHEA); ephedra/ephedrine; vitamins.

Additional Reading

Babcock, Charles R. "Stimulant Propels Diet Empire: Herbal Coalition Fights FDA's Proposed Safety Regulation." *Washington Post,* 24 May 1999, A1.

"Be Wary of Chinese Herbs, American-Style." *Environmental Nutrition,* April 2000, 8.

Cowley, Geoffrey, and Jamie Reno. "Mad About Metabolife: Some Call It a Dieter's Dream; Others Say It's a Health Hazard. But Americans Can't Get Enough of This Herbal Weight-Loss Remedy." *Newsweek,* 4 October 1999, 52–53.

Gugliotta, Guy. "A Neutral Comment, a Company's Tough Reaction." *Washington Post,* 23 July 2000, A16.

"No Category Is More Faddish Than Weight Loss." *Chain Drug Review,* 24, no. 4 (18 February 2002): 48.

Wallace, Phil. "Jury Decides for Plantiffs in Metabolife Product Case." *Food Chemical News* 44, no. 41 (25 November 2002): 15.

Webb, Marion. "Metabolife to Appeal Court's Defamation Ruling." *San Diego Business Journal* 20, no. 47 (22 November 1999): 4.

National Weight Control Registry

The National Weight Control Registry is a database of people who have been successful at losing large amounts of weight and being able to maintain that weight loss. It was founded in 1993 as a collaborative venture between researchers at the University of Colorado and the University of Pittsburgh. By identifying such a large group of people who have been successful at maintaining weight loss (60 percent of registrants have lost an average of 60 pounds and have kept it off for five years), researchers are able to draw some conclusions about actions and motivations.

The registry contains names of more than 2,000 people from the United States who have met the minimum criterion of having lost at least 30 pounds and having maintained that weight loss for at least one year. Registrants much be at least eighteen. It's free to register and names of registrants are kept confidential. New registrants are asked to fill out questionnaires when first enrolling and all participants are sent annual questionnaires. The Web site mentions some of the characteristics these registrants share:

"Successful weight losers report making substantial changes in eating and exercise habits to lose weight and to maintain their losses. On average, registrants' report consuming about 1400 kcal/day (24 percent calories from fat) and expending about 400 kcal/day in physical exercise. Walking is the most frequently cited physical activity....Two-thirds of these successful weight losers were overweight as children and 60 percent report a family history of obesity. About 50 percent of participants lost weight on their own without any type of formal program or help."

Additional Reading

http://www.uchsc.edu/nutrition/nwcr.htm

Nutri/System

Nutri/System is a weight-loss and weight-maintenance program that comes with its own food. Dieters choose from over 100 prepackaged meals and snacks for a daily calorie count of about 1,000. Recently, Nutri/System made the successful transition to an online weight management program called Nutrisystem.com, restructuring itself as a publicly traded Internet company. However, success has not always come easily to the company.

In 1991 Nutri/System faced nearly 200 lawsuits charging that the diet had caused gallbladder damage in users because it did not follow minimum requirements for safe weight loss as established by the American Medical Association (AMA). The AMA recommends that a person lose no more than 2 percent of his or her total body weight per week. According to the suit, plaintiffs in the Nutri/System case were losing 15 to 20 percent of total body weight within a week without medical supervision. The franchiser eventually won all of the eighteen suits that went to trial and settled hundreds more, according to a 1993 article in the *Wall Street Journal*.

The Nutri/System program is divided into two sections: weight loss, followed by weight maintenance. Participants who enroll in the program are asked to fill out a health questionnaire. No physical exam is required to begin the diet, although a doctor's permission is needed for dieters who suffer from serious conditions such as diabetes, ulcers, heart disease that limits activity, kidney disease, anorexia, and bulimia.

In the first phase, dieters eat Nutri/System foods seven days a week and supplement their prepackaged meals with fresh fruits, vegetables, and skim milk. The time spent in the weight loss portion depends on individual goal weights. The company estimates that dieters lose an average of two to two-and-a-half pounds each week. Described as a reduced-calorie diet, the plan follows a general breakdown of 60 percent carbohydrates, 20 percent protein, and 20 percent fat. Company literature suggests that this follows the U.S. Department of Agriculture (USDA) Food Guide Pyramid and meets the USDA Recommended Dietary Allowance standards for nutrients.

A sample 1,200-calorie meal plan begins with one Nutri/System breakfast entrée such as apple cinnamon oatmeal or frosted oats cereal, along with a Nutri/System milk alternative or 8 ounces of fat-free milk or yogurt. The morning snack is a prepackaged milk alternative or fat-free milk or yogurt. Lunch includes one Nutri/System lunch entrée, a piece of fruit, salad, and the company's fat-free salad dressing. Lunch choices range from black beans and rice to chicken cacciatore to pasta salad with ham. One piece of fruit serves as a late afternoon snack. Dinner is one prepackaged dinner entrée of beef teriyaki with rice, fish fillets, beef stew or Mexican-style chicken with rice, two regular vegetable servings or one starchy vegetable serving, along with one teaspoon of margarine or oil and a prepackaged skim milk alternative or 8 ounces of fat-free milk or yogurt followed by a prepackaged serving of dessert, chocolate chip cookies, fudge brownies, or lemon crisps.

The maintenance section lasts one year, during which dieters eat Nutri/System foods two days a week but choose regular foods the other five days to learn how to maintain their weight loss. Nutri/System's meals are not required purchases, unlike the Jenny Craig program. Yet many clients of the company say the prepackaged meals make a huge difference in their success at following the menu plans and at losing weight. Still, dieting experts criticize the meals as a crutch that can lead to long-term problems because they fail to teach dieters about food preparation or selection. Satisfied dieters, on the other hand, call the prepackaged meals convenient and say they are helpful in controlling portion size. Still, health professionals all agree that learning proper food selection and developing healthy eating habits are both important to long-term success. Including the initial fee, the purchase of food during weight loss as well as during maintenance, the cost of losing 30 pounds and keeping it off for one year could add up to $2,000.

Incorporated in 1972 and taken public in 1981, Nutri/System was developed by Harold Katz, a Philadelphia native who got the idea for the program from his mother after she had tried every kind of diet from pills to low-calorie foods to behavioral counseling. Katz put together a program geared for the individual, a departure from other early diet programs like Weight Watchers that worked with groups. The concept was immediately successful.

But a leveraged buyout in 1986 that brought heavy debt, along with a series of lawsuits from dieters and a class-action suit by shareholders, created difficulties for the company. Finally, in 1993, debt forced Nutri/System, Inc., to file for Chapter 11 bankruptcy and to close its headquarters, shut down some 300 company-owned clinics, and discontinue support to over 800 franchised centers. Jenny Craig centers seized the opportunity to gain customers and released a series of advertisements to enroll Nutri/System clients at "no additional service fee," according to a 1993 *Time* magazine article. Weight Watchers representatives also sought to sign disgruntled Nutri/System dieters while Nutri/System centers were closed.

Just five years earlier in 1988 the *New York Times* reported that Nutri/System had earned $230 million; Weight Watchers was the nation's largest weight loss program that year with earnings of $500 million, and Jenny Craig profited by $120 million. Yet, by the time the company filed for bankruptcy Nutri/System's debt was reported to be in excess of $40 million. The company emerged from bankruptcy as Nutri/System, LP, but sales remained sluggish and the company was sold in 1997 to Complete Wellness Centers.

Shortly before the 1997 sale, Nutri/System faced another public relations problem. The Food and Drug Administration (FDA) withdrew a drug called phentermine from the market in 1997 after dieters suffered permanent heart-valve damage and others died from a rare lung complication. Those problems were thought to occur when phentermine was used together with fenfluramine, a combination known as fen-phen. Nutri/System centers had been dispensing fen-phen to dieters, and immediately stopped just before the FDA withdrawal of fenfluramine. The centers turned instead to Prozac, and created something called the NutriRx phen-Pro program.

But that drug combination drew strong criticism from the Eli-Lilly Company, makers of Prozac. The conflict arose after Nutri/System centers began marketing the Prozac and phentermine combination. Nutri/System officials claimed the two drugs together were a clinically tested prescription medication that helped control hunger. However Lilly officials released a statement saying that the company did not "in any way, market or endorse the use of Prozac in combination with phentermine as an obesity or weight control medication." According to a story in the 1997 *Philadelphia Business Journal,* Lilly's action followed a statement by the Nutri/System vice president for scientific affairs who said the combination appeared to be an effective and safe drug regimen to help people lose weight.

In an effort to get products to customers after the 1997 sale and closing of its many centers, the company began taking orders over the phone and shipping directly to dieters. From there it developed the logistics to take orders over the Internet and Nutrisystem.com was launched in 1999. The online company now offers counseling via private chat rooms where dieters can talk to Nutri/System employees as well as registered dietitians at the company's headquarters in Horsham, Pennsylvania. The online counseling and informational resources are a computer version of its earlier weekly meetings, when nutrition specialists met with dieters to guide them through the program. Company officials say the Internet also provides privacy the centers did not, which has resulted in increased sales to men who may have been too self-conscious to go to the weight-loss centers. Other recent advertising strategies include a 2001 agreement signed with QVC, giving it exclusive rights to promote Nutri/System's weight-loss products on its television programs in the United States.

Earlier advertising practices were not always successful for Nutri/System. The Federal Trade Commission (FTC) cited Nutri/System, along with Jenny Craig and several other diet firms in 1993, for false advertising after investigators asserted the programs made misleading claims about weight loss and weight-loss maintenance. Nutri/System and the other companies eventually signed agreements with the FTC to stop the ads and to gather and offer scientific data as proof that customers were able to lose the desired pounds in a set amount of time, then keep it off for a specified time with no extra cost for dieters.

Today the Web site makes no mention of how many dieters experience long-term success, but a 1990 article in *Prevention* magazine quoted Nutri/System claims that over 90 percent of clients who comply with the diet, maintain their weight loss for at least a year. Still, critics complain that whether prepackaged food is sold from centers or via the Internet, it still gives short shrift to developing the patterns of eating and exercise that experts say are crucial in keeping weight off.

See also:

Jenny Craig; fen-phen; Food Guide Pyramid; Weight Watchers.

Additional Reading

Davis, Riccardo A. "Weight of One Lawsuit Off, Nutri/System Gains Another." *Philadelphia Business Journal*, 10, no. 28 (16 September 1991): 12.

Donahue, Peggy Jo. "Inside America's Hottest Diet Programs." *Prevention*, February 1990, 55.

Farhi, Paul. "Three Diet Firms Agree to Stop Disputed Ads." *Washington Post*, 30 September 1993, D11.

"Feeding Frenzy." *Time*, 17 May 1993, 21–22.

Goldman, Kevin. "Ads Dished Up for Nutri/System Dieters." *Wall Street Journal*, 7 May 1993, B8.

Janofsky, Michael. "Nutri/System's Shrinking May Put Jenny Craig on a Gravy Train." *New York Times*, 28 May, 1993, D4.

Key, Peter. "Nutrisystem.com Looks to Fatten Up." *Philadelphia Business Journal*, 19, no. 9 (7 April 2000): 3.

Rosenberg, Hilary. "Nutri/System after the fall." *Financial World*, 15 August 1983, 38–40.

Waters, Craig. "Slim Pickings, Harold Katz and Nutri-System Inc." *INC.*, May 1985, 94–100.

Nutrition Facts Label

Since the government passed the National Label Education Act in 1990, packaged foods in the United States are required to have a Nutrition Facts label on them. These labels provide information on certain nutrients and are one of the best sources of understanding the quality of your diet. The labels must contain information about calories, fat, carbohydrates, fiber, sodium, cholesterol, and vitamin and mineral content of the food. The labels may contain more information—such as breaking down the fat counts to polyunsaturated fat and monounsaturated fat. They may also list essential vitamins and minerals beyond the required ones. Here's what you can learn from a Nutrition Facts label:

Calories

A calorie is a measurement of heat needed to raise 1 kilogram of water 1 degree Centigrade. Since food "stokes the furnace" of our bodies, foods have assigned calorie values. Fat and alcohol are high in calories. Foods high in both sugars and fat contain many calories but often are low in vitamins, minerals, or fiber. There are numerous calorie counters readily available—online and often in cookbooks. If you reduce your caloric intake, you'll lose weight. If you increase the amount of calories you consume, you'll gain weight. But that doesn't mean that a low-calorie diet is the best way to lose weight. That's how those awful grapefruit and black-coffee diets originated. Sure, if you starve yourself for a week, you'll lose weight. But if you return to your old eating habits, you'll put the weight right back on again. A pound equals 3,500 calories. So to lose a pound in, say a week, you'll either have to eat 3,500 calories less or burn off 3,500 calories in exercise or some combination of the two.

Exercise burns calories. For example, walking briskly can burn off about 100 calories per mile. Bicycling for a half hour at nearly 10 mph will burn about 195 calories. The specific number depends on the person's weight and the intensity of the activity. A variety of interactive exercise counters, available on the Internet, allow you to plug in your weight, age, and change variables such as the length of time and intensity of the activity.

The following formula will help you determine the approximate number of calories you need per day to maintain your body weight. Moderately active males should multiply their weight in pounds by 15. For example, if you weigh 170 pounds, you need about 2,500 calories per day. Moderately active females should multiply their weight by 12. A 130-pound female needs about 1,560 calories per day. However, the number of calories needed per day decreases as the level of activity does. Relatively inactive men should multiply their weight by 13 pounds and women in that category should multiply their weigh by 10. So that 170-pound man who is relatively inactive needs only 2,210 calories and the 130-pound inactive woman needs only 1,300 calories to maintain body weight.

The information on nutrition labels is based on a 2,000-calorie-per-day diet. Keep that in mind if the caloric intake you need to maintain your weight is significantly higher or lower.

Calories from Fat

Numerous health and government authorities, including the U.S. Surgeon General, the National Academy of Sciences, the American Heart Association, and the American Dietetic Association, recommend reducing dietary fat to 30 percent or less of total calories. However, that doesn't mean you have to pass by all high-fat food products. For example, peanut butter with sugar added has 190 calories in a 2-tablespoon serving. Of those, 130 calories are from fat—68 percent. Add that peanut butter to two slices of whole-wheat bread, which have 120 calories and 20 calories from fat and the equation is different: now the fat is down to about 48 percent. It's still higher

than the recommendation, but by adding a glass of skim milk and an apple, you start to bring it down a healthy level.

Total Fat

This is measured in grams. For someone eating a 2,000-calorie-per-day diet, daily fat intake should not exceed 65 grams. Fatty foods are always high in calories. Despite its bad image, though, fat isn't all bad. Some fat is needed because fats supply energy and help the body absorb fat-soluble vitamins A, D, E, and K. Fats contain both saturated and unsaturated fatty acids. Saturated fat raises blood cholesterol more than other forms of fat. Limiting saturated fats to less than 10 percent of calories will help lower your blood cholesterol level. High levels of saturated fats and cholesterol in the diet are linked to increased blood cholesterol levels and a greater risk for heart disease.

While polyunsaturated and monounsaturated fats could help lower blood cholesterol levels, the recommendation still holds that total fat account for no more than 30 percent of daily calorie intake.

Cholesterol

Your body makes cholesterol, but it is also obtained from food. Animal products, such as egg yolks, higher-fat milk products, poultry, fish, and meat are high in cholesterol—and usually also in saturated fats. The daily value for cholesterol should be 300 milligrams. There are two kinds of cholesterol: LDL, the so-called "bad cholesterol" and HDL, or "good cholesterol." LDL stands for low-density lipoproteins. If there's too much LDL cholesterol in the bloodstream, it can build up within the walls of the arteries and contribute to the formation of plaque, which can ultimately clog the arteries. That blockage could affect the flow of blood to the heart, and cause a heart attack, or to the brain, and result in a stroke. Doctors can measure the level of LDL in the blood—ideally it should be below 130.

High-density lipoproteins (HDL) is the "good" cholesterol because experts believe HDLs can carry cholesterol away from the arteries and to the liver, where it's passed from the body. HDL levels typically range from 40 to 50 milligrams/dL for men and 50 to 60 milligrams/dL for women. Levels below 35 milligrams/dL are abnormally low and a risk factor for cardiac problems. Low HDL levels can be caused by cigarette smoking, obesity, and physical inactivity.

Sodium

Sodium is a trace mineral that helps maintain body fluid balance. Salt is an excellent source of sodium. One-quarter teaspoon, the typical serving, provides 540 milligrams of sodium, or 25 percent of the daily recommended allowance. Milk and processed foods are other sources. Sodium intake should stay below 2,400 milligrams. That might sound like a lot, but realize how quickly these sources add up. A frozen turkey pot pie, single serving, contains about 29 percent of the recommended daily intake. Hot dogs typically have at least 21 percent of the daily total of sodium per hot dog. Even a tablespoon of ketchup has 190 milligrams of sodium or 8 percent of the daily value. Lower sodium intake could help people avoid or control high blood pressure—a risk factor in heart disease and strokes. If you eat many processed, packaged foods and are exceeding the sodium intake, start looking for ways to duplicate the foods you like while cooking them fresh. Many herbs and spices have no sodium and can add tremendous flavor to foods. These include garlic, basil, pepper, parsley, chives, vinegar, sage, cinnamon, nutmeg, and cloves.

Total Carbohydrates

Carbohydrates provide energy for the brain, central nervous system, and muscle cells. They are found largely in sugars, fruits, vegetables, and cereals and grains. Meats generally have no carbohydrates. There are simple carbohydrates, such as sugars, and complex carbohydrates, such as breads and pastas, that the body breaks down into sugars. Someone with a 2,000-calorie-per-day diet should limit carbohydrates to 300 grams. Someone with a 2,500-calorie-per-day diet can consume up to 375 grams of carbohydrates. A medium baked potato with skin has 51 grams of carbohydrates. An apple has about 21 grams of carbohydrates, a tablespoon of sugar has 12 grams and a slice of pie can pack 60 or more grams of carbohydrates.

Carbohydrates are divided into three kinds: monosaccharides or simple sugars, such as glucose and fructose; disaccharides—composed of two monosaccharides—such as maltose, sucrose and lactose; and polysaccharides which are starches and glycogen.

On the Nutrition Facts label, total carbohydrates are broken down into two categories: fiber and sugar.

Dietary Fiber

Fiber helps the body digest food. Soluble fiber, combined with a low-fat diet, may reduce levels of "bad cholesterol." The RDA for fiber is 25 grams. Generally, grains, such as oat, wheat, and rice products are good sources of fiber, as are some vegetables. But some foods that might seem as though they would be high in fiber, such as cereals, in fact have very little. High-sugar cereals often have just 1 gram of fiber; a high-fiber hot wheat cereal could have 5 and a 100 percent bran cereal could have up to 8 grams or more. Some fruits, such as an apple (3.5 grams), a banana (2.4 grams), three prunes (3 grams), and a half grapefruit (3.1 grams) also have high fiber content.

Sugar

Sugars in foods are the monosaccharides and disaccharides described above. In some foods, carbohydrate makeup is almost entirely sugar. For example, a tablespoon of fruit preserves, sweetened only with fruit juices, derives 9 of its 10 grams of carbohydrates from sugar. Breads and pastas, on the other hand, have much high polysaccharide contents. One pita bread pocket, for example, has 2 grams of sugar out of its 24 grams of total carbohydrates. Looking at the Nutrition Facts label becomes especially important if you're seeking to cut down on the simple sugars. Take breakfast cereals, for example. Let's look at two boxes of General Mills cereal designed to appeal to children. One is Kix; the other Apple Cinnamon Cheerios. Both have 120 calories per serving and similar carbohydrate totals. But of the 25 carbohydrate grams in Apple Cinnamon Cheerios, 13 are sugar and 11 are "other," and there's 1 gram of dietary fiber. Of the 26 carbohydrate grams in Kix, only 3 are sugar and 22 are "other." There's also 1 gram of dietary fiber there.

Protein

Protein is actually a combination of twenty-two amino acids. Your body makes thirteen of these amino acids on its own. These are called nonessential amino acids. But nine of the amino acids—essential amino acids—must come from the foods you eat. Protein builds up and maintains the tissues in your body. Protein comprises much of your muscles, your organs, even some hormones. Protein also makes hemoglobin, the part of the red blood cells that carries oxygen around the body. Protein also makes antibodies to help fight off infections and disease. Protein is found in meat, chicken, fish, eggs and nuts, dairy products, and legumes.

Vitamins and Minerals

These are expressed on Nutrition Facts labels as the percentage the Recommended Dietary Allowance (RDA). If you're eating a varied diet most days, and not severely limiting your calories, chances are good that you do not need additional vitamin or mineral supplements.

Some foods are enriched with additional nutrients. For example, enriched flour and bread contain added thiamine, riboflavin, niacin, and iron; skim milk, low-fat milk, and margarine are usually enriched with vitamin A; and milk is usually enriched with vitamins A and D. The ingredient list on packaging will let you know which nutrients are in the food. In a nutshell, vitamin A is found in fruits and dark-green and deep-yellow vegetables, such as carrots, pumpkins, and spinach. Vitamin A is important to your vision and healthy skin. Vitamin B actually refers to a group of vitamins—B^1, B^2, B^6, B^{12}, niacin, folic acid, biotin, and pantothenic acid. These vitamins play a role in making red blood cells, which carry oxygen to all the parts of your body. In other words, the B vitamins help with energy. Fish, beef, pork, chicken, whole-wheat grains, green leafy vegetables, dried beans, and enriched breads and cereals are sources of vitamin B. Vitamin C strengthens bones and muscles and also has some infection-fighting capabilities. However, large doses can result in kidney problems. Good natural sources of vitamin C are citrus fruits, strawberries, melons, sweet potatoes, cabbage, broccoli, tomatoes, and peppers. Vitamin D contributes to strong healthy bones and teeth and it also helps the body absorb calcium. You can get vitamin D through fortified milk products, egg yolks, and fish. Another great source for vitamin D is sunshine. Vitamin E helps form red blood cells, muscles, and other tissues throughout the body. Vitamin E also helps your body store vitamin A. It's found in vegetable oils and dark-green leafy vegetables, nuts, poultry and seafood, and wheat germ and fortified cereals. Vitamin K is essential for blood clotting. It's also found in dark-green vegetables, whole grains, potatoes and cabbage, and cheese.

Calcium

Calcium warrants special attention because new research is pointing to an even more crucial role than previously thought and because calcium requirements are highest for young people whose bones are developing. Calcium is used in building bone mass and also plays a role in the proper functioning of the heart, muscles, and nerves maintaining blood flow. Adequate calcium can also reduce the risk of osteoporosis, a weakening of the bones that can occur late in adulthood. Calcium is found naturally in dairy products and in dark, green leafy vegetables.

Iron

Iron is a trace mineral found in red meat, liver, fish, green leafy vegetables, enriched bread, and some dried fruits such as prunes, apricots, and raisins. Recommended iron intake for young women is 15 milligrams per day; for boys aged 15 to 18, it's 12 milligrams per day, decreasing to 10 milligrams per day after age 19. The level of iron required for women stays the same until menopause. Blood loss, such as menstrual cycles, is a major cause of iron deficiency. Low iron levels can result in iron-deficiency anemia. Iron supplements can be taken, and you can eat more foods that are higher in iron content. Vitamin C can help iron absorption, while coffee, tea, wheat bran, eggs, and soy inhibit iron absorption. Medications such as antacids, for example, can also interfere with iron absorption.

Iron demands are typically highest for pregnant women. The requirement for iron doubles in the second trimester and triples in the third as blood volume increases and the fetus grows dramatically.

Obesity

Obesity is defined as having a body mass index (BMI) of over 30. Roughly, it's being about 30 pounds overweight. The obesity rate in the United States in 2000 was 19.8 percent. The obesity rate in the United States showed an alarming 61 percent increase in the preceding decade, from 12 percent in 1991.

According to a massive study released by the American Cancer Society (ACS) in April 2003, obesity is second only to smoking as the main cause of cancer. Thus, researchers say that according to their results, weighing too much is second only to smoking as a preventable cause of cancer.

The ACS team studied more than 90,000 people nationwide for sixteen years to provide what they are calling a definitive understanding of the role of obesity in causing cancer. The results show that being overweight increases the risk of virtually every form of cancer and the more overweight, the greater the risk. The study relied on the body mass index using heights and weights reported by study participants. Brain, bladder, and skin cancers were among the very few cancers that were not found to be related to excess weight.

In addition to the obesity rate, more than half the U.S. population is overweight. Being overweight is defined as being more than 10 to 20 percent over one's ideal weight. And 27 percent of Americans did not participate in any physical activity during the 1990s, according to the Centers for Disease Control and Prevention (CDC).

In order to control the obesity epidemic, the CDC suggested the following in a 2001 press release: health care providers must counsel their obese patients; workplaces should offer healthy food choices in their cafeterias and provide opportunities for employees to be physically active on site; schools should offer more physical education that encourages lifelong physical activity; urban policy makers should provide more sidewalks, bike paths, and other alternatives to cars; and parents should reduce their children's TV and computer time and encourage outdoor play. In addition to

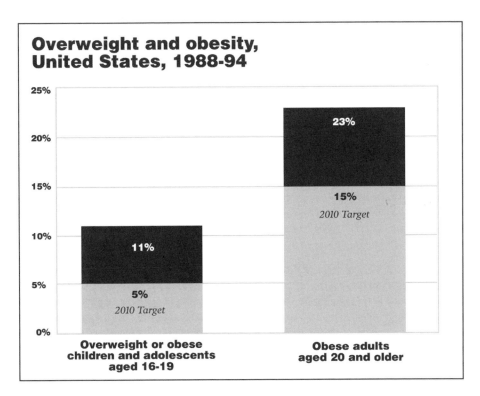

Figure 3 Overweight and Obesity, United States, 1988–94
Source: Healthy People 2010, U.S. Department of Health and Human Services.

proper nutrition, it is important to restore physical activity to daily routines to promote health. Just 30 minutes each day of moderate physical activity improves health.

Obesity is a contributing factor to chronic conditions, including heart disease, high blood pressure, and Type 2 diabetes. The number of Americans who have Type 2 diabetes increased from 4.9 percent of the population in 1991 to more than 7 percent in 2000. In 1997, the health-care costs associated with diabetes were $98 billion.

The government's Healthy People 2010 initiative calls for reducing the percentage of obese adults and children. During 1988 to 1994, 11 percent of children and adolescents (6- to 19-year-olds) were overweight or obese. Twenty-three percent of adults were considered obese. The target rates for 2010 are to get those obesity rates down to 5 percent for children and adolescents and down to 15 percent for adults.

The Healthy People 2010 report notes, "More than half of adults in the United States are estimated to be overweight or obese. The proportion of adolescents from poor households who are overweight or obese is twice that of adolescents from middle- and high-income households. Obesity is especially prevalent among women with lower incomes and is more common among African American and Mexican American women than among white women. Among African Americans, the proportion of women who are obese is 80 percent higher than the proportion of men who are obese. This gender difference also is seen among Mexican American women and men, but the percentage of white, non-Hispanic women and men who are obese is about the same."

Total costs related to obesity, calculated by direct medical costs and lost productivity, totaled an estimated $99 billion in 1995.

See also:

body mass index; childhood obesity; Healthy People 2010.

Obesity Surgery

Obesity surgery, also called bariatric surgery, is the last resort for severely obese people who have tried weight loss and exercise programs and have repeatedly failed. The different procedures include gastric-bypass surgery, the lap band procedure, vertical banded gastroplasty, and jejuoileal bypass. The theory behind all types of obesity surgery is simple: if the volume the stomach holds can be reduced, bypassed, or shortened, people will not be able to consume or, in some cases, to absorb as many calories. With obesity surgery the volume of food the stomach can hold is typically reduced from about four cups to about a half a cup. But these procedures are not a magic solution. There is a long-term failure rate of up to 50 percent, additional surgery is necessary in some cases, and many patients face daily complications like intolerance to foods high in fats, lactose intolerance, vomiting, diarrhea, and intestinal discomfort.

Gastric-bypass surgery, developed in the 1960s, is a procedure where surgeons sew the stomach shut to a fraction of its original size, then reattach that portion directly to the small intestine, limiting room for food and time for absorption. Patients must be carefully screened physically and psychologically for the operation, which is suggested only for people with 100 or more pounds to lose, and always as a last resort. The operation can be risky; stomach perforations, infection, allergic reaction to anesthesia, or excessive bleeding or blood clots in the lungs, and heart attacks are among the serious or even fatal complications. And because the surgery can affect absorption in the intestine, all gastric-bypass patients have to take vitamins for the rest of their lives.

After the procedure patients need to follow a lifelong diet, exercise, and behavior modification program, keeping in mind how important their food choices are now that they can literally fill up on a single piece of bread. Once patients return to eating solid food, poor choices leave them without necessary nutrients and can even make them physically ill. Foods to avoid include carbonated beverages, popcorn, nuts, fried foods, red meat, and sugar, meaning no pie, cookies, or cake. Still, some surgery patients experience a 10- to 20-pound weight gain once the new stomach stretches a bit, while others who do not adopt the necessary lifestyle and dietary changes find themselves returning to their preoperation weight.

The American Society of Bariatric Surgery (ASBS) reports that up to five patients in 1,000 die from gastric-bypass surgery. On the other hand, complications from obesity, such as diabetes, high blood pressure, and arthritis cost consumers millions of dollars in related health-care costs each year. Still, many health insurance companies do not cover the cost of the operation, which can range from $20,000 to $25,000. Figures from the National Institutes of Health say that almost 90 percent of dieters who use other methods regain the weight they lost within five years. But a 1995 study cited by the Gainesville, Florida-based chapter of the ASBS reported that fourteen years after the surgery most bypass patients

have managed to keep off more than 50 percent of their original weight loss, over 100 pounds in most cases.

The success rate for the surgery may be one reason the number of gastric-bypass operations performed in the past several years has jumped by as much as 25 percent. But this increased popularity can also be attributed to publicized surgeries like the operation on Carnie Wilson, daughter of the Beach Boys' Brian Wilson and a member of the singing group Wilson Phillips. Wilson was morbidly obese and after trying and failing at all sorts of diets, she dropped 150 pounds and almost twenty dress sizes following gastric-bypass surgery in August 1999. She even had the procedure broadcast live on the Internet as a way to educate people about the reality of morbid obesity.

The less invasive lap band procedure (short for laparoscopic adjustable gastric band), approved in June 2001 by the Food and Drug Administration, is intended for people with smaller weight loss requirements and involves the surgeon wrapping a band around the top part of the stomach to restrict how much food it can hold. The procedure is cheaper and faster than gastric-bypass surgery, and requires a shorter hospital stay. Lap band surgery takes less than an hour and requires an overnight stay, compared to the more extensive bypass surgery that lasts two to three hours and requires a three-day hospital recuperation. The adjustable silicon band with a balloon at the end, used in the lap band procedure, can be adjusted or even removed if the patient experiences serious side effects, a reversal not possible with the gastric-bypass procedure.

Other obesity surgery procedures include vertical banded gastroplasty, where an artificial pouch is created using staples in a different section of the stomach. Plastic mesh is sutured into part of the pouch to prevent it from dilating. In this surgery, like the gastric-bypass operation, the food enters the small intestine farther along than it would enter normally, reducing the time available for absorption of nutrients and calories. Jejuoileal bypass, now rarely performed, involves shortening the small intestine. This procedure has a high occurrence of serious complications, such as chronic diarrhea and liver disease, and is thought to be the least effective of any of the procedures. It is rarely performed now and has been replaced by safer procedures.

Following obesity surgery, most patients are restricted to a liquid diet for up to three weeks. Patients then graduate to a diet of puréed food for about a month or two until they can tolerate solid food. High-fat food is especially hard to digest and causes diarrhea. Patients must also be careful not to eat too quickly or to ingest too much food or they can experience nausea, vomiting, and intestinal "dumping," when undigested food is shunted too quickly into the small intestine, causing pain, diarrhea, and dizziness.

Meanwhile, researchers continue to study the complex system of brain and body chemicals that govern weight and appetite. Exciting new studies on the growth hormone ghrelin have some scientists suggesting that an effective weight loss drug is closer than ever before. The development and use of obesity drugs came under close scrutiny in 1997 when the FDA ordered the withdrawal of the drug combination fen-phen when it was discovered to have dangerous effects on the heart. Still, doctors say it may be a long time before obesity surgery becomes obsolete and at this time it remains the best option for some patients who have tried everything else and failed.

See also:

fen-phen; ghrelin.

Additional Reading

Abouzeid, Nehme E. "Insane Growth in Inquiries About Surgeries for Obesity." *Boston Business Journal,* 21, no. 39 (2 November 2001): 39–40.
Crawford, Dan, and Jeff Bell. "This Lap Band is No Opening Act at Polaris." *Business First-Columbus,* 17, no. 48 (20 July 2001): A3.
Davidson, Tish. "Obesity Surgery." In *Gale Encyclopedia of Medicine,* ed. Jacqueline L. Longe and Deidre S. Blanchfield, 1st edition. Detroit: Gale Research, Inc., 1999: 2079–80.
Desloge, Rich. "Appetite for Thinness." *St. Louis Business Journal,* 21, no. 46 (20 July 2001): 8.
Haire, Pat. "Extreme Measures: Gastric-Bypass Surgery Is the Last Resort of the Overweight, but Iris Starr Says the Results More Than Justify the Risks." *Sarasota Magazine,* November 2001, 211–16.
Lemonick, Michael D. "Lean and Hungrier: Is a Recently Discovered Hormone the Reason Why Folks Who Lose Weight Can't Keep It Off?" *Time,* 3 June 2002, 54.

Ohsawa, George

George Ohsawa (b. October 18, 1893, in Kyoto, Japan; d. April 23, 1966, in Tokyo, Japan) is credited with introducing macrobiotics to the West. He was born Yukikazu Sakurazawa to Magotaro and Setsuko Sakurazawa. As a young man he attended a commercial high school to prepare for a career in business, a placement that exposed him to Western culture and opened his thinking to Western ideas.

At age 18 Sakurazawa was diagnosed with tuberculosis, a fatal disease at that time. During his illness he turned to the writings of Sagen Ishizuka. A Japanese

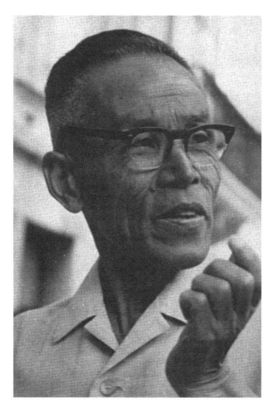

George Ohsawa introduced macrobiotics to the Western world with the publication of his book *Zen Macrobiotics* in 1965. A macrobiotic diet is believed by followers to create health by balancing the yin and yang of food. Ohsawa devoted his life to lecturing around the world and to writing on the macrobiotic philosophy and its application. He died of a heart attack in Tokyo in 1966 at age seventy-three. (George Ohsawa Macrobiotic Foundation, Inc.)

army doctor, Ishizuka had established his theory of nutrition and medicine based on the traditional Asian diet, which he tied to the Western medical sciences of chemistry, biology, and physiology. Ishizuka's diet theories were published in two books, *Chemical Theory of Longevity,* in 1896, and *Diet for Health,* in 1898.

Sakurazawa responded well to Ishizuka's diet and regained his health. He then went on to become president of the Shoku-Yo-Kai, an association founded by Ishizuka before his death in 1910. In the years that followed, Sakurazawa became a prolific author, devoting his life to writing about the teachings of Ishizuka and lecturing around the world. He also began to develop his own ideas that expanded on Ishizuka's earlier work by incorporating the concepts of yin and yang into his twelve principles of macrobiotics. Yin and yang represent the two basic universal tendencies in Asian philosophy. According to Ishizuka, health problems were caused by the imbalance of yin and yang. Ohsawa carried this connection further when he linked yin with potassium and yang with sodium.

After World War II Sakurazawa, to further his work in the West, changed his name to George Ohsawa and officially named his philosophy *macrobiotics*, or "all-embracing life." After years of world travel, he and his wife Lima Ohsawa, moved to New York in 1959 to join Michio Kushi and a small group of followers. Kushi, a teacher and founder of the East West Foundation and the Kushi Institute, originally met Ohsawa through the World Federalist Movement, an American peace movement and the precursor to the United Nations. It was through this organization that Ohsawa arranged for Kushi to go to the United States, and Kushi then used that opportunity to introduce macrobiotics in North America.

During his life Ohsawa wrote more than 300 books and pamphlets in languages from Japanese and French to English and German. He also published a monthly magazine for more than forty years. Ohsawa died at the age of seventy-four in 1966. The George Ohsawa Macrobiotics Foundation, Inc., a nonprofit organization, was founded in 1961 by Kushi and

Herman Aihara, and continues to educate the general public about the principles and health benefits of a macrobiotic diet.

Macrobiotics calls for people to balance their overall intake of yin and yang foods and, by doing so, to establish a harmony within the body. Yin foods are thought to be foods like vegetables, grains, beans, and seaweed. Animals and animal products are considered yang foods. In later years, Kushi liberalized the diet by emphasizing a more relaxed approach to food, a shift away from the strict, cereal-based diet espoused by Ohsawa. Kushi also encouraged less salt or sodium in the diet. Contemporary critics say the current macrobiotic diet can improve health mostly because those who follow it stop eating refined foods, and cut back substantially on meat, milk, and other animal products. They suggest that followers improve not because of the foods they take in, but because of the foods they leave out.

Additional Reading

Kotzsch, Ronald E. *Macrobiotics: Yesterday and Today.* Tokyo: Japanese Publications, 1985.

Melton, J. Gordon, Jerome Clark, and Aidan A. Kelly. *New Age Encyclopedia.* Detroit: Gale Research Inc., 1990.

Ohsawa, George. *Zen Macrobiotics: The Art of Rejuvenation and Longevity.* Reprint. Chico, Calif.: George Ohsawa Macrobiotic Foundation, 1995.

Wells, Patricia. "Macrobiotics: A Principle, Not a Diet." *New York Times,* 19 July 1978, C1–9.

Ornish, Dean

Dr. Dean Ornish (b. July 16, 1953, in Dallas) is an innovative physician who has developed a scientifically proven system to reverse heart disease without drugs or surgery, replacing those invasive techniques

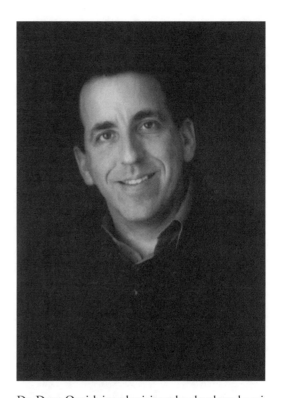

Dr. Dean Ornish is a physician who developed a scientifically proven diet plan to reverse heart disease. As director of the Preventive Medicine Research Institute in California, he has written numerous best-selling books promoting an eating plan that focuses on beans, fruits, vegetables, and whole grains, and recommends that dieters derive only 10 percent of their calories from fat. Ornish has published research findings in medical periodicals that show that his diet can slow down, stop, and even reverse heart disease. While critics claim that his diet is too severe to follow, a number of major health insurers now reimburse the cost of his program for heart patients. (Preventive Medicine Research Institute)

with a very-low-fat diet, exercise, and stress management. And unlike many diet book authors, Ornish has published research findings about his program in medical journals such as the *Journal of the American Medical Association* and the *American Journal of Cardiology.*

The doctor, whose best-selling books include *Dr. Dean Ornish's Program for Reversing Heart Disease: The Only System*

Scientifically Proven to Reverse Heart Disease without Drugs or Surgery (1990); *Eat More, Weigh Less: Dr. Dean Ornish's Life Choice Program for Losing Weight Safely While Eating* (1993); *Stress, Diet and Your Heart* (1982), first gained attention from the medical community in 1989 when he released data showing a reduction in overall heart blockages in his patients. What was unusual was that the improvement came not from the standard treatment of drugs or surgery, but instead from a high-fiber, low-fat, vegetarian diet along with stress-management techniques. Founder and president of the Preventive Medicine Research Institute of the University of California at San Francisco, Ornish champions what other cardiologists at first labeled "radical" ideas. Many in the medical establishment still continue to insist Americans will never find a soy and plant diet acceptable.

Ornish wasn't always a maverick. Growing up in Dallas, he was a straight-A student in high school. While at Rice University, he came down with a case of mononucleosis and returned to his parents' home to recuperate. There he met the Swami Satchidananda, who was staying with the Ornish family during a lecture tour. Under the swami's influence, Ornish said in a March 1987 *Discover* magazine interview that he started to practice yoga, meditate, and eat a vegetarian diet. Following his recovery, Ornish transferred from Rice to the University of Texas at Austin and graduated first in his class in 1975.

His next move was to the Baylor College of Medicine in Houston, and it was there that Ornish said he began questioning the standard treatment for heart patients. At the time, the Baylor-affiliated Texas Medical Center was a world leader in coronary-bypass operations. Yet years later Ornish told *Discover* that "having a bypass without changing your lifestyle is like trying to mop up the floor around an overflowing sink without turning off the faucet." In 1977 Ornish conducted his first medical experiment, a study titled "The Effects of Stress Management and a Low-Cholesterol Diet on Heart Disease." That study showed that after only thirty days on his plan, subjects said their chest pain was somewhat alleviated and more blood was flowing to their hearts. After graduating from Baylor, Ornish started his internship and residency at Massachusetts General Hospital, a Harvard University affiliate. By the time Ornish left Harvard in 1984 he had completed his internship and residency, conducted more original research, and published his first book, *Stress, Diet and Your Heart.*

In the summer of 1984 Ornish moved to San Francisco and established the Preventive Medicine Research Institute with Shirley E. Brown, whom he later married. The institute is based in Sausalito and is affiliated with the University of California at San Francisco, where Ornish joined the faculty as an assistant clinical professor of medicine. National recognition came in 1988 and 1989 following another Ornish study, the results of which he presented at a meeting of the American Heart Association and which eventually won him grants from the National Institutes of Health among other major research organizations.

His work continued to achieve mainstream success when the Mutual of Omaha Insurance Company in 1993 agreed to provide full reimbursement to patients enrolled in Ornish's program for reversing heart disease. In the spring of 2000 the Health Care Financing Administration announced a demonstration project involving the Ornish program as an alternative to conventional medical treatments for selected Medicare patients. Meanwhile, dozens of health insurers now reimburse the cost of Dr. Ornish's program for selected patients. Today the idea of a low-fat diet is more acceptable to mainstream cardiologists who recommend that patients make food choices based on the U.S. Department of Agriculture Food Guide Pyramid or the so-called Mediterranean diet, which is rich in fruits, vegetables, and whole grains.

Ornish admits that there is nothing new about his approach that, in fact, is similar to the low-fat food plan developed in the 1970s by the late Nathan Pritikin, the California inventor, author, and founder of the Pritikin Longevity Centers. In the late 1950s Pritikin was diagnosed with heart disease following an angina attack. Dissatisfied with the standard treatment, Pritikin began to experiment with his diet. After seeing favorable results from his regime, he wrote several books, including his best sellers, *The Pritikin Program for Diet and Exercise* (1979) and *The Pritikin Promise: 28 Days to a Longer, Healthier Life* (1983). Pritikin, like Ornish, promoted a diet filed with fresh fruits, vegetables, and whole grains, with only 10 percent of calories from fat. And like Ornish, Pritikin was also criticized by some doctors who called his diet unnecessarily severe.

Dr. John McDougall is another physician who developed a low-fat, vegetarian eating program, similar to the Ornish plan. McDougall established the St. Helena Health Center in 1987, located in California's Napa Valley. He is also the author of several best-selling diet books, including *The McDougall Plan* (1985), *The McDougall Program for Maximum Weight Loss* (1994), and *The McDougall Program for a Healthy Heart* (1996).

Ornish continues to break new ground in his research. In the 1998 book *Love and Survival: The Scientific Basis for the Healing Power of Intimacy,* he offers readers clinical and anecdotal evidence as well as research findings to support his newest theory that having deeply intimate, loving relationships can be invaluable in preventing and treating heart disease. The book classifies love broadly from the love of a mate to the love of family, friends, and God. But the overall message, along with his dedication to Molly, whom he married in 1998, remains that love and intimacy are among the most powerful factors in determining a person's health or illness.

See also:

Food Guide Pyramid; Life Choice diet; McDougall Program; Pritikin, Nathan.

Additional Reading

Brink, Susan. "The Low-Fat Life." *U.S. News & World Report,* 12 July 1999, 56.
Condor, Bob. "Lifestyle Changes Can Go Right to the Heart." *Chicago Tribune,* 13 February 2000, 3.
Cowley, Geoffrey. "Healer of Hearts." *Newsweek,* 16 March 1998, 50–57.
"Dean Ornish." *Contemporary Authors Online.* Detroit: Gale Group, 2001.
Grady, Denise. "Can Heart Disease Be Reversed?" *Discover,* March 1987, 54–66.
Perlmutter, Cathy. "Heal Your Heart With Love: America's Favorite Doctor Dean Ornish Gives Advice on Preventing Heart Attacks." *Prevention,* August 1998, 118–25.
Ornish, Dean. "Healing Broken Hearts." *Nutrition Action Healthletter,* 26, no. 5 (June 1999): 1.

Osteoporosis

Osteoporosis is a skeletal disease, in which bones lose mass and density, pores enlarge, and bones become fragile. The National Osteoporosis Foundation estimates that the disease causes some 1.5 million bone fractures each year in the United States. The disease is four times more common in women than in men due to differences in bone density. Lack of exercise and low calcium intake during childhood, adolescence, and early adulthood are all risk factors for the disease.

Overeaters Anonymous

Overeaters Anonymous (OA) is not a diet club; it doesn't advertise and there are no weigh-ins, no dues or fees, no special frozen meals, and no recipes to swap. Modeled after the Alcoholics Anonymous program, OA is an organization for people who eat compulsively. Groups meet in church basements, community rooms, private homes, anywhere they can gather to share their experiences and strength and hope for recovery from what can be a crippling addiction to food.

Overeaters Anonymous looks at compulsive overeating as a physical, emotional, and spiritual disease. OA members include an eclectic group, from those who are extremely overweight, morbidly obese, of average weight or moderately overweight, to those who are underweight or those who cannot control their compulsive eating. Symptoms that members experience are as varied as the individuals. Those symptoms include obsession with body weight, size, and shape; eating binges or grazing; preoccupation with reducing diets; starving; laxative, or diuretic abuse; excessive exercise; inducing vomiting after eating; inability to stop eating certain foods after taking the first bite; vulnerability to quick-weight-loss or fad diets; constant preoccupation with food.

While not a diet club, members often lose weight when they gain control over their overeating. Participants are treated much like recovering alcoholics; OA offers its members support in dealing with their problem one day at a time through the implementation of an eating plan under the guidance of an experienced sponsor. However, OA does not endorse, recommend, or distribute any specific diet or food plan; instead, anyone seeking nutritional guidance to lose weight is advised to talk to a doctor. Those members who don't find success in achieving their weight loss goals may still experience recovery in other parts of their lives.

The individual eating plans are as diverse as each member and each plan is based on an honest appraisal of past experiences, current individual needs, and knowledge of "trigger foods" or situations that may contribute to an episode of overeating. The sponsor, a veteran member, helps new members work out a food plan and stick with it as part of the sponsor's commitment or obligation to OA. Critics of the organization say the rigid food plans, rules for sponsorship, and other techniques for avoiding "trigger" foods may actually reinforce obsessive food behavior, which can be a problem for a compulsive overeater.

Founded in 1960, OA held its first meeting in Los Angeles, when a woman named Rozanne met with a few friends in an effort to change her life and her weight. OA is now a worldwide organization with over 8,000 groups meeting in some sixty countries and a headquarters in Rio Rancho, New Mexico. The program is based on the 12 Steps and 12 Traditions of Alcoholics Anonymous. The Traditions describe attitudes early members thought were important to group survival. Anonymity is considered by OA to be the foundation of all of the other Traditions, which include: common welfare comes first since personal recovery depends on OA unity; group leaders are trusted servants but they do not govern; God is the ultimate authority; the only requirement for membership is a desire to stop eating compulsively; each group should carry its message to any compulsive overeater still suffering from an addiction to food; every OA group should be fully self-supporting and should decline outside contributions; and the OA public relations policy must be based on attraction rather than promotion.

The 12 Steps, considered the heart of the OA recovery program, originated in Alcoholics Anonymous but were adapted for use with food addiction. Those steps include that members recognize they were powerless over food until they came to believe a greater power could restore their health. OA members are also expected to make a list of all persons they harmed and try to make amends; to take personal inventory and, when wrong, promptly admit it; pray for knowledge of God's will and also admit to God the exact nature of any wrongdoing. Members are required to ask God to remove any shortcomings and they should have a spiritual awakening as a result of the Steps. This will make it possible to carry their message to other compulsive overeaters.

Like other 12-Step groups, OA stresses that talk of spirituality has nothing to do with any structured religion. According to the OA Web site, the group "does not practice any religion in the meetings." Persons of all faiths are welcome: agnostics, Catholics, atheists, Jews, and Protestants. Recovery and spiritual growth are said to depend only upon any member's willingness to practice the principles and rules of the program on a daily basis.

While weight loss groups like Weight Watchers or TOPS have regular weigh-ins and pounds are an important part of the discussion, OA members often talk about a variety of issues, since many join as a last resort to solving emotional troubles that go far beyond coping with excess pounds. So members place their faith and trust in the group itself, which underscores why member anonymity is so important. This reassures members that anything shared with the group will be held in the strictest confidence and will not be discussed outside of the meetings. OA says another important aspect of anonymity is that all members are considered equal in the program: outside status, wealth, or social standing has no bearing.

See also:

TOPS, Take Off Pounds Sensibly; Weight Watchers.

Additional Reading

Fletcher, Anne M. "Inside America's Hottest Diet Programs." *Prevention,* May 1990, 46.

Seligman, Jean. "Helping Fight Extra Helpings: Food Junkies Are Turning to OA to Kick Their Habit." *Newsweek,* 5 December 1988, 78.

Wilson, Gail O. "Overeaters Anonymous Offers Help, Hope and Recovery." *Alcoholism & Addiction Magazine,* October 1989, 34.

Phenylpropanolamine (PPA)

Phenylpropanolamine (PPA) is an amphetamine-like substance used until recently as an appetite suppressant or as a nasal decongestant. It disrupts hunger signals to the brain and dries out the mouth, making food taste bland and unappetizing, and it also clears nasal congestion by narrowing or constricting the blood vessels. It has been the main ingredient in several weight-loss products sold over the counter, including Dexatrim and Acutrim. In November 2000 the U.S. Food and Drug Administration (FDA) issued a public health warning cautioning consumers against taking such products. The FDA also asked manufacturers of products containing PPA to voluntarily replace it with alternative active ingredients.

The FDA determined that PPA was not safe for over-the-counter use based on the results of the Hemorrhagic Stroke Project, a study conducted between 1994 and 1999 by the Yale University School of Medicine that showed an increased risk of stroke in people taking drugs containing PPA. This action was aimed at diet products and also at over-the-counter allergy and cold medications.

In response, many cold and cough recipes switched from PPA to pseudoephedrine, an ingredient already used in products like Sudafed. However, pharmacologists say there is no FDA-approved alternative to PPA for over-the-counter diet pills, only herbal ingredients which are considered dietary supplements and are not subject to FDA regulations under the Dietary Supplement Health and Education Act of 1994. Dexatrim manufacturers have withdrawn their PPA-containing product and introduced Dexatrim Natural, an herbal alternative containing ephedra. However, researcherscontinue to study the possibility that the human body may convert ephedra to PPA. In a November 2000 study published in the *New England Journal of Medicine,* researchers linked dietary supplements containing ephedra to serious side effects, including heart attacks, strokes, and seizures.

See also:

ephedra/ephedrine; Dexatrim; Dietary Supplement Health and Education Act (DSHEA); Food and Drug Administration (FDA).

Additional Reading

Brink, Susan. "Diet Drugs: What a Pill." *U.S. News & World Report,* 20 November 2000, 74.
"By the Way, Doctor—What's the Story with PPA?" *Harvard Women's Health Watch,* 8, no. 9 (May 2001).
Haller, C. A., and N. L. Benowitz. "Adverse Cardiovascular and Central Nervous System Events Associated with Dietary Supplements Containing Ephedra Alkaloids." *New England Journal of Medicine,* 343, no. 25 (21 December 2000): 1833–38

Phytochemicals

Phytochemicals are disease-fighting substances found in plant foods. These substances and antioxidants help reduce the risk of cancer, heart disease, and Alzheimer's disease. Some research suggests that phytochemicals may even slow down the aging process.

Anthocyanins are antioxidants that help control high blood pressure and protect against diabetes-related circulatory problems. The best naturally occurring sources of this phytochemical are found in black or blue fruits such as blackberries, elderberries, black currants, and purple grapes. Red fruits and vegetables are also good sources of anthocyanins. Eat red raspberries, sweet cherries, strawberries, cranberries, beets, red apples, red cabbage, red onion, and kidney beans.

Phenolics and anthocyanins also help reduce the risk of heart disease, cancer, and Alzheimer's, and may even slow down the aging process. The best naturally occurring sources of phenolics are prunes, eggplant, raisins, and plums.

Indoles help protect against breast cancer and prostate cancer. Indoles are found in broccoli, cauliflower, cabbage, and brussels sprouts.

Lutein is an antioxidant that has been connected with better eye health. Lutein helps reduce the risk of forming cataracts and macular degeneration, both of which can cause vision loss in older people. Lutein is found in green leafy vegetables.

Beta carotene is another antioxidant linked to a reduced risk of cancer and heart disease as well as giving an overall boost to the immune system. Beta carotene is found in orange vegetables, such as carrots.

Bioflavanoids work together with vitamin C to improve overall health and heart health, to reduce the risk of cancer, to strengthen bones and teeth, and to promote more rapid wound healing. Orange- and yellow-colored fruits and vegetables supply both bioflavanoids and vitamin C.

Allicin may help lower cholesterol and blood pressure as well as work as an anti-infective for the body. It's found in garlic and onions.

Lycopene helps reduce the risk of several types of cancer. It's found in watermelons, pink grapefruits, and fresh tomatoes and tomato-based products, such as spaghetti sauce and tomato juice.

Additional Reading

Fukushima, Rhoda. "The Top Ten." *St. Paul Pioneer Press,* 7 April 2002, F1.
Stieg, Bill, and Lisa Jones. "Guy-Friendly Food." *Men's Health,* June 2002, 44.
"Stronger than C." *Vegetarian Times,* May 2002, 13.
"10 Foods That Pack a Wallop: Eat, Drink and Be Healthy! Scientists Are Rapidly Identifying the Natural Chemicals That Give Preventive Punch to a Rainbow of Ordinary Edibles." *Time,* 21 January 2002, 76.

Prediabetes

Prediabetes is a condition affecting 16 million Americans who could develop Type 2 diabetes within ten years. Prediabetes diagnosis means blood glucose levels are higher than normal but not yet diabetic. A March 27, 2002, press release from the American Diabetes Association reported that Health and Human Services Secretary Tommy G. Thompson warned that people with prediabetes are at significant risk for developing Type 2 diabetes and their risk for heart disease is increased by 50 percent.

However, with changes in diet and physical activity, the onset of diabetes can be prevented. The health agency and the American Diabetes Association are calling on physicians to begin screening overweight people age fourty-fave and older for prediabetes, particularly if they have a family history of diabetes, low HDL cholesterol and high triglycerides, high blood pressure, a history of gestational diabetes or if a woman has given birth to a baby weighing more than 9 pounds, or belong to a minority group. African Americans, Native Americans, Hispanic Americans/Latinos, and Asian American/Pacific Islanders are at increased risk for Type 2 diabetes.

A clinical trial run by the HHS involving more than 3,000 people found that diet and exercise resulting in a 5 to 7 percent weight loss lowered incidence of Type 2 diabetes by 48 percent. The press release stated that participants lost weight by cutting fat and calories in their diet and by exercising (most chose walking) at least 30 minutes a day, 5 days a week.

See also:

diabetes; insulin; obesity.

Additional Reading

American Diabetes Association press release: "HHS, ADA Warn Americans of 'Pre-Diabetes,' Encourage People to Take Healthy Steps to Reduce Risks." Washington, D.C., 27 March, 2002.

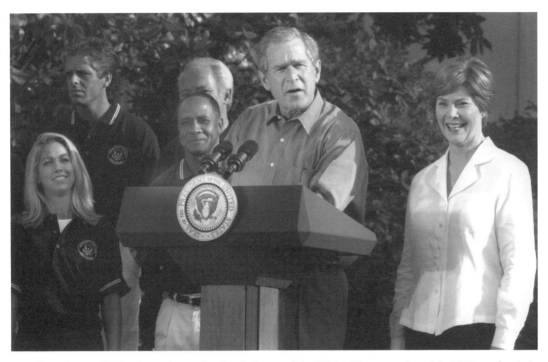

President George W. Bush speaks on the South Lawn of the White House on June 20, 2002, as first lady Laura Bush, right, looks on, prior to touring the White House fitness expo. Overseeing an exercise fair under way in the backyard of the White House, Bush said poor health weakens the nation. Standing with Bush are fitness expert Denise Austin, left, and Lynn Swann, to the President's immediate right, chairman of the President's Council on Physical Fitness and Sports. (AP/Wide World Photos)

President's Council on Physical Fitness and Sports

The President's Council on Physical Fitness and Sports (PCPFS) was founded on July 16, 1956, by President Dwight D. Eisenhower after a study showed American children were less physically fit than children in other countries. Originally named the President's Council on Youth Fitness, the agency name was changed to its current name four years later in 1960 by President John F. Kennedy to reflect an expanded mandate to serve Americans of all ages. And in 1968 President Lyndon B. Johnson added the word *sports* to the council title in a move to emphasize the importance of participation in sports. Johnson also began the tradition of pre-senting Presidential Physical Fitness Awards in 1966; the Presidential Sports Award program was created in 1972.

The PCPFS is made up of twenty members appointed by the President. Assisted by the U.S. Public Health Service, the PCPFS provides guidance to the President and to the Secretary of Health and Human Services on how to encourage more Americans to be physically active. In its efforts to educate Americans about the benefits of physical fitness, the Council develops and distributes publications and pamphlets, and works with individual citizens, civic groups, private enterprise, community organizations, and others to promote fitness for all Americans. The PCPFS encourages and supports the development of community recreation and sports programs and works with business, industry, government, and labor organizations to set up workplace physical fitness programs. The Council also works with agencies to encourage research in sports medicine, physical fitness, and sports performance.

Pritikin, Nathan

Nathan Pritikin (b. August 29, 1915, in Chicago; d. February 21, 1985, in Albany, New York) was a self-taught nutritionist and an inventor who championed the concept that a low-fat, high-fiber diet of natural foods like fruits, vegetables, and whole grains, combined with regular aerobic exercise, could prevent and treat heart disease and other diseases of affluent society. He wrote six books, including the first, *Live Longer Now* (1974) and his best-selling *Pritikin Program for Diet and Exercise* (1979). Other titles included *The Pritikin Permanent Weight-Loss Manual* (1982), *The Pritikin Promise: 28 Days to a Longer, Healthier Life* (1983), *The Official Pritikin Guide to Restaurant Eating,* co-authored with wife Ilene (1985), and *Diet for Runners* (1985). Newer titles authored by Nathan Pritikin's son Robert Pritikin include *the New Pritikin Instinct* (1998) and *the Pritikin Principle: The Calorie Density Solution* (2000). In late 1984 Nathan Pritikin was hospitalized due to complications related to cancer treatment, and, fully aware that he was deteriorating rapidly, took his own life in early 1985.

Although Pritikin received little formal education (he dropped out of the University of Chicago to work on the Nordon bombsight), he began his lifelong study of human anatomy and physiology as a youth. During World War II, Pritikin began to develop his theory concerning the causes and cures of heart disease. Scientific thinking at that time held that

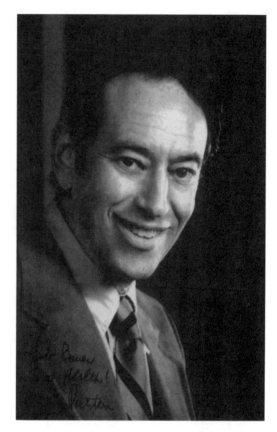

Nathan Pritikin was an inventor and self-taught nutritionist who began to advocate a low-fat diet and aerobic exercise in the 1970s. His experiences battling his own heart disease prompted him to write his best-seller *The Pritikin Program for Diet and Exercise*. Early critics argued that there were no connections between fats in the blood and the risk of heart disease, and charged that the Pritikin plan was too impractical to follow. (Pritikin Longevity Center)

heart disease was caused, in large part, by stress. Yet in looking over statistics on the civilian populations of Europe, he noticed that death rates due to heart attack had fallen during the stress-filled war years. In a 1991 interview in *Vegetarian Times,* Pritikin's son Robert said that his father had also noticed that while stress was high, rationing during the war meant people were eating very little meat and few dairy products. After the war, when rationing ended but stress subsided, Pritikin noted that the rates of heart disease went right back up.

Pritikin's years of research were put to the test in 1956 when he had his own cholesterol checked. It was over 300. He then underwent a stress electrocardiogram, which showed coronary insufficiency. A second cardiologist and second testing confirmed that Pritikin's arteries were clogging up. He was diagnosed with substantial coronary heart disease. He was forty-one years old. A prestigious team of cardiologists gave him the standard prescription of the day: stop all exercise, stop climbing stairs, take it easy, and take naps in the afternoon. But Pritikin's readings of population studies had convinced him that dangerous arterial plaque would form at any cholesterol level over 160. If he could get his cholesterol level down with dietary measures, he figured he might have a chance of surviving. By April 1958, he had become a vegetarian. He had also started running three to four miles daily. By May, his cholesterol had fallen to 162. By January 1960, his cholesterol had dropped to 120, and a new electrocardiogram showed his coronary insufficiency had disappeared.

Encouraged by the results of his diet and exercise program, Pritikin launched several research projects over the next twenty-five years that validated the efficacy of his program. But the medical establishment was at first slow to accept Pritikin's theory that heart disease could be cured through dietary changes and exercise. Groups like the American Heart Association and the American Medical Association initially dismissed his claims and criticized the diet, saying it did not show lasting benefits and it was too restrictive as a lifelong program. Pritikin ignored the criticism. His studies on heart disease, diabetes, hypertension, and nutrition were published in several key medical journals, including the *New England Journal of Medicine,* the *Journal of the American Medical Association,* and *Circulation.* Pritikin's theories and practices are similar to the low-fat, high-fiber diet recommended by Dr. Dean Ornish, a physician whose medical studies have also shown significant reduction in heart disease when patients are treated through diet, exercise, and stress reduction. Dr. John McDougall is another physician who developed an eating program sharing the common theme of low-fat and high-fiber foods. Like Pritikin and Ornish, McDougall also established his own health facility, the St. Helena Health Center.

The Pritikin diet calls for a menu rich in natural foods: fruits, vegetables, whole grains, all varieties of legumes (such as pinto beans, black beans, and lentils), moderate amounts of nonfat dairy products like nonfat milk and nonfat yogurt, and small amounts of poultry, lean meat, and seafood. Limited, too, are salt, sugar, and other refined carbohydrates like white flour. On a typical day an individual following the Pritikin diet would eat three meals and three snacks consisting of many different foods, such as hot oatmeal with banana and strawberries for breakfast; fresh fruit and yogurt for a midmorning snack; pasta with marinara sauce, fruit, and steamed vegetables for lunch; soups such as minestrone, lentil, or gazpacho for an afternoon snack; for dinner, broiled seafood, a large green salad, steamed asparagus, and a baked potato; and for dessert or an evening snack, popcorn or frozen yogurt.

Pritikin went public with his program through lectures, his presentations to medical communities, and the establishment of his Pritikin Longevity Center in 1975 in Santa Barbara, California, an in-residence program of nutrition, exercise, and lifestyle education that has attracted people from all over the world. The Pritikin Longevity Center in Florida continues to operate as both a lifestyle-training program and a research center, with a laboratory that works to investigate the relationship between diet, exercise, and disease prevention.

Pritikin also established the Pritikin Research Foundation, a nonprofit organization that both conducts and funds research examining the relationship between diet and disease. Robert Pritikin, Nathan's son, was named director of the Pritikin Program in 1985. In 1984, shortly before Nathan Pritikin's death, the National Heart, Lung, and Blood Institute announced that lowering blood cholesterol reduced the risks of heart attacks and coronary disease, vindicating Pritikin's earlier dietary recommendations.

Years before Pritikin first learned of his heart disease, he had been diagnosed with leukemia, an illness that would eventually lead to his death. Pritikin suspected that radiation he had been exposed to during World War II had contributed to his contracting leukemia. For decades, the leukemia was in remission. In 1984 the cancer reappeared. Pritikin suffered complications caused by his cancer treatments and grew increasingly weak. Even though his health was failing, Pritikin continued to work on new technology designed to remove fats from the blood without the use of drugs. Pritikin held more than two dozen patents in physics, chemistry, and electrical engineering, and marketed his inventions to companies including Honeywell, General Electric, Bendix, and Corning. Following his death, Pritikin's autopsy showed a heart and arteries that were in extraordinarily healthy condition, "like that of a 16-year-old," noted the supervising pathologist. Nathan Pritikin was buried in Santa Monica, California.

See also:

Life Choice diet; McDougall Program; Ornish, Dean; Pritikin Program for Diet and Exercise.

Additional Reading

Almanac of Famous People, 6th ed. Farmington Hills, Mich.: Gale Research, 1998.

Barnard, Neal D. "The Pritikin Legacy." *Vegetarian Times,* May 1991, 64–73.

Hoover, Eleanor. "When his Health Deserted Him, Diet and Fitness Guru Nathan Pritikin Turned to Suicide." *People Weekly,* 11 March 1985, 57–59.

Pritikin, Nathan. *The Pritikin Program for Diet and Exercise.* New York: Grosset and Dunlap, 1979.

Scribner Encyclopedia of American Lives. Volume 1: 1981–85. Farmington Hills, Mich.: Gale Group, 1998.

Shute, Nancy. "A Childhood Without Twinkies: Young Pritikin Modifies His Father's Draconian Fat-Free Message." *U.S. News & World Report,* 12 January 1998, 62.

Pritikin Program for Diet and Exercise

The Pritikin Program for Diet and Exercise by Nathan Pritikin, a self-taught nutritionist and inventor, is a program Pritikin developed while treating his own heart disease. The four-week program is based on a low-fat, high-fiber diet and exercise plan available through the Pritikin Longevity Center, also spelled out in Pritikin's many best-selling books, including *The Pritikin Program for Diet and Exercise* (1979), and in his son Robert Pritikin's books. Pritikin called his diet "a declaration of war against the American dependence on processed foods, fats, sugars, proteins, salt, caffeine, alcohol, and nonfoods." It focuses on complex carbohydrates, fresh fruits and vegetables eaten raw or cooked. The Pritikin Diet advocates a fat level that averages no more than 10 percent of total calories daily. The average American diet may run from 30 to 40 percent fat while the U.S. Department of Agriculture (USDA) Dietary Guidelines for Americans recommend eating no more than 30 percent or less of daily calories from fat.

Unlike many fad diets, the Pritikin Program does not limit specific food groups but instead divides foods into those to use versus those to limit or avoid altogether. In his book *The Pritikin Permanent Weight-Loss Manual,* dieters who want more structure are advised to find daily menu plans outlining four different calorie-intake levels. Most breakfast menus contain some grain foods to help dieters meet important nutritional requirements and also because whole grains are filling and provide a substantial start for the day. Breakfast grains include hot cereals of cracked wheat, rolled oats, or cornmeal, plus recommended cold cereals like Shredded Wheat or Grape-Nuts.

The Pritikin diet strongly encourages snacking between meals, saying the body functions best when food is eaten more frequently during the day. People who attend the Pritikin Longevity Center eat seven to eight meals a day with few restrictions on quantity of food eaten. Good snack choices include low-fat, high-fiber soups like minestrone and other bean-based varieties, whole fruits, vegetables, and salads. Lunch and dinner often include pasta dishes, seafood rich in omega-3 fatty acids, Asian rice and vegetable entrées, Mexican dishes like burritos and enchiladas, and a wide variety of salads and soups. Pritikin called fresh fruit the best dessert but his book also features other dessert recipes. He cautioned that many of his recipes did contain generous amounts of fruit juice sweeteners and should be restricted or reserved for only

occasional use. Each of Pritikin's books also contains daily menu ideas as well as many recipes.

A typical breakfast on the Pritikin Program menu includes hot oatmeal, sliced bananas and blueberries, nonfat milk, half a grapefruit, and a cup of green tea. Lunch might include a large green salad with nonfat dressing, a veggie or garden burger on whole-wheat bread topped with onion and tomato, an ear of corn, fresh fruit, and herbal tea or mineral water. A typical dinner would be poached salmon, roasted new potatoes, steamed asparagus, a green salad with balsamic vinegar or nonfat dressing, fruit salad, and a glass of wine or herbal tea. Snacks throughout the day would include fat-free plain yogurt mixed with fresh fruit, fresh vegetables like carrots and cherry tomatoes, popcorn, salsa with baked tortilla chips, or baked potatoes with fat-free sour cream.

The Pritikin program also emphasizes foods, like fruits and vegetables, that are low in calorie density, in other words, nutrient-rich foods that fill you up with the least amount of calories. These foods include most fruits; vegetables; nonfat dairy products; many unrefined carbohydrates, such as pasta, hot cereals like oatmeal, brown rice, yams, and corn; beans, peas and lentils; and lean animal protein like seafood, chicken breast, and turkey breast.

Pritikin cautioned against high-protein diets such as the Scarsdale Medical Diet and Dr. Atkins's Diet Revolution. He said high-protein, low-carbohydrate diets had immediate as well as long-term adverse effects, including nausea; constipation; vitamin and mineral depletion; mineral imbalances; accumulation of toxic substances such as ketones, uric acid, and ammonia; elevated blood cholesterol that narrows arteries; increased kidney malfunction; and possible increased risk of colon disease. In his book

The Pritikin Program for Diet and Exercise, he wrote, "There is nothing good that can be said for high-protein diets. I am against them because of their inherent dangers, because they discourage people from adopting healthy and satisfying eating habits and because they are of dubious effectiveness even in the short term."

Pritikin did encourage people to exercise daily, and said a good exercise program would improve well-being, build resistance to heart disease, and help any weight loss effort. Pritikin was himself an avid jogger, and followed a regular exercise routine until the last year of his life.

See also:

Atkins Nutritional Approach; Dietary Guidelines for Americans; ketones/ketosis; Scarsdale diet.

Additional Reading

American National Biography, New York: Oxford University Press, 1999.

Barnard, Neal D. "The Pritikin Legacy." *Vegetarian Times,* May 1991, 64–73.

Pritikin, Nathan. *The Pritikin Program for Diet and Exercise.* New York: Grosset and Dunlap, 1979.

———. *The Pritikin Permanent Weight-Loss Manual.* New York: Grosset and Dunlap, 1981.

Protein Power

The Protein Power plan is a high-protein, low-carbohydrate plan developed by Dr. Michael Eades and Mary Dan Eades. The concept behind the Protein Power plan is that reducing intake of carbohydrates will reduce the amount of insulin released into the body. Protein Power also suggests avoiding "bad fats," which include fried foods, hydrogenated fats, and trans fats such as margarine.

The Protein Power Web site offers minimum requirements for protein, depending on your level of activity and "lean body mass." For example, a sedentary person needs only 0.5 grams of protein per pound of lean body mass compared to a very active person (one who exercises an hour or more at least five times a week) who needs 0.8 grams of protein per pound of lean body mass.

In calculating carbohydrates, the Eades use the "effective carbohydrate content." This is the total carbohydrates in a food, minus the dietary fiber. In other words, high-fiber carbohydrate foods have a lower carbohydrate rating than a simple sugar might, even if the total carbohydrates listed on the Nutrition Facts label are the same.

Low-carbohydrate, high-protein diets have become increasingly popular in recent years. An article in the *Journal of the American Dietetic Association* suggested that carbohydrates became the dieters' taboo "because the low-fat diets of the 1980s and 1990s failed consumers who mistakenly believed that consumption of low-fat products was license to eat voraciously while paying no mind to the amount of sugar and energy being consumed. Many people find irresistible the basis of low-carbohydrate diets: eating as much protein as desired—including steaks, eggs, and other fatty foods that they had previously been told by media reports and medical practitioners to shun—and still losing weight, so long as intake of carbohydrates is strictly limited."

Yet many critics of these restrictive carbohydrate plans say severely limiting carbohydrates is not good either. All high-protein, low-carbohydrate plans put the dieter at risk of loss of vitamin B, calcium, and potassium, resulting from lack of carbohydrates in the diet, and risk of coronary heart disease from eating more high-protein foods that are also high in fat.

While a low-carbohydrate diet will help a dieter lose weight initially, critics say the dieter will feel lethargic. Because there are so few carbohydrates to burn as energy, the body begins to burn lean muscle mass for energy. The Eades respond on the Web site, noting, "In the first seven to ten days, some people may feel tired. This is because it may take a week or two for your body to manufacture the necessary enzymes to effectively handle your new nutritional structure. Your body will make the enzymes it needs, but there is a short lag in the time it takes to do so. During this period, you may feel slightly fatigued, but that should quickly pass. Be sure that you are taking your potassium supplement. You should try to pamper yourself in the first couple of weeks on the plan. Get some extra rest. Take it easy on any hard-core exercise."

Nonetheless, most nutritionists and physicians would recommend a carbohydrate-moderating diet, not a severe reduction.

See also:

ketones/ketosis.

Additional Reading

Eades, Michael R., and Mary Dan Eades. *Protein Power: The High Protein/Low Carbohydrate Way to Lose Weight, Feel Fit and Boost Your Health—In Just Weeks.* New York: Bantam Books, 1997.

———. *The Protein Power Lifeplan.* New York: Warner Books, 2001.

Gotthardt, Melissa Meyers. "The New Low-Carb Diet Craze." *Cosmopolitan*, February 2000,148.

Stein, Joel. "The Low-Carb Diet Craze." *Time*, 1 November 1999, 71–79.

Stein, Karen. "High Protein, Low-Carbohydrate Diets: Do They Work?" *Journal of the American Dietetic Association,* 100, no. 7 (July 2000): 760.

Turner, Richard, and Joan Raymond. "The Trendy Diet That Sizzles: A Counterintuitive Program Reaches Critical Mass." *Newsweek International,* 13 September 1999, 62.

Wilgoren, Jodi. "Low-Carb Diet: Lose the Bun, Not the Burger." *New York Times,* 11 January 2000, D7.

www.eatprotein.com

Relaxacisor

The Relaxacisor was a handheld device designed to help people firm and tone their muscles by delivering a mild electric shock through contact pads. The shocks caused muscle spasms, which were supposed to firm and tone and tighten problem areas in a woman's figure. The Relaxacisor was billed as an easy solution to being "out-of-shape"; Relaxacisor, Inc., sold more than 400,000 of the machines from 1949 until 1970 when the FDA banned them as ineffective and dangerous. According to Stephen Barrett and William Jarvis, authors of *The Health Robbers,* it took years of investigation and a five-month court battle to eventually produce the federal ban on the devices.

In his final decision, federal Judge William P. Gray said the Relaxacisor could cause miscarriages and could aggravate many preexisting medical conditions, including hernia, ulcers, varicose veins, and epilepsy. Following the decision, many who had purchased the devices wrote requesting refunds while the firm filed an appeal. The appeal was dismissed and the FDA promptly sent posters to all U.S. post offices warning against use of the devices. The government also warned that the sale of secondhand Relaxacisors was illegal. Owners were encouraged to either destroy them or make them inoperable to

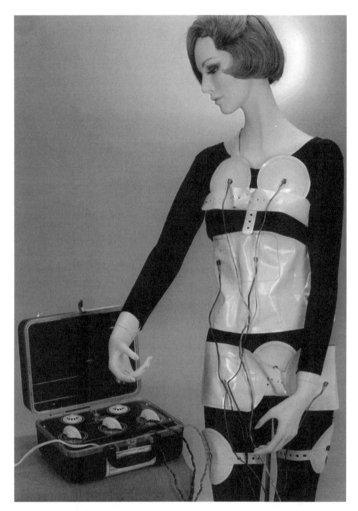

Relaxacisor was a handheld device designed to firm and tone muscle through mild electric shock that produced muscle spasms in problem areas. The device was banned by the Food and Drug Administration as ineffective and dangerous. Electrical muscle stimulators, or EMSs, are similar devices with limited usefulness in physical therapy for people with spinal cord injuries. (National Archives)

avoid the possibility of harm to "unsuspecting users."

The standard model had three control knobs and six pads to exercise six muscles at a time. The deluxe model was twice as large. A 1956 magazine advertisement for the device promoted it as passive exercise. "It's a modern mode of NO-EFFORT exercise that you can concentrate on the areas that need it most. Relaxacisor, for example, can exercise just the muscles of your tummy while the rest of you RESTS!" Magazine advertisements in the 1950s and 1960s pictured shapely models reclining with a book or magazine. The pads were visible, attached to hips, thighs, buttocks and stomachs and each woman appeared completely relaxed.

Known as electrical muscle stimulators, or EMSs, these devices have limited usefulness in physical therapy for people with spinal cord injuries who can no longer voluntarily control their muscles, according to doctors. They are also still used to reduce muscle shrinkage in bed-ridden patients.

Additional Reading

Barrett, Stephen, and William T. Jarvis. *The Health Robbers: A Close Look at Quackery in*

America. Buffalo, N.Y.: Prometheus Books, 1993.

"Eminently Suitable Affair: Relaxacisor." *Vogue,* 1 March 1968, 88.

Gilbert, Susan. *Medical Fakes and Frauds.* New York: Chelsea House Publishers, 1989.

Simon, Stephanie. "A Gaggle of Quackery Going Mainstream." *Los Angeles Times,* 4 February 2002, A12.

Registered Dietitian (RD)

Only registered dietitians—those who have completed an academic program accredited by the American Dietetic Association, and gained related experience—can use the letters "RD" after their name. Registered dietitians must keep up with continuing professional education to maintain their certification.

In some states, dietitians are licensed by the state, and only state-licensed dietetics professionals are permitted to provide nutrition counseling. Not all states require licensing, however. Some states have less restrictive certification or registration regulations. According to the American Dietetic Association, "Consumers in these states [without licensing requirements] who are seeking nutrition therapy assistance need to be more cautious and aware of the qualifications of the provider they choose."

Resting Metabolic Rate

Resting metabolic rate is the rate at which your body consumes calories during rest. Your body burns up calories simply to support its basic functions. To create a baseline for the appropriate overall calorie intake, it might be helpful to know your resting metabolic rate. Once you determine it, you can multiply it by another factor, depending on your activity level, to calculate an approximate daily calorie need.

Men and women use different formulas to calculate their resting metabolic rate.

For women, start with 655, then add your weight × 4.3, add you height in inches × 4.3, and subtract your age in years × 4.7.

Here's an example for a twenty-year-old female, 5′4″ or 64 inches tall, weighing 130 pounds.

$$655 + (130 \times 4.3 = 559)$$
$$+ (64 \times 4.3 = 275) - (20 \times 4.7 = 94)$$

or

$$655 + 559 + 275 - 94 = 1{,}395.$$

That means this young woman's resting metabolic rate is about 1,395 calories per day.

For men, the formula is this:

$$66 + (\text{weight} \times 6.2) + (\text{height in inches} \times 12.7) - (\text{age in years} \times 6.8)$$

Our example here is a twenty-two-year-old male, 5′10″ (or 70 inches) weighing 190 pounds.

$$66 + (190 \times 6.2 = 1178)$$
$$+ (70 \times 12.7 = 889) - (22 \times 4.7 = 150)$$

or

$$66 + 1178 + 889 - 150 = 1{,}983.$$

Knowing your resting metabolic rate is just a starting point in determining the amount of calories to consume. Your active metabolic rate, or the amount of calories you burn while moving around and doing other physical activities, will obviously be higher. About 65 to 80 percent of the calories your body burns up are consumed while your body is at rest. One rule of thumb is that sedentary people should multiply their resting metabolic rate by 1.2; moderately active people can multiply it by 1.4; and serious athletes can multiply it by 1.8.

Rotation Diet

The Rotation Diet, written in 1986, is Dr. Martin Katahn's answer to helping people lose up to a pound per day and, most importantly, never gain it back. Katahn was director of the Vanderbilt University Weight Management Program near Nashville at the time he wrote his best seller. When first released, the Rotation diet was so popular it grew into a citywide fad, with more than 75,000 Nashville residents dieting collectively to shed 1 million pounds in 12 weeks. As the Rotation diet gained popularity, people began joining the "Melt-a-Million" at their local Kroger grocery stores. The supermarket chain served as diet headquarters, giving away thousands of sample rotation menus and running weekend public weigh-ins. Nashville restaurants, fearing huge business losses even added Rotation diet specials to their menus. Nashville was "rotating."

The basic rotation plan calls for dieters to eat less fat and more fish, and walk or incorporate other exercise into their daily routine. What makes it different is the rotation aspect, which requires both men and women to vary the number of calories they consume during a three-week period. After the three weeks, dieters are encouraged to take a diet vacation and return to normal eating habits for anywhere from a week to a month. Katahn then suggests that those who need to lose more weight can follow another three-week rotation, completing the cycle as many times as it takes to reach a target weight.

The rotation theory is based on Katahn's belief that the majority of diets routinely fail because people tire of eating the same, boring foods and because metabolism gradually slows during any diet that strictly limits calories. Katahn's other theory, that hormone and enzyme levels increase after dieting and send signals to the body to regain and store any lost weight, have been bolstered by recent research on ghrelin, an appetite-stimulating hormone. Research published in a May 2002 issue of the *New England Journal of Medicine* showed that ghrelin is present in the stomach and increases following weight loss.

Katahn insists that his program will deliver permanent weight loss because dieters who follow the plan keep their metabolism at a consistent level and avoid regaining weight when they return to eating what they consider normal amounts of food. But he warns users that the Rotation Diet is forever, and was quoted in a 1986 *People* interview as saying, "If you go back to eating the way you did before, you're going to gain your weight back." Katahn also cites research conducted using participants in the Vanderbilt Weight Management Program. He said Vanderbilt studies show there was no reduction in metabolic rate for participants who followed the Rotation Diet. Instead, he says their metabolic rate increased, meaning dieters were able to eat normally after the diet without any weight gain.

Critics of the diet caution that losing 3 to 4 pounds a week is excessive and they questioned the safety of eating only 600 calories per day. The daily calorie count for women using this plan rotates between 600, 900, and 1,200, and men eat 1,200, 1,500, or 1,800 calories daily. By following Katahn's suggested menus, the first three days for women are at the lowest calorie level, 600. Female dieters then increase their calories to 900 per day for four days. The entire second week for women calls for a daily level of 1,200 calories and the third week rotates back to the 600 and 900 limits. Men follow the same schedule, substituting slightly higher calorie allowances. During the maintenance period dieters are encouraged to gradually increase their intake of calories until they reach a point where they can eat and not regain any weight.

The menu for men and women on the Rotation Diet is basically the same, but men eat an additional two grain servings, 50 percent larger portions of meat, fish, or fowl and three extra-safe fruits. A typical 600-calorie breakfast is half a grapefruit, one slice of whole wheat bread with an ounce of cheese and a no-calorie beverage, usually water. In fact, Katahn recommends that dieters drink eight 8-ounce glasses of water per day and he discourages the consumption of artificially sweetened drinks. The Rotation Diet allows up to two cups of coffee or tea per day and suggests a beverage of low-salt bouillon for a change of pace.

A Rotation Diet lunch might include a protein food such as salmon, tuna, or cottage cheese along with unlimited free vegetables, salad, crackers, or a slice of bread. Dinner ideas range from baked chicken and salad to poached fish served with a variety of steamed vegetables and fruit desserts. To soothe hunger pangs, especially during low-calorie days, dieters are allowed to eat unlimited amounts of free vegetables and fruits.

Katahn classifies free vegetables as anything that has so few calories it can be eaten in unlimited quantities: spinach, watercress, cucumber, celery, endive, lettuce, parsley, and asparagus are all free vegetables and allowed as snacks. Safe fruits— fruits that are low in calories and high in fiber—include apples, berries, grapefruit, melon, oranges, peaches, pineapple, and tangerines. The Rotation Diet book includes recipes for dishes like Almond Chicken, Royal Indian Salmon, Baked or Broiled Rainbow Trout, Gingered Beets, and Braised Carrots and Celery.

The Rotation Diet program, sponsored by the Nashville Kroger stores, eventually generated millions of dollars in free TV, radio, and newspaper publicity, as other supermarket chains jumped on the diet bandwagon. Stores, from Bi-Lo to Farm Fresh Supermarkets, Publix, and Wegman's offered in-store programs and promotional efforts. Every chain reportedly contacted the state health department before endorsing or recommending the diet and hired professional nutritionists, home economists, or dietitians to answer any diet-related questions, according to a 1986 article in *Supermarket News.* Despite the success of the Rotation Diet, some Nashville supermarkets did not offer the diet in their stores, stopping short of promoting this specific diet. Instead, they urged customers to follow a healthy eating plan based on the Dietary Guidelines for Americans, devised by the U.S. Department of Health and Human Services and the U.S. Department of Agriculture.

The author's theory came from his own personal experience of losing 70 pounds in 1963 following a heart attack at the age of 35. Katahn said in a 1986 *People* interview that it took him eighteen months to lower his weight to 154 from 230 pounds by following his own rotation principle, and by adding a daily physical exercise program. The Rotation Diet recommends up to 45 minutes of daily exercise, from walking to jogging, tennis, or swimming.

Katahn wrote some fourteen diet manuals, including *The T-Factor 2000 Diet,* a revised edition of his original 1989 *T-Factor Diet; The Tri-Color Diet: A Miracle Breakthrough in Diet and Nutrition for a Longer, Healthier Life* (1996); *The Cancer Prevention Good Health Diet* (2000); and *How to Quit Smoking Without Gaining*

Weight (1994). *The T-Factor Diet,* another best-seller, resembles Katahn's rotation plan and was among the early diet books that promoted reducing dietary fat as a practical way to lose weight.

Both the Rotation and T-Factor diets contain the same elements and similar menu suggestions, but the T-Factor system only counts daily fat intake, not total calories. In his T-Factor plan Katahn argues that the source of calories eaten is more important than the total number of calories ingested. By understanding the "T-factor," or thermogenic effect, in which carbohydrate calories are burned faster than fat calories, Katahn believes dieters can successfully lose weight. In his T-Factor books Katahn explains how to choose foods that naturally maximize the T-Factor level and activate the body's hidden fat-burning potential. The plan also provides two daily diet menus—one for people who want moderate weight loss and another for those who want quick results. Critics raised concerns about the rapid weight loss and called the fat and fiber counter in the book difficult to use, with foods listed according to type instead of alphabetically by name.

Katahn retired from his position at Vanderbilt University in 1991 and is now involved in promoting chess for children in Tennessee public schools.

See also:

Dietary Guidelines for Americans; ghrelin; T-Factor Diet.

Additional Reading

Chu, Dan. "Nashville Hopes to Shrink Its Population by a Million—A Million Pounds, That Is." *People Weekly,* 10 March 1986, 52–55.
Davis, Tim, and Rachel Kaplan. "Rotation Diet: A Heavy-Weight Promotion; Stores Get Publicity and Traffic Increases." *Supermarket News,* 18 August 1986, 1–3.
Katahn, Martin. *The Rotation Diet.* New York: W. W. Norton & Company, 1986.
———. *The T-Factor 2000 Diet.* New York: W. W. Norton & Company, 1999.
Stoddard, Maynard Good. "The Diet That Consumed Nashville." *Saturday Evening Post,* July–August 1986, 26–29.
Toufexis, Anastasia. "Hey, Are You Rotating?" *Time,* 14 April 1986, 108.
Zilberter, Tanya. "To Count or Not to Count? The T-Factor and Rotation Diets." www.chasefreedom.com. Accessed 10 June 2003.

Scarsdale Diet

The Complete Scarsdale Medical Diet (1987), by Herman Tarnower, MD, and Samm Sinclair Baker became an instant best-seller and dieters were losing up to 20 pounds per week with this high-protein, low-carbohydrate, and low-calorie regime.

The Scarsdale diet was designed to be followed precisely and it contained no "bewildering array of choices." Instead, users merely followed an exact list of menus for fourteen days and then were advised to stop. Dr. Tarnower explained in the book that it worked well because people had such specific directions, plus the short duration made the rigid regime less daunting. As the doctor noted, "You won't develop any vitamin or mineral deficiency in two weeks, even on a starvation diet." But he cautioned dieters that it was important to stop the diet at the two-week mark. At that point users would follow the Scarsdale maintenance diet for one or two weeks. His suggested timetable for success was two weeks on the diet, two weeks off, and then two weeks back on.

In the book Tarnower discussed the mind of an obese person who is desperately trying to lose weight and failing. He wrote, "The more you worry about food, the more you even think about it while you're on a diet, the more difficult and tiresome the whole process can become." The Scarsdale diet also maintained that quantities of foods were less important than the chemical reactions between them. Yet, the meals were very low calorie, designed to average 1,000 calories or less per day with triple the amount of protein recommended by the U.S. Department of Agriculture's Dietary Guidelines for Americans.

Breakfast each day was the same and included half a grapefruit or fruits in season; one slice of protein bread, toasted with no spread, and coffee or tea with no sugar, cream, or milk. Lunch included assorted cold cuts, such as chicken, turkey, beef, or tongue, plus tomatoes and coffee, tea, or diet soda. Because all food choices were allowed in any amount desired, Tuesday's dinner, for example, called for "plenty of steak," tomatoes, lettuce, celery, olives, cucumbers, or brussels sprouts. Sunday's dinner was the same minus the tomatoes, lettuce, and olives. Thursday's dinner included two eggs, cottage cheese, cabbage, and a slice of dry protein toast. Protein bread was any bread with a high-protein content, such as gluten or whole-wheat bread. The diet suggested the bread be chewed in little bites so that it would be more satisfying, and no margarine, spreads, or jams were allowed.

Substitutions were taboo except for one "official" lunch substitution: 1/2 cup low-fat cottage cheese mixed with 1 tablespoon of low-fat sour cream, sliced fruit and 6 halves of walnuts or pecans sprinkled over the fruit. That could be eaten any day in place of an afternoon meal. All foods were prepared without butter; all salads without dressings except lemon and vinegar. No alcohol was allowed and the only approved between-meal snacks were raw carrots and celery.

Critics of high-protein reducing plans strongly disagree with this style of high-protein, low-calorie, and low-carbohydrate diets. Scientists with the USDA and the American Dietetic Association say carbohydrates are essential for providing energy for the body and without them the body will burn its own fat, reacting to what it perceives as starvation. Problems develop because the body does not burn this fat completely, causing substances called ketones to form. They are eventually released into the bloodstream, which increases the levels of uric acid in the blood. Doctors say abnormally high ketone levels in the blood cause ketosis, which can trigger kidney disease, gallstones, gout, or cardiac complications in some people. However, abnormally high ketone levels in the body make dieting easier because they decrease appetite by causing nausea, weakness, dehydration, headaches, and constipation or diarrhea.

Tarnower maintained that his carefully designed combination of foods increased the fat-burning process and provided rapid weight loss. In answer to concerns about the lack of carbohydrates, he suggested that dieters who produced ketones were "enjoying fast fat metabolism," a desired state. And he wrote that ketones were a good thing because they acted to curb the appetite, making the dieting process "less burdensome and cutting down any need for appetite-depressing drugs." The book told readers that ketones are washed out through the urine, which is a helpful, cleansing part of the increased fat-burning process.

Researchers suggest that a gradual loss of 1 pound per week is a healthy goal in contrast to the Scarsdale diet average of 1 pound per day. The position of the ADA on weight management recommends a gradual, incremental weight loss, a far cry from the quick, dramatic losses experienced by Scarsdale dieters. Instead, the ADA suggests that prospective dieters reduce their focus on actual weight loss and food, and instead establish a more constructive focus in life. And the American Heart Association continues to caution dieters about the problems associated with protein-rich regimens like the Scarsdale diet. They recommend following the USDA Food Guide Pyramid, a model that includes moderate amounts of lean protein foods as well as fresh fruits and vegetables and complex carbohydrates. They caution against foods full of saturated fat and cholesterol that can increase the risk of heart disease.

See also:

Dietary Guidelines for Americans; Food Guide Pyramid; ketones/ketosis; Tarnower, Herman.

Additional Reading

Dullea, Georgia. "The Sensational Scarsdale Diet." *New York Times,* 7 July 1978, 10.
Tarnower, Herman, and Samm Sinclair Baker. *The Complete Scarsdale Medical Diet.* New York: Rawson, Wade Publishers, Inc., 1978

Sears, Barry

Barry Sears (b. June 6, 1947, Long Beach, California) is a biochemist and the author of *Enter the Zone: A Dietary Road Map.* His controversial nutritional theory recommends a daily intake of 40 percent carbohydrates, 30 percent fat, and 30 percent protein. Sears maintains that his own studies show that food has a potent, drug-like effect on the hormonal system and

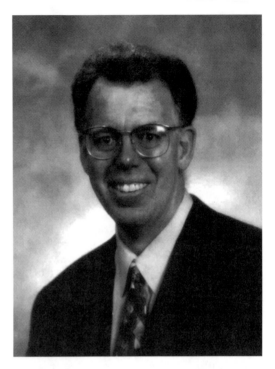

Barry Sears, a biochemist and the author of a dieting plan called The Zone, recommends a daily intake of 40 percent carbohydrates, 30 percent fat, and 30 percent protein. His interest in dietary theory followed his father's early death from heart disease. (John F. Wagner/Wagner Studios)

eating the right combination of foods leads to a "zone" metabolic state in which the body works at peak performance while decreasing hunger, increasing energy, and losing weight.

His interest in dietary theory followed his father's death from heart disease at age 53. In fact, Sears's grandfather, father, and three uncles all died of heart attacks before the age of 54. In his book Sears describes how this personal tragedy changed the focus of his research as he sought to understand the role of fat in heart disease. That research became his first best-seller, written in 1995 in collaboration with professional health writer Bill Lawren. Sears followed with the sequel, *Mastering the Zone* (1997), which spent eleven weeks on the best-seller list. Other titles include: *The Anti-Aging Zone* (1999); *The Soy Zone* (2000); *Zone Perfect Meals in Minutes* (1997); *Zone Food Blocks: The Quick & Easy, Mix & Match Counter for Staying in the Zone* (1998); and *A Week in the Zone* (2000).

Following an undergraduate degree from Occidental College, Sears earned a doctorate in biochemistry in 1971 from Indiana University. A lanky six-foot-five he described himself in a 1997 *Time* magazine article as a "pointy-headed scientist." His book jackets list him as a "former MIT researcher," where he was a technical staff member at the Francis Bitter Magnet Laboratory at MIT, a facility that studies condensed matter physics, not nutrition. As a practicing biochemist, Sears also holds twelve patents for biomolecular inventions from the 1970s and 1980s. Those inventions involve systems for delivering cancer and heart-disease drugs into the bloodstream on a fat-molecule carrier.

An avid entrepreneur, Sears has been supported in various business ventures by his widowed mother Betty as well as his younger brother Doug, who is also his business partner, as is Sears's wife Lynn. The couple have two children, Kristin and Kelly. In southern California, Sears's diet book has grown from a lifestyle choice into an industry. Life Zone is one of several health clubs, which will, for a fee, enroll members on Zone diets. Plus, area restaurants like the L.A. Farm offer Zone menu choices where a five-course Zone meal goes for at least $45. All this has made Sears a millionaire but brings with it skeptics who dispute the scientific foundations of The Zone.

Those critics include the American Cancer Society (ACS), which recommends that people adopt a diet high in fruits and vegetables, but low in meat and fat. And ACS studies show that high-fat, high-protein foods may be associated with up to one-third of the 500,000 cancer deaths in the United States each year from colorectal, stomach, lung, mouth, throat, larynx, esophagus, prostate, and possibly breast cancer. But Sears writes in his book that he believes the opposite—that a high-carbohydrate diet brings with it cardiovascular risks and medically approved low-cholesterol, low-fat diets actually cause heart disease.

Criticism of The Zone and Sears from the medical community seems to have enhanced Sears's image as a crusader fighting the national nutrition and medical establishment. Many celebrities and professional athletes have followed his diet, including Madonna, Janet Jackson, Arnold Schwarzenegger, former president Bill Clinton, and 1992 Olympic gold medal swimmer Jenny Thompson.

See also:

The Zone.

Additional Reading

Norris, Eileen. "High-Protein Diets: Where's the Beef?" *Harvard Health Letter*, 22, no. 3 (January 1997): 1–3.

"Don't Look for Magic Bullets." *Consumers' Research Magazine*, July 2000, 24.

Ratnesar, Romesh. "Against the Grain: The Low-Carb Zone Diet Rises from Fad to Fixture." *Time*, 15 December 1997, 86.

Seigel, Jessica. "Zoned Out: The Medical Miracles Promised by Barry Sears, Diet Guru of the Moment, Are Sometimes Hard to Swallow." *Los Angeles Magazine*, February 1997, 34–42.

Shamblin, Gwen

Tennessee dietitian Gwen Shamblin founded the Weigh Down Workshop,

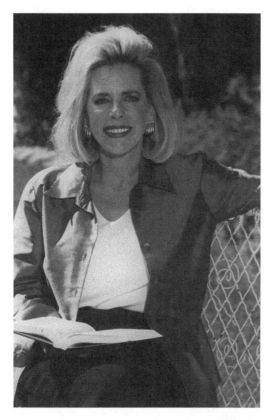

Gwen Shamblin is a Tennessee dietitian who founded the Weigh Down Workshop in 1986 based on her belief that healthy eating and a healthy relationship with God go hand in hand. Despite the diet's popularity, critics call it nutritionally superficial. (The Weigh Down Workshop)

Inc., in 1986 using the principles she developed as part of her own successful weight loss. "I was a thin eater growing up," she confessed in her 1997 best-seller, *The Weigh Down Diet*. But with college came the familiar freshman weight gain and the beginning of her self-described battle with food.

A registered dietitian, Shamblin graduated from the University of Tennessee with a master's degree in food and nutrition. Following graduation she was employed by health departments in Ten-

nessee and Mississippi but later began a weight control consulting practice in 1980 in Memphis. During that time she started counseling people toward the spiritual dimension of weight loss and away from a focus on food. After several years she launched the Weigh Down Workshop, which tailored her weight loss program for church-sponsored classes. It's centered around a ten-week program that starts by teaching participants what hunger is. The idea is to help dieters understand the difference between being physically hungry and being spiritually hungry. By beginning the diet with a fast, participants can feel hunger pangs—something to which they are probably unaccustomed. Critics of the diet plan say that it does not provide enough nutritional guidance, especially not for people with poor eating habits.

Shamblin's latest book, *Rise Above,* also focuses on the spiritual dimension of weight loss, and her diet programs are now held in more than 30,000 churches across the country.

According to Shamblin, most overeaters eat to fill the void in their lives and some develop an unhealthy passion for food. She suggests participants fill that emptiness with a passionate relationship with God. Critics charge she combines the superficial nutritional advice of diet personalities like Susan Powter with the evangelistic fervor of televangelists such as Jimmy Swaggart. In recent years Shamblin's theological beliefs have also created some controversy when various church leaders questioned her views on the Trinity. Their concerns were based on comments Shamblin posted on her Weigh Down Web site.

See also:

Weigh Down Diet.

Additional Reading

Mulrine, Anna. "A Godly Approach to Weight Loss." *U.S. News & World Report,* 5 May 1997, 12.

Shamblin, Gwen. *The Weigh Down Diet.* New York: Doubleday, 1997.

Smith, Pam. *The Diet Trap.* Washington, D.C.: LifeLine Press, 2000.

"The Weigh Down Diet." *Publishers Weekly,* 244, no. 8 (24 February 1997): 8.

Winner, Lauren F. "The Weigh & the Truth." *Christianity Today,* 4 September 2000, 50.

Simmons, Richard

Richard Simmons (b. July 12, 1948, New Orleans) reached the status of popular-culture icon in the 1980s with his zeal for dancing off the pounds.

Simmons's father, Leonard, and mother, Shirley, were both in show business; his mother was a successful dancer and club performer. In his autobiographies and numerous press interviews, Simmons details the humiliation of being an overweight child and his conflicted relationship with his father. By second grade, he was seriously overweight and a doctor put him on a diet. He cheated, he wrote in his autobiography, *Still Hungry —After All These Years,* adding, "My best shot lasted three days."

He documented the years of dieting struggles, from diet pills supplied to him by friends in middle school to practically starving himself while in art school in Italy. During that time, he stopped eating altogether and lost 112 pounds in less

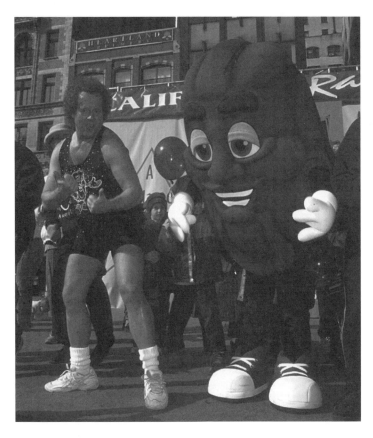

Exercise guru Richard Simmons presents the unveiling of the next generation of the "California Raisin & Grapevine Line" dance in 2002 to promote the California Raisin Marketing Board and to benefit the American Cancer Society Camp Adventures program. (Zuma Press/NewsCom)

than three months. He ended up in the hospital and soon after was excluded from military service.

Most of his experiences with weight loss, however, were followed by periods of serious weight gain. He listened as others described their tricks—diet shakes, laxatives, bulimia, and HCG—a hormone derived from the urine of pregnant women.

In California, he once attended a workout session—but unlike other gyms, the exercise regimen was based on dancing. He loved it, but the women in the class felt uncomfortable with him there. Simmons described his frustration at not being able to find an appropriate gym when he came to Los Angeles in 1973. On his Web site, he wrote, "I immediately started searching for an exercise class to help me maintain my 123-pound weight loss. As I stood in line waiting to join the most popular, trendy gym in the city, I heard one the trainers refusing to sell a membership to an overweight woman in front of me, saying she was an insurance risk. Well, as you can imagine, I was horrified! I left the line *and* the gym, and I found the woman outside and said, 'Here's my card. I'm going to open a gym, and you can come to *my* gym any time you want!'"

Shortly after, he created Slimmons, his own gym with an attached salad bar called Ruffage—so people could get exercise and eat healthy foods. In his book, he recalls that because he couldn't afford a piano player, he brought in his own records. Simmons still teaches one exercise class per week at the studio.

The idea took. Simmons's encouragement, self-deprecating humor, and high energy were attractive to many. Slimmons became popular in Beverly Hills and, soon afterward, Simmons was playing the role of an aerobics exercise instructor on the soap opera *General Hospital*. After four years on *General Hospital,* he became host of his own show, *The Richard Simmons Show*. In his autobiography, he recalls that he had his mother on as a regular guest to do some of the cooking segments.

By 1986, Simmons was running infomercials on television, and his diet Deal-A-Meal and more recent FoodMover plans and exercise videos, including *Sweatin' to the Oldies*, were well known. Simmons, with his Afro hairstyle and his uniform of short shorts and tank top, is part funny-man, part motivational speaker, and part exercise guru. His publicity appearances can be unusual—such as his February 2000 workout session with hundreds of children and adults and a life-sized California Raisin character, sponsored by the California Raisin Marketing Board as part of its campaign to spread the word that raisins are a healthy food.

Today, the Richard Simmons Web site lists the more than thirty videos he's developed. These include the *Sweatin' to the Oldies* series, "Dance Your Pants Off," "Groovin' in the House," "Blast Off the Pounds," and "Sit Tight"—a special workout program for people in wheelchairs or anyone else who needs to remain sitting during an exercise session. He also personally participates in a seven-night special session on Carnival Cruise Lines called "Cruise to Lose" He also markets his FoodMover program, a combination of a cookbook, video, calorie charts, and an instructional booklet. Plus, the Web site offers his newest Slim Away Every Day program—a 30-day plan to help dieters get into good habits.

The combination of eating less—a minimum of 1,200 calories—and exercise has earned Simmons's programs favorable comments from most dietitians. Some criticize the recent addition of nutritional supplements into Simmons's lineup, however.

One of the characteristics that has most endeared Simmons to his followers is his genuine concern for them. In his autobiography, he wrote, "One thing I've always done throughout my career has been my daily telephone calls—talking to people about their weight issues and offering them all the encouragement I can, and helping them to get started on a program of healthy eating and exercising." Since the mid-1970s, Simmons has been making 40 to 50 calls per day, even while traveling. On busy days, he wrote, he can make as many as 100 calls. And most days are busy days. The Web site notes that Simmons makes about 300 appearances a year.

Additional Reading

Dalka-Prysby, Sandra, and Richard Simmons. *Slow But Sure: How I Lost 170 Pounds With the Help of God, Family, Family Circle Magazine and Richard Simmons.* New York: Signet, 2001.

Emmons, Steve. "Clown Prince of Weight Loss Takes Big Interest in Fans." *Los Angeles Times,* 14 July 1991, E2.

"Dancing Raising Turn to Aerobics." May 2000, www.preparedfoods.com/archives/2000/2000_05/0005marketwatch.htm. Accessed 12 June 2003.

Simmons, Richard. *Richard Simmons' Never-Say-Diet Cookbook.* New York: Warner Books, 1985.

———. *The Richard Simmons Farewell To Fat Cookbook.* New York: Good Times Publishing, 1996.

———. *Still Hungry—After All These Years: My Story.* New York: GT Publishing, 1999.

Stewart, Susan. "Richard Simmons Holds Nothing Back." Knight-Ridder/Tribune News Service. 21 January 1994.

Wedlan, Candace A. "Exercising Discipline." *Los Angeles Times,* 1 May 1996, E3.

Weinraub, Judith. "Richard Dishes Up Dessert." *Washington Post,* 14 January 1998, E1.

www.richardsimmons.com

Slim-Fast

Slim-Fast is synonymous with easy weight loss to millions of dieting Americans. Considered a dominant player in the growing $1.3 billion diet products market, Slim-Fast had net sales of were $611 million in 1999, according to industry figures, with sales growth of more than 20 percent.

The company's advertising efforts have continuously put Slim-Fast in the public eye, thanks to commercials featuring celebrities like baseball manager Tommy LaSorda, television entertainer Kathy Lee Gifford, and actresses Elizabeth Ashley and Shari Belafonte. In 1992 Slim-Fast scored a national marketing coup, thanks to residents of the small town of Pound, Wisconsin, who took part in a Slim-Fast weight reduction plan for four months and lost a combined 2,800 pounds.

A Slim-Fast diet averages about 1,200 calories a day, some 500 calories less than the typical American woman eats and at least 1,000 calories less than the typical American male consumes. One of the most common meal replacement diets available, the plan requires a shake for breakfast and lunch along with a sensible dinner. Slim-Fast markets its own canned shakes as well as powdered Slim-Fast formula that can be mixed with one cup of low-fat milk twice a day. Dieters following the Slim-Fast plan are also allowed two additional pieces of fruit as well as a Slim-Fast Bar for snacks during the day.

A sensible meal, according to the Slim-Fast program, looks something like this: 4–6 ounces of poultry, fish, or lean meat;

half a baked potato; three steamed vegetables; and fruit for dessert. Basically, the plan controls calorie intake and reducing calories means losing weight. Nutrition experts say the program is not a good choice for long-term dieting but Slim-Fast can be an acceptable supplement if dieters remember to eat fruits, vegetables, and whole grains as part of their one daily meal. But critics say dieters must also remember that the shakes and bars are processed foods and while they contain added vitamins and minerals, they still lack important fiber, antioxidants, and the other health benefits associated with eating fresh foods.

Americans can buy the familiar diet drink everywhere; Wal-Mart stores sell an estimated $100 million worth of Slim-Fast products each year. However, liquid diet products have not always been that popular. Slim-Fast was first introduced in 1977, the same year some fifty-eight dieters died as the result of following very low-calorie liquid protein diet products. Although Slim-Fast was not involved in the deaths, it was pulled from shelves that same year as sales all but disappeared. It was reintroduced again in the early 1980s by originator S. Daniel Abraham. At the same time that Slim-Fast was returning to store shelves, concerns were being raised about PPA, phenylpropanolamine, an ingredient now banned by the Food and Drug Administration (FDA) after studies linked it to an increased risk of stroke. The FDA action was aimed at diet pills containing PPA, like Dexatrim and Metabolife, and also at over-the-counter cold and allergy remedies. Partly due to consumer concerns over PPA, sales of the reintroduced Slim-Fast showed dramatic improvement from $149 million in 1983 to $197 million in 1984.

Embracing computer technology and use of the Internet, Slim-Fast Foods now promotes an online "Buddy Program" over its Web site and matches up dieters according to ages and preferences in food and exercise for weekly, e-mail messages. According to the Web site, the purpose of the program is to provide mutual, nonjudgmental support over e-mail for the some 14,000 online Slim-Fast customers. A recent study by Brown University found that dieters who received weekly, personal e-mail messages from behavioral therapists lost three times as much weight in six months as those receiving only general information on the Internet, but far less than dieters with fact-to-face supervision. In response to concerns about the risk of encouraging bad or unhealthy food habits or eating disorders through the online buddy program, the company assured critics that the site does block out teens and it works to warns adult users against potentially dangerous eating behaviors.

Slim-Fast faced a minor public relations problem in 1999 when it was discovered that some of the ready-to-drink diet shakes were filled with diluted cleaning solution. The statement released by the company said only a few cans were involved but as a safety precaution about 192,000 cans of Ultra Slim-Fast shakes were pulled off the shelves. The recalled cans were from Arizona, California, Colorado, Michigan, New York, Ohio, Oregon, Utah, Virginia, and Wisconsin. In 2000 Unilever PLC acquired Slim-Fast Foods Company for $2.3 billion in cash. Industry analysts say the move reflects Unilever's commitment to developing its burgeoning functional foods business.

See also:

liquid protein diets; phenylpropanolamine (PPA).

Additional Reading

Berman, Phyllis, and Amy Feldman. "An Extraordinary Peddler." *Forbes,* 9 December 1991, 136–39.

Eder, Rob. "Unilever Purchases Slim Fast Foods." *Drug Store News,* 22, no. 7 (22 May 2000): 31.

Harrison, Joan. "Unilever Joins Other Food Giants Scrambling to Get Healthy." *Mergers & Acquisitions,* June 2000, 19.

Johnsen, Michael. "Slim Fast Gets a New Look, Focuses on Snack Replacement." *Drug Store News,* 24, no. 3 (4 March 2002): 35.

"Slim Fast Recalls a Batch of Shakes." *New York Times,* 18 April 1999, 27.

Somers, Suzanne

Suzanne Somers (b. October 16, 1946, in San Bruno, California), the actress best known for playing the "ditzy blonde" character of Chrissy on the 1970s comedy series *Three's Company,* has developed a successful career writing diet books following years as a model, actress, and owner and spokesperson for ThighMaster exercise equipment. Her eating plan, called "Somersizing," requires dieters to follow a two-part system of weight loss and maintenance where proteins and fats are eaten together but never with carbohydrates. Although Somers brings no nutrition credentials to bear on her books, she credits endocrinologist Dr. Diana Schwarzbein with helping her develop the low-carbohydrate, controlled–sugar intake program. Schwarzbein, who first self-published her own book for her diabetic patients, has written the foreword for Somers's best-selling title *Suzanne Somers' Eat Great, Lose Weight.* Other best-selling books by the actress include *Get Skinny on Fabulous Food; 365 Ways to Change Your Life;* and *Eat, Cheat and Melt the Fat Away.*

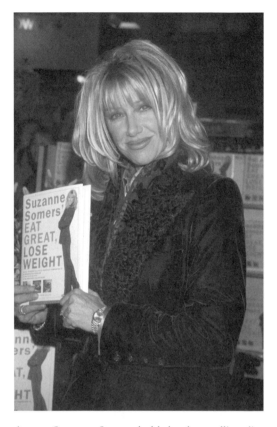

Actress Suzanne Somers holds her best-selling diet book *Suzanne Somers' Eat Great, Lose Weight.* Her eating plan calls for food combining and the elimination of what she labels Funky Foods. Recently the actress drew criticism for disclosing that she underwent liposuction following treatment for breast cancer. (Zuma Press/NewsCom)

Somers got her first taste of acting while appearing in a high school musical. In the spring of 1977 she won the part of Chrissy in *Three's Company* and became a television star. Somers left the show in 1982. She first hit the lecture circuit after her 1988 best-selling autobiography *Keeping Secrets,* detailing her childhood plagued by her alcoholic father's all-night rages. She published a book of interviews with people from abusive families titled *Wednesday's Children* (1992), and founded the Suzanne Somers Institute for the Effects of Addiction on Families to set up outpatient centers to treat addicts and family members of addicts.

The actress then moved into the fitness business when she and her husband Alan Hamel invested in the company that made ThighMaster exercise equipment. Somers was pictured on the box and also starred in infomercials touting its benefits. Thigh-Master quickly became part of American pop culture, mentioned on television shows like *Saturday Night Live*. Somers wrote in her second autobiography, *After the Fall: How I Picked Myself Up, Dusted Myself Off, and Started All Over Again* (1998), that in a move to revitalize her entertainment career she appeared in Las Vegas and in 1991 costarred in a new sitcom, *Step by Step*. She also produced and starred in a television movie based on her autobiography.

Somers wrote in her first diet best-seller, *Suzanne Somers' Eat Great, Lose Weight*, that she reached a nutritional turning point at age forty when her struggle to stay slim intensified. That was when she developed her eating plan based on the concept of food combining. In her book she emphasizes the importance of eliminating sugar and foods high in starch, then combining foods to aid in weight loss and digestion. Those who follow the "Somersize" plan stop eating what she calls Funky Foods, all sugars from white and brown sugar to corn syrup, molasses, and honey along with maple syrup, beets, and carrots. Starches to avoid are anything made with white or semolina flour, pasta or couscous, white rice, corn, popcorn, sweet and white potatoes, pumpkin, winter squashes, and bananas. She also cautions again eating nuts, olives, liver, avocados, coconuts, low-fat or whole milk, and any tofu or soy milk. Her plan also eliminates caffeine and alcohol, except in cooking, which burns off the alcohol but leaves the flavor behind.

The rest of the food choices are separated into "Somersized food groups" for mixing and matching. Somers maintains that when proteins and carbohydrates are eaten together, their enzymes create a halt in the digestion process and cause weight gain. She says her book is different from similar high-protein diet programs, such as The Zone, Sugar Busters!, and the Atkins diet, because those plans encourage dieters to eat animal proteins and fats, as long as very few carbohydrates are eaten. Somers's plan does allow such carbohydrates as whole-grain bread, cereal, and pasta but never at the same meal as proteins and fats. In *Eat, Cheat and Melt the Fat Away* she praises Atkins for having "the courage to take on the medical establishment and, in doing so, has paved the way for a new way of thinking."

Critics of Somers's plan, however, don't see many differences between it and the other high-protein diet programs. The American Institute for Cancer Research (AICR), cautions that the high amounts of cholesterol and saturated fat prescribed in these protein-packed eating plans increases the risk of heart disease and possibly some cancers. There is also recent evidence that a diet featuring excessive protein may leach valuable calcium from the bones. A 1997 AICR report, *Food, Nutrition and the Prevention of Cancer: A Global Perspective,* identified numerous studies possibly linking a high fat intake with increased risk of several cancers and other chronic diseases.

Pleased with her own weight-loss success, the actress has made several workout videos as well. More recently, Somers drew criticism for disclosing that she underwent liposuction following treatment for breast cancer. Her cancer was discovered in April 2000 during a routine mammogram. Doctors performed a lumpectomy and followed with radiation treatments. Somers told radio and TV personality Larry King during an interview the following April that the liposuction was performed to counteract the effects of swelling from radiation.

During the interview she also admitted rejecting conventional follow-up chemotherapy for an alternative treatment of daily Iscador injections, an herb made from mistletoe. And in an April 30, 2001, *People* magazine story, Somers's doctor, Melvin J. Silverstein, voiced concern over her decision not to undergo chemotherapy and advised her to give up the plant-based estrogen he says she takes to replace hormones lost because of menopause. Conventional medical wisdom, he says, holds that estrogen speeds up the growth of cancer cells. However, Somers was quoted in that same article as saying her decision to stay on the estrogen was prompted by "a gut feeling." Her doctors report that she is currently cancer free. But for the woman who built a fortune on diet and fitness, any future health concerns or unorthodox treatment plans will have doctors, nutritionists, and her fans paying close attention.

See also:

Somersizing.

Additional Reading

Breu, Giovanna. "Let the Patient Beware: Cancer Expert Barrie Cassileth Warns That Alternative Treatments May Pose Serious Dangers." *People Weekly*, 30 April 2001, 77.
Newsmakers 2000. Issue 1. Detroit: Gale Group, 2000.
Pierce, Ellise. "On Tour with Suzanne Somers." *People Weekly*, 3 March 1997, 42.
Quinn, Judy. "Science of Sugar Brings Sweet Diet Book Sales." *Publishers Weekly*, 246, no. 31 (2 August 1999): 21.
Schneider, Karen S., and Elizabeth Leonard. "A Matter of Choice: Coping with Breast Cancer and the Controversy Over her Unorthodox Treatment Plan, Suzanne Somers Faces the Future with Serene Self-Assurance." *People Weekly*, 30 April 2001, 72–78.
Wolfson, Nancy. "The Suzanne Somers Diet." *Good Housekeeping*, July 2000, 110–12.

Somersizing

Somersizing, the weight-loss and lifestyle plan created by actress Suzanne Somers, focuses on the principles of food combining, not on counting calories or weighing and measuring fat grams or foods. The actress published her plan in her first best-selling diet book, *Suzanne Somers' Eat Great, Lose Weight*. Since its publication in 1997, she has gone on to write several other million-dollar diet books. The plan is low in sugar and carbohydrates but permits many types of fruits when eaten on an empty stomach. It also allows dieters to combine vegetables with proteins and fats, but never proteins and fats with carbohydrates. Somers maintains that her plan is far healthier than other anti-carbohydrate plans, which encourage dieters to eat animal proteins and fats, as long as very few carbohydrates are eaten. Somers's plan does allow whole-grain bread, cereal, and pasta, but never at the same meal as proteins and fats.

The seven Somersizing steps include: eliminate what she calls Funky Foods, described below; eat fruits alone and on an empty stomach; eat proteins and fats with vegetables; eat carbohydrates with vegetables but no fat; keep proteins and fats separate from carbohydrates; wait three hours between meals if switching from a meal of proteins and fats to a carbohydrate meal or vice versa; and eat three meals a day and eat until comfortably full. A sample menu would include a cheese omelet for breakfast then a carbohydrate and vegetable lunch of whole-grain pasta and plain tomato and basil sauce with a cucumber tomato salad without dressing. The afternoon snack would be fruit followed three hours later by a dinner of proteins and fats, such as roast chicken with sausage stuffing and gravy, along with steamed vegetables and salad.

Funky Foods, according to Somers, include all sugars from white and brown sugar to corn syrup, molasses, and honey, along with maple syrup, beets, and carrots. Starches to avoid are anything made with white or semolina flour, pasta or couscous, white rice, corn, popcorn, sweet and white potatoes, pumpkin, winter squashes, and bananas. She also cautions again eating nuts, olives, liver, avocados, coconuts, low-fat or whole milk, and any tofu or soy milk. And Somersizing means no caffeine and alcohol, except in cooking, which burns off the alcohol but leaves the flavor behind.

Critics of the Somers plan say it closely resembles other high-protein, low-calorie diets like Protein Power, Dr. Atkins's New Diet Revolution, and the New Beverly Hills Diet. The American Institute for Cancer Research (AICR), cautions that the high amounts of cholesterol and saturated fat prescribed in these protein-packed eating plans increases the risk of heart disease and possibly some cancers. There is also recent evidence that a diet featuring excessive protein may leach valuable calcium from the bones. A 1997 AICR report, *Food, Nutrition and the Prevention of Cancer: A Global Perspective,* identified numerous studies possibly linking a high fat intake with increased risk of several cancers and other chronic diseases.

Critics also disagree with Somers's claim that when proteins and carbohydrates are eaten together their enzymes interrupt the digestive process. The fact is that the human body contains many different enzymes and each of them are specifically keyed to individual proteins, carbohydrates, and fats. Nutritionists say these enzymes do not cancel each other out because they remain in different areas of the digestive tract. The AICR and other health organizations argue that food combinations have no nutritional basis and amount to magical thinking. Dr. Diana Schwarzbein, who provided much of the scientific data used by Somers in her books, recognizes that the effectiveness of food combining has not been established in medical or nutritional studies. She writes in the forward to *Suzanne Somers' Eat, Cheat and Melt the Fat Away,* that while she supports Somersizing, "her [Somers's] thoughts on food combining are outside the scope of my own research."

Like other fad diets, Somers's eating plan, if followed over an extended period of time, can lead to an unbalanced diet and give rise to health risks, critics say. By restricting carbohydrates, dieters fail to ingest enough fiber; as a result, they may experience constipation and other gastrointestinal difficulties, as well as running the obvious risks from high amounts of cholesterol and saturated fat, which may increase their risk of heart disease and possibly some cancers. Another concern among nutrition specialists is that Somers does not emphasize the need for portion control or increased exercise. Nutritionists recommend that any long-term program of weight loss and maintenance include increased exercise and decreased portion sizes to be successful. According to organizations like the AICR, the healthiest food choices for anyone, whether they are overweight or not, include more carbohydrates from plant-based foods and less protein and fat from animal-based foods.

Additional Reading

Eberle, Girard. "Go Ahead, Order the Combo Plate: The Rules of Food Combining Are an Unforgiving Master, But Is That Tangerine After Lunch Really Evil Incarnate?" *Women's Sports and Fitness*, 19, no. 5 (June 1997): 78–80.

Quinn, Judy. "Science of Sugar Brings Sweet Diet Book Sales." *Publishers Weekly*, 246, no. 31 (2 August 1999) :21.

Scheider, Karen S., and Elizabeth Leonard. "A Matter of Choice: Coping with Breast Cancer and the Controversy Over Her Unorthodox Treatment Plan, Suzanne Somers Faces the Future with Serene Self-assurance." *People Weekly*, 30 April 2001, 72–78.

Somers, Suzanne. *After the Fall: How I Picked Myself Up, Dusted Myself Off, and Started All Over Again*. New York: Crown, 1998.

———. *Suzanne Somers' Eat, Cheat and Melt the Fat Away*. New York: Random House, 2001.

Wolfson, Nancy. "The Suzanne Somers Diet." *Good Housekeeping*, July 2000, 110–12.

Starch Blockers

Starch blockers are a so-called miracle weight-loss cure that claims to block the absorption of starches or carbohydrates. The theory behind starch blockers, an extract made from a protein in various beans, is simple. Essentially an enzyme in the beans prevents the breakdown of starch molecules. This, according to their manufacturers, allows dieters to lose weight even as they fill up on pizza, pasta, and bread. Starch blockers were marketed heavily in the 1970s but were finally forced off drugstore shelves by the Food and Drug Administration (FDA) in 1983, when the FDA ordered more than 200 manufacturers and distributors to stop selling the pills pending further investigation into their long-term effects.

The FDA made its ruling after receiving more than 100 reports of problems associated with starch blockers, side effects ranging from abdominal pain and diarrhea to vomiting and other extreme reactions. Problems developed with the pills when undigested starch ended up being dumped into the colon. And while dieters suffered no permanent damage, they did not enjoy permanent weight loss either.

Following the FDA ruling, there was a flurry of legal wrangling between the government and starch blocker manufacturers as they sued to get the ban overturned. At one point the FDA seized a shipment of starch blocker pills valued at $480,000, as some distributors attempted to defy the government ban on their sale.

The manufacturers argued that the pills were food supplements and did not need to be proven safe and effective under the law. However, the FDA pushed to classify the pills as a drug, meaning the product was intended to affect the function of the body and anything labeled a drug falls under government purview. At that time there were only two categories of products—food or drugs. Now, following the passage of the Dietary Supplement Health and Education Act of 1994, manufacturers have another category for products, that of dietary supplement.

Critics of the pills include health organizations, such as the American Medical Association (AMA). Physicians with the AMA's Department of Foods and Nutrition, quoted in *Newsweek*, stated that there are no clinical studies that prove starch blockers actually help people lose weight. In fact, researchers suspect that starch blockers do not work for two possible reasons. Either the protein-digesting enzyme breaks down the bean extract before it can act to block the starch, or there are more enzymes secreted than needed and they lead to carbohydrate absorption in spite of the starch blocker. Either way, scientists, nutritionists, and health care professionals say pills like starch blockers or fat blockers continue to cast doubt over the credibility of the dietary supplements industry.

See also:

Dietary Supplement Health and Education Act (DSHEA); fat blockers.

Additional Reading

Barrett, Stephen, M.D. "Be Wary of Calorie-Blockers." www.quackwatch.com. Accessed 10 June 2003.

Biddle, Wayne, and Margot Slade. "FDA Outlaws 'Starch Blockers.'" *New York Times,* 4 July 1982, E9.

Seligmann, Jean. "Starch Blockers: How Safe?" *Newsweek,* 12 July 1982, 83.

Sugar Busters!

Sugar Busters! makes this attention-grabbing point: "Sugar is toxic." Not in the sense that sugar can kill you instantly. But the four authors, three of whom are MDs, argue that significant amounts of refined sugar can cause digestive and metabolic problems, as well as being a major factor in weight gain. That is because sugar stimulates production of the hormone insulin. Insulin regulates blood sugar levels but overproduction of insulin causes the body to store excess sugar as fat and stimulates the liver to make cholesterol.

Sugar Busters! is the name of the *New York Times* number-one best-seller, authored by H. Leighton Steward, Morrison C. Bethea, MD, Sam S. Andrews, MD, and Luis A. Balart, MD. Sugar Busters menu options are available at some restaurants. The underlying principle is that sugar contributes to weight gain and overall poor health. The authors point out that refined sugar became a part of the diet only around the 1700s and in the past century our consumption of it has grown exponentially. In 1980, Americans consumed 124.6 pounds of sugar per year and in 1994, that figure was up to 149.2 pounds. "Sugar just may be the number-one culprit in lowering quality of life and causing premature death," the authors state. However, their sugar-busting doesn't stop at the sugar jar on the kitchen counter. Since carbohydrates are turned into sugars in the body, some carbohydrates are to be avoided on this diet plan. In particular, Sugar Busters requires you to avoid potatoes, corn, white rice, bread from refined flour, beets, carrots, refined sugar, corn syrup, molasses, honey, sugared colas, and beer.

Instead, the Sugar Busters menu encourages eating high-protein foods, such as meats, nuts, and some vegetables. Because these high-protein foods supply very little glucose to the body, the liver biosynthesizes glucose in a process called gluconeogenesis. Glucagon is a hormone that stimulates the mobilization of previously stored fat cells.

The fundamental point of Sugar Busters is that sugary foods, including many carbohydrates, promote production of insulin, which causes the body to store excess sugar as fat, while protein foods prompt the body to use up previously stored fat cells.

The book contains a 14-day menu and various recipes, developed at New Orleans restaurants, following the principles of the plan. The menu typically calls for a whole-grain cereal or hot oatmeal for breakfast. Lunch is often a sandwich on whole-grain bread with meat, lettuce, tomato, and mayonnaise. Dinners are grilled or baked meat, such as pork tenderloin, salmon or other fish, chicken, veal, steak, or lamp chops. These are generally accompanied by a whole-wheat pasta, brown rice, salads, and fresh steamed vegetables. Suggested drinks are limited to milk, water, tea, coffee, and diet drinks. Desserts are on the menu about every other night, and are typically a dozen almonds or other nuts, two thin slices of cheese, sugar-free ice cream or frozen yogurt, or a Sugar Busters chocolate mousse recipe.

Throughout the book, the foods that raise the most concern are sugary or high-carbohydrate foods. The authors dispute the "myths" surrounding traditional weight-loss regimens, discounting the dangers of fats and foods high in cholesterol, contending that calorie counting isn't necesssary, and even downplaying the role that exercise plays in weight control. While they acknowledge that most Americans eat a diet too high in saturated fats, they make the point of distinguishing among different types of fat. While they agree that very high cholesterol levels are "significantly related" to coronary artery disease, they don't believe that total cholesterol alone is a reliable indicator for the risk of heart disease. About calories, they write, "Our view is that calories per se are not as important as the types of food we eat…What we do know is that normal, even significant, amounts of the proper types of food can be consumed for indefinite periods without causing weight gain." And exercise, while good for the body, isn't necessary for weight loss.

The book and the Web site (www. sugarbusters.com) contain plenty of success stories, from overweight noninsulin-dependent diabetics who lost weight and were able to control their diabetes with diet alone, to people who were unable to control their weight through any other diet plan. In fact, short of serious athletes or exercise "fanatics," who need higher levels of sugary foods for immediate energy, the authors say this food-choice lifestyle will work for anyone.

However, the Sugar Busters plan has its critics. The Physicians Committee for Responsible Medicine gives the book only two stars out of a possible five, rating it "not satisfactory." The group states that Sugar Busters "menus are low in fiber and high in fat and cholesterol with cheese, eggs, butter, yogurt, and cream not restricted in the meal plans. These foods squeeze out others that are higher in fiber and lower in fat."

Some dietitians and endocrinologists have suggested that the reason people lose weight on the Sugar Busters plan is that they limit overall calories, not insulin production. They argue that the body does not distinguish between carbohydrates from milk and carbohydrates from chocolate bars. And the downside of the plan is that the high-in-fat, low-in-fiber menu options limit variety, the basis of a healthy diet.

Additional Reading

Gorman, Christine. "Sugar Busters! What You Should Know About the New Diets That Blame Insulin, Not Calories, for Your Extra Girth." *Time,* 6 July 1998, 1.

Grieger, Lynn. "Sugar Busters—Truth or Bust?" *Nutrition Guide,* 27 May 1999.

Kenney, Jay. "Do Potatoes Inhibit Weight Loss?" *Communicating Food for Health,* January 1999, 1–5.

Steward, H. Leighton, Morrison C. Bethea, Sam S. Andrews, and Luis A. Balart. *Sugar Busters!* New York: Ballantine Publishing Group, 1998.

"Sugar Myths—A Trick or Treat." American Dietetic Association Web site, http://www.eatright.org. Accessed 12 June 2003.

T-Factor Diet

The T-Factor diet, written in 1989 by Dr. Martin Katahn, calls itself a scientific breakthrough and promises dieters they can lose weight safely and quickly without cutting back or counting calories. The thermogenic effect, or "T-factor," according to Katahn, is the way the body generates heat by burning carbohydrates, fats, and proteins at different rates. The author points to studies that he says suggest that fat in the diet turns into body fat more easily than do carbohydrates. By getting dieters to eat a much higher proportion of carbohydrates to fats, Katahn maintains that, over time, without extra fat coming in, excess pounds will simply melt away. In other words, eat less fat, store less fat, and lose weight.

In his book, *The T-Factor 2000 Diet,* Katahn tells dieters that the source of calories eaten is more important than the total number of calories taken in. He instructs dieters to choose foods that naturally maximize the T-factor level and activate what he calls the body's hidden fat-burning potential. This simply means dieters must choose low-fat foods instead of fat-laden favorites; choose a baked potato instead of french fries.

The diet itself earns high marks for being well balanced, with plenty of fruits, vegetables, and whole grains. Yet critics point to the plan's strictness, saying it is too difficult to follow, since it recommends that only 15 to 20 percent of daily calories come from fat. Other low-fat, high-fiber diets, like the eating plans by Dr. Dean Ornish, Dr. John McDougall, and Nathan Pritkin, have been criticized for being too difficult to follow because they are also very low in fat. Americans traditionally consume closer to 40 percent of their calories as fat and nutritionists note that many people have difficulty dropping that to the newest American Heart Association recommendation of a 30 percent level.

The T-factor formula for weight loss is 20 to 40 grams of fat per day for women and 30 to 60 grams of fat per day for men. People wishing to lose weight quickly should cut their fat intake to the bottom limit of the recommended range—20 grams of fat for women and 30 grams of fat for men. Katahn also tells dieters to compensate for the reduction of fat in their diet with "whatever increase in carbohydrate foods feels good and satisfies your appetite." The book offers lists of fruits, vegetables, and grain foods that have little or no fat and can be eaten in unlimited amounts, as well as a fat substitution guide that suggests that dieters substitute foods like ground turkey for ground beef, bouillon for fatty sauces, skim milk for whole milk or cream, and water chestnuts for nuts in some dishes.

Sample menus in the book are basic and easy to follow. Breakfast for a typical day includes a banana or fresh fruit, dry cereal, 1 cup of skim milk, and coffee or tea, for a fat total of 3 grams. Lunch weighs in at 4 grams, with half a cup of cottage cheese, assorted raw vegetables, 5 whole-wheat crackers, and fresh fruit. Dinner includes up to 10 grams of fat with a small serving of baked chicken, brown or wild rice, a tossed salad with fat free dressing, and fruit. Snacks are plain, nonfat yogurt, fresh fruit, or low-fat crackers. This particular example adds up to a daily total of 20 grams of fat.

The T-Factor Diet was published a few years after Katahn's best seller *The Rotation Diet* in 1986. That diet, which measures calories, instructed women to complete a dieting cycle by eating 600, 900, and then 1,200 calories per day in rotation. But Katahn writes in his diet book that the T-factor plan is an improvement over his earlier effort. "When I created the Rotation Diet, I was unaware of the direct relationship between the fat content of your body and the fat content of your diet." He adds that the rotation plan, "unfortunately failed many people in maintenance," and also did not adequately stress the importance of continuing to control fat intake when dieters reached goal weight.

The T-Factor diet, like the Rotation Diet was heavily promoted in Katahn's hometown of Nashville, although the T-factor program fell short of the earlier rotation craze. In 1986, the author had the entire city "rotating," as some 75,000 residents collectively dieted to shed 1 million pounds in twelve weeks as part of a "Melt-a-Million" program sponsored by the Nashville Kroger grocery stores.

Katahn also includes what he calls "an advance over the Rotation Diet," a concept called the Quick Melt, where dieters can get the quick weight loss they desire by following the T-Factor diet and then cutting calories. In this way, he writes, "By cutting calories, not just substituting carbohydrates for fat, you create a deficit that pulls even more fat from your fat cells." The menus he provides have a daily calorie count for women of 1,100 to 1,300 and 1,600 to 1,800 calories for men. However, the rotation theory is absent from the Quick Melt and dieters are not instructed to vary calorie intake to prevent their metabolism from slowing down, as they were in the rotation plan. Instead, they are cautioned to add calories back slowly and to increase exercise after such a restricted diet to prevent any rapid weight gain.

However, unlike the Rotation diet, the T-factor book does devote a chapter to the importance of exercise in weight loss and in maintaining that loss. The author divides activities into "carb burners" and "fat burners." The carbohydrate-burning activities are what he calls start-stop choices like tennis, football, or calisthenics classes. The steady-state activities, or fat burners, require continuous whole-body movement like jogging and swimming and, according to Katahn, these aerobic activities burn fat more efficiently. The author lost 75 pounds on his diet and during that time became a strong supporter of daily exercise as a way to achieve fitness and a healthy weight.

See also:

McDougall Program; Ornish, Dean; Pritikin, Nathan; Rotation Diet.

Additional Reading

Katahn, Martin, Ph.D. *The Rotation Diet.* New York: W. W. Norton & Company, 1986.
———. *The T-Factor Diet.* New York: W. W. Norton & Company, 1989.
———. *The T-Factor 2000 Diet.* New York: W. W. Norton & Company, 1999.
"Successful Weight Loss Includes an Understanding of Thermogenesis." *Better Nutrition,* 58, no. 3 (March 1996): 12.
"The T-Factor Diet." *Tufts University Diet & Nutrition Letter,* 7, no. 6 (August 1989): 6.
Toufexis, Anastasia. "Hey, Are You Rotating?" *Time,* 14 April 1986, 108.

TOPS, Take Off Pounds Sensibly

TOPS, Take Off Pounds Sensibly, founded in 1948 by Milwaukee housewife Esther Manz, was the first of the weight-watching organizations to successfully advocate the use of praise for weight loss. According to the organization's official Web site, TOPS was born around a kitchen table when Manz and three other women gathered to support each other in an effort to lose weight for health reasons. There are now some 10,500 chapters, located in the United States and in Canada. Manz saw obesity as a disease and believed sufferers should not face their problem alone. She conceived of the idea of a mutually helpful group, much like the support meetings of Alcoholics Anonymous. Years later, Overeaters Anonymous began, another nonprofit organization that offers group support and recommends seeing a doctor or health professional for an eating plan. According to its Web page, TOPS does endorse a standard exchange diet like the one offered by Weight Watchers, Inc.

TOPS differs from the Weight Watchers program, founded in 1963, in several significant ways. With its brand-name diet foods and other products Weight Watchers, Inc., is a profitable business. However, TOPS remains a nonprofit and noncommercial group. Leaders are volunteers and each chapter is designed to offer individuals support, encouragement, and educational opportunities that focus on healthy eating and lifestyles.

Members who reach their goal weight become honored KOPS, Keep Off Pounds Sensibly. Any TOPS money left over from member dues is used for research into the causes of obesity. The group has contributed over $4 million to obesity research, much of it to the TOPS Center for Metabolic Research at the Medical College of Wisconsin, which includes the Esther Manz Laboratory and the Ronald K. Kalkhoff Library. The late Dr. Kalkhoff was TOPS' original medical advisor. Manz, the organization's founder, died at age 88 in 1996.

See also:

Overeaters Anonymous; Weight Watchers.

Target Heart Rate

Fitness experts refer to a target heart rate—an optimum number of beats per minute—during aerobic exercises. There are several ways to figure out your target heart rate—and online calculators that can help determine it—but they're based on figuring out your maximum heart rate and working at about 75–80 percent of that. The prevalent formula for figuring out your maximum heart rate is subtracting your age from 220. So a 20-year-old would have a maximum heart rate of 200 (220–20) and a target heart rate of 160. A 40-year-old would have a maximum heart rate of 180 (220–40) and a target heart rate of 146. But these are ballpark figures and may not be useful if you are not "average"—either quite sedentary or extremely fit.

So use these numbers as a general guide. If you can't maintain an exercise routine at your "target" heart rate, slow down. You shouldn't push yourself to exhaustion—essentially your maximum heart rate. But you do need to push yourself at least hard enough to get your heart pumping. A minimum heart rate for exercise could be considered one-half of your maximum heart rate. Therefore, the 20-year-old, with the maximum heart rate of 200, should be exercising at a level that at least brings the heart rate up to 100. Remember, the target is around 160.

How do you know your heart rate? The least expensive way is to measure it yourself or have a friend do it for you. Place your index and middle finger over the pulse—the inside of your wrist. Count the number of beats in a 10-second interval and multiply by 6 to get your heart rate per minute. Take the pulse as soon as you finish exercising or even in the middle of a workout. Your heart rate begins to slow down quickly as soon as you stop exerting yourself.

To get the maximum benefit from your exercise routines, the American College of Sports Medicine recommends exercising at an intensity of 60–90 percent of your target heart rate for 20 to 60 minutes, three to five days a week. This doesn't mean taking a brisk hour-long walk every day. Exercise intervals can be as short as ten minutes to get the benefit. Just do them three times a day or more.

Tarnower, Herman

Herman Tarnower (b. March 18, 1910, in New York; murdered March 10, 1980) was a physician and cardiologist who achieved worldwide fame on the basis of his book *The Complete Scarsdale Medical Diet* (1978). By the time of Tarnower's death in 1980, over 2 million copies of his book had been sold. The Scarsdale diet and the 1973 Dr. Atkins's Diet Revolution were forerunners of the high-protein, low-carbohydrate regimens popular in newer diets like The Zone and Protein Power. Tarnower said in his book that his diet's success came from a metabolic change brought on when dieters restricted carbohydrates and filled up on protein.

An internist and cardiologist for over forty years, Tarnower never followed the diet himself but he did counsel heart patients about losing weight. The actual Scarsdale diet began as a list he created of good and bad foods for his patients. Over the years the list was passed by word of mouth until friends from the publishing business suggested that Tarnower write a book selling his diet to a larger audience. He worked with Samm Sinclair Baker, author of the popular *Dr. Stillman's 14-Day Shape-up Program*. The Scarsdale book included recipes, successful case histories, and Tarnower's thoughts on weight, eating, and health.

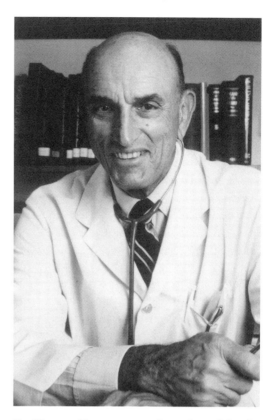

Dr. Herman Tarnower was the author of the diet book, *The Complete Scarsdale Medical Diet,* a high-protein, low-carbohydrate plan he wrote with Samm Sinclair Baker. The book became an instant best-seller and dieters were losing up to 20 pounds per week on the plan. Tarnower dedicated the book to his close friend Jean Harris who was later convicted of his murder. At the time of his death in 1980, over 2 million copies of his book had been sold. (© Bettmann/CORBIS)

Tarnower, the son of Jewish immigrants Dora and Harry Tarnower, received his MD degree in 1933 from Syracuse University in New York and completed his internship and residency in internal medicine at Bellevue Hospital in New York. He traveled abroad in 1936 and 1937 on a New York Academy of Medicine fellowship and following World War II was selected as one of only two doctors to head a study of the possible aftereffects of radiation suffered by Japanese civilians in Nagasaki and Hiroshima. He was a founder and senior staff member of the Scarsdale Medical Group and was a clinical professor of medicine from 1975 until his death at the New York Medical College in New York City.

A bachelor described as a balding man of medium height, Tarnower died at the hands of Jean S. Harris, a longtime companion whom he credited with helping research and write the Scarsdale diet book. At the time of the shooting, the fifty-six-year-old Harris was headmistress of the Madeira School, a prominent private high school for girls in the Washington, D.C., area. During her trial Harris maintained that she meant to take her own life but Tarnower grabbed the gun and it went off, striking him as he attempted to wrestle it from her.

Newspaper accounts of the murder depict Harris as a jilted lover, angry over Tarnower's relationship with his nurse, Lynn Dryfaros. Tarnower had been shot four times when police found him lying on the bedroom floor. Harris was arrested minutes later, leaving the scene in her car. She was tried and convicted of second-degree murder and sentenced to fifteen years to life at the Bedford Hills Correctional Facility, a maximum-security prison in New York. She was the author of two books during her incarceration and was finally pardoned in 1992 by New York Governor Mario Cuomo.

See also:

Atkins Nutritional Approach; Scarsdale Diet; The Zone.

Additional Reading

Biographical Directory of the American College of Physicians. New York: R. R. Bowker Co., 1979.

Feron, James. "Scarsdale Diet Doctor is Slain; Headmistress is Charged." New York Times, 12 March 1980, A1.

Trilling, Diana. Mrs. Harris: The Death of the Scarsdale Diet Doctor. New York: Harcourt Brace Jovanovich, 1981.

Trans Fatty Acids

Trans fatty acids are just about everywhere in the typical American diet. They are created through the hydrogenation process that turns liquid oils into stick margarines or shortening and they are used in foods like crackers, cookies, and doughnuts. They make pie crusts flakier and french fries crispier. Trans fats are helpful to food manufacturers because they increase the shelf life and flavor stability of products. Unfortunately, gram for gram they may be even more damaging than saturated fat. In other words, french fries cooked in partially hydrogenated vegetable shortening have as much artery-clogging potential as potatoes fried in lard or beef tallow.

Although nutritionists are still studying how a diet high in trans fats compares to one heavy in saturated fats, there is growing concern that those trans fats may be raising concentrations of the so-called bad form of cholesterol, or LDL, in the body while lowering levels of HDL, the good cholesterol, setting the stage for heart disease. In 1993 investigators from Harvard reported the results of a study using female nurses. Even after accounting for other heart disease risk factors, women who consumed the most trans fatty acids had one and a half times more heart attacks than those who consumed the least trans fat. A 1994 Harvard study of men also found that those who ate large amounts of trans fats had more than twice the number of heart attacks as men who ate small amounts.

Unfortunately, trans fats are nearly invisible to consumers because food labels list the amount of saturated fat per serving, but not the trans fat. That's due in part to the continuing debate and delay over a proposed law that would require food manufacturers to list the percentage of trans fat in their foods. The Food and Drug Administration (FDA) has been considering this change in label requirements for fat since 1999 when controversy arose over its specifics. Groups like the Center for Science in the Public Interest (CSPI) petitioned the FDA for the label change so consumers would see how much artery-clogging fat was in different products. Even though the measure has stalled for years, the FDA declared in a 2002 statement that reaching a final decision on the trans fatty acid rule remains a top priority for the agency.

As it stands the rule would require processors to list the number of grams of trans fats and then to combine it with the grams of saturated fat on food labels. The FDA would also require manufacturers to list the specific amount of trans fatty acids per serving. The American Dietetic Association (ADA) has publicly supported this proposal but opposes the efforts to combine the trans and saturated fat into one category. The ADA said this might lead consumers to believe that trans fats are saturated fats, an idea they say is scientifically inaccurate and misleading.

The strongest opposition to the rule comes from groups like the National Frozen Pizza Institute (NFPI). In a statement the NFPI called the rule premature, since no consensus exists on the effects of trans fatty acids on heart health. The NFPI criticized the proposal, arguing, "The FDA has offered no consumer research showing that labeling of trans fatty acids will help achieve this goal" of a healthier diet.

Until food labels list grams of trans fat, consumers trying to avoid them in foods can follow several suggestions: read ingredients lists and stay away from products with the words "partially hydrogenated oil" (if this is one of the first ingredients listed, the product likely has lots of trans fat); when buying margarines and spreads, the softer the spread the lower in trans fats; use olive or canola oil instead of butter, margarine, or shortening whenever possible; avoid deep-fried foods; buy and eat low-fat foods, since the lower the fat per serving, the lower the trans fat will be; shop in natural-food stores whenever possible, since the majority of their product lines are trans-free; read labels and look for hidden trans fats in all kinds of foods, including whole-wheat breads and peanut butters, prepared mixes for muffins, cakes, and cookies, and boxes of macaroni and cheese.

The wide variety of names and types of fats continues to confuse American consumers. Basically, different categories of fats get their names from their patterns of hydrogen atoms. All fatty acids, which make up fats, contain chains of carbon atoms, with hydrogen atoms attached to some or all of the carbon atoms. Fats with one double bond are called monounsaturated; those with more double bonds are called polyunsaturated. Both monounsaturated and polyunsaturated fats are considered good fats by nutritionists. Good fats, the heart-healthy kind, include olive oil, canola oil, walnut oil, peanut oil, nuts, and avocados plus omega-3 fatty acids from fatty fish. These fats provide the HDL or high-density lipoprotein cholesterol that protects artery walls by carrying away the LDL cholesterol back to the liver, where it is excreted into the intestines and out of the body.

Saturated fats, those found in animal fats, palm oil, and processed foods like margarine and pastries, don't have what scientists call double bonds. Saturated fats, considered the bad fats, promote high blood-cholesterol levels because they encourage the body to make more LDL cholesterol than it normally does. These LDL or low-density lipoproteins, damage artery linings and form deposits on artery walls, eventually slowing blood flow.

When early research linked saturated fats to a variety of health problems like heart disease, high blood pressure, and diabetes, consumers switched to unsaturated fat products, going from butter to margarine. At first, trans fatty acids, because they contain a type of unsaturated fatty acid, were not considered a health risk. But nutritionists now say studies show that when vegetable oils are changed into semisolid or solid substances, those newly created trans fats act like saturated fats, or worse, and increase the blood level of LDL.

With so many confusing categories of fats, consumers look to health organizations like the ADA and the FDA for recommendations on healthy eating. According to a 2002 article in *The Journal of the American Dietetic Association*, the 1995 Dietary Guidelines for Americans recognized that based on research released in a 1993 National Cholesterol Education Program Pubication, trans-fatty acids may raise blood cholesterol levels. The newest updated Dietary Guidelines, 2000, contain a stronger recommendation including the following statement that urges Americans to moderate trans-fat consumption. "Foods high in trans fatty acids tend to raise blood cholesterol. These foods include those high in partially hydrogenated vegetable oils, such as hard margarines and shortenings. Foods with a high amount of these ingredients include some commercially fried foods and some bakery goods."

Food producers, especially in Europe, are working on ways to lower the trans fat content of foods by diluting hydrogenated oil with liquid or by avoiding hydrogenation altogether. A research team with the USDA is also experimenting with hydrogenated soybean oil, using a solvent known as supercritical carbon dioxide. They have reported that their method has produced hydrogenated oils that are solid enough for use in foods, like margarine, but with lower amounts of trans fats. Although this new technique is more expensive, it could create products with less than 10 percent trans fatty acid content, a level that everyone agrees would be more healthful for consumers. And health associations like the ADA hope that as more data comes to light about health problems associated with trans fats, food manufacturers may even voluntarily replace trans fats with better, newer ingredients. The ADA also estimates that if the FDA's new labeling proposal is passed, in the first decade alone it would prevent from 7,000 to 17,000 cases of coronary heart disease and avert over 5,000 deaths annually by helping consumers translate food label information on fats into healthier food choices.

See also:

cholesterol; dietary fat; Dietary Guidelines for Americans.

Additional Reading

Dausch, Judith G. "Trans-Fatty Acids: A Regulatory Update." *Journal of the American Dietetic Association*, 102, no. 1 (January 2002): 18–20.

Gorman, Jessica. "New Studies Add to These Fats' Image Problem." *Science News*, 10 November 2001, 300–302.

"Headless FDA Begins 2002 with Broad Agenda." *Food Chemical News*, 43, no. 47 (7 January 2002): 3.

"Heart-Healthy Eating." *Harvard Heart Letter,* 11, no. 2 (October 2000), 00279002.

McCord, Holly, and Gloria McVeigh. "How to Shop Trans-Free." *Prevention,* April 2000, 70.

Wootan, Margo, Bonnie Liebman, and Wendie Rosofsky. "Trans: The Phantom Fat." *Nutrition Action Healthletter,* 23, no. 7 (September 1996): 1–6.

Television

Why is there an entry on television in this volume? For the simple reason that watching television might be related to childhood obesity and overall poor quality diets. A study published in the June 2002 issue of *Pediatrics,* the journal of the American Academy of Pediatrics, found that young children who had televisions in their bedrooms were more likely to be overweight than those who did not. About 40 percent of the children in the study had a television in their room, and these children spent 4.6 hours more per week watching TV/video than children without a TV in their bedroom.

Furthermore, watching television may be linked with an overall decline in the

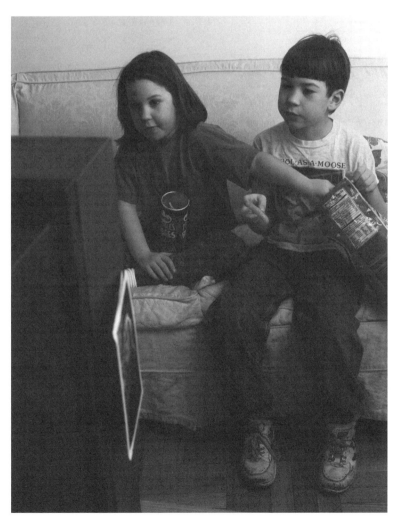

Ten-year-old Nathan and seven-year-old Rachel eat unhealthy food as they watch television. Nutritionists suspect that a steady diet of commercials for fast-food restaurants and unhealthy snacks may be a risk factor for the rapidly growing obesity rates in this country, especially among children and teens. The rising obesity rate among youngsters brings with it an increase in childhood diabetes. Doctors say the incidence of childhood diabetes has doubled during the last two decades. (© Laura Dwight/CORBIS)

quality of the diet. A press release issued by the North American Association for the Study of Obesity noted that, "Children who watched television during dinner and snacked while watching television—practices that are greatly influenced by their parents—consumed less milk, fruits and vegetables than those who turned off the television at dinnertime and didn't snack while watching television."

Other studies have shown that, in older children, body mass index tends to increase along with the number of hours spent watching television.

The number of hours Americans watch television has been creeping upward. According to Census Bureau numbers, in 1993, the average American over eighteen years of age spent 1,535 hours per year watching television. By 1998, that figure had increased to 1,573. The average was expected to increase to 1,610 hours per person per year in 2003.

The authors of the *Pediatrics* study concluded, "This study extends the association between TV viewing and risk of being overweight to younger, preschool-aged children. A TV in the child's bedroom is an even stronger marker of increased risk of being overweight. Because most children watch TV by age 2, educational efforts about limiting child TV/video viewing and keeping the TV out of the child's bedroom need to begin before then."

In a May 2000 press release issued by the Bassett Healthcare Research Institute in Cooperstown, New York, quotes Dennison as saying that children who watched less than 5 hours a week of TV were the least likely to be overweight, while the prevalence of obesity was 37 percent among children who watched 30 hours or more of TV per week.

See also:

childhood obesity; obesity.

Additional Reading

"Bassett Study Reports Early Childhood Obesity Not Recognized By Most Parents." Bassett Healthcare Research Institute press release, 22 May 2000.

Dennison, Barbara A., Tara A. Erb, and Paul L. Jenkins. "Television Viewing and Television in Bedroom Associated with Overweight Risk Among Low-Income Preschool Children." *Pediatrics*, 109, no. 6 (June 2002): 1028–35.

"Watching TV May Be Related to Poor Quality Diet and Increased Risk of Child Obesity." North American Association for the Study of Obesity press release, 10 October 2001.

Vegetarian Diet

A vegetarian diet is a plant-based diet that does not include meats. The number of vegetarians in the United States varies widely, depending on which organization is doing the survey. A 1998 Cornell University news release reported that an estimated 14 million Americans consider themselves vegetarians and about 1 million people adopt a vegetarian diet every year. Yet a Zogby poll in 2000, commissioned by the Vegetarian Resource Group estimated that there are about 4.8 million vegetarian adults (over 18) in the United States. Another 2 percent of youth (aged 6 to 17) also considered themselves vegetarian.

This variety in polling numbers does not indicate a sudden drop in those eating a vegetarian diet, but rather reflects the differing audiences (all Americans as opposed to American adults). It also reflects the variety in vegetarian diets themselves. For example, lacto-ovo-vegetarian, a popular type, describes a diet that includes milk, cheese, yogurt, and eggs. This is easiest in terms of menu planning and you will also find food choices in most restaurants and fast-food restaurants. Those who eat dairy but not eggs are called lacto-vegetarians. Those who eat eggs but no dairy, by contrast, are called ovo-vegetarians. And those who choose to eat no animal products at all are called vegans. Vegan diets are based on vegetables, fruits, grains, legumes, nuts, and seeds, and exclude all meat, fish, poultry, dairy, and eggs. Many vegans are also philosophically opposed to animal products, such as wool, leather, honey, and cosmetics and soaps from animal products. A raw foodist eats uncooked nuts, fruits, vegetables, and sprouted seeds. Fruitarians are people who eat only raw fruits, nuts, and berries. A pollo-vegetarian eats a diet similar to lacto-ovo but incorporates poultry. A pesca-vegetarian eats fish and seafood along with the lacto-ovo diet.

Many nutritionists and doctors acknowledge the health benefits of a plant-based diet when compared to a meat-based diet high in cholesterol and saturated fat. Research shows that, on the whole, vegetarians eat a more healthy diet than nonvegetarians and consume about two to three times as much fiber as their meat-eating counterparts. And a diet high in fiber can actually lower the chances of developing certain cancers, particularly colon cancer, according to the National Cancer Institute.

In fact, the National Cancer Institute, the American Dietetic Association (ADA), the American Heart Association, and the U.S. Department of Health and Human Services now support a well-planned vegetarian diet and its associated health benefits. The ADA stated in a 1997 position paper, "Appropriately planned vegetarian diets are healthful, are nutritionally adequate, and provide health benefits in the prevention and treatment of certain diseases." The paper also stated that vegetarian diets have been used successfully to reverse severe coronary artery disease as well as offer protective benefits from hypertension and some cancers.

But health concerns are not the only reason that young adults give for changing their diets. Some make the choice out of concern for animal rights. When faced with the statistic that some 90 percent of animals raised as food live in confinement, many teens give up meat to protest those conditions. Others turn to vegetarianism to support the environment. Meat production uses vast amounts of water, land, grain, and energy while creating problems with animal waste and subsequent pollution. It takes more than three times as much fossil fuel to feed a meat eater as it does to feed a person who eats no meat or dairy products, according to EarthSave, an organization founded in 1988 to educate people about the environmental benefits of a plant-based diet. Whatever the reason you choose to become a vegetarian, your choice brings with it questions from parents about your health and nutrition. By becoming an educated vegetarian, you can achieve good nutrition as well as support a more humane and ecological world and do your part to reduce global hunger.

A vegetarian diet does not have to be bland, brown, and boring. The plant kingdom is a multicolored world of crunchy, chewy, creamy, and meaty textures. From portabello mushrooms to polenta, from summer corn to seitan, there are wonderful tastes to try. In fact, you are already familiar with many basic and classic meatless dishes: eggplant parmesan, spaghetti with marinara sauce, pasta with pesto sauce,

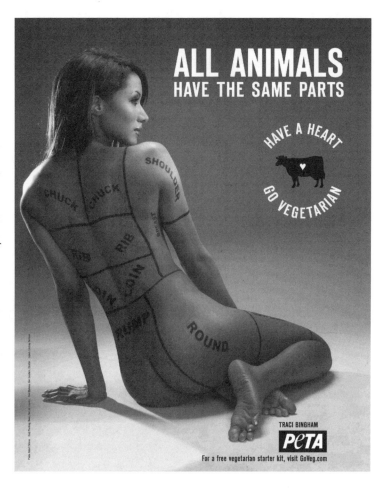

ALL ANIMALS HAVE THE SAME PARTS

HAVE A HEART
GO VEGETARIAN

SHOULDER

CHUCK   CHUCK

RIB

LOIN

RUMP

ROUND

TRACI BINGHAM

PeTA

For a free vegetarian starter kit, visit GoVeg.com

Ex-*Baywatch* babe Tracy Bingham strips naked and bares all to promote vegetarianism for the animal rights group People for the Ethical Treatment of Animals (PETA). The actress is pictured in a provocative pose that mimics a butcher's diagram and highlights the various cuts of meat on her body. The advertisement, launched by PETA, carries the slogan "All Animals Have the Same Parts. Have a Heart. Go Vegetarian." The actress further helped promote the PETA campaign by turning up at a nightclub in New York's meatpacking district wearing nothing but a lettuce bikini. She said, "By exposing myself, I hope to expose others to the many benefits of a vegetarian diet." (Photographers Showcase/NewsCom)

bean burritos, stuffed peppers, split pea soup, vegetable lasagna, and baked potatoes with broccoli and cheese sauce. Gourmet cuisine is also part of the vegetarian experience, with foods like roasted pepper and tomato soup; fassolada, a Greek bean soup; and mango raita, a fruity yogurt sauce. Or maybe you would prefer your fresh mango in a couscous salad or fajita wraps with salsa verde and chocolate rum cake. Many Italian dishes are vegetarian naturals and pasta in its myriad forms makes numerous meatless meals. Mexican cooking is often meatless as well, using tortillas, beans, and cheese. Other ethnic cuisines have made a culinary art out of vegetables, like the Greek spinach

dish, spanakopita. Asian stir-fries are another example of delicious meatless cooking, as are Indian curries and Ethiopian dishes of assorted vegetables and beans. Overall, a vegetarian diet is an indulgence in good food and in good health.

Well-known vegetarians include Leonardo da Vinci, Albert Einstein, Benjamin Franklin, Charles Darwin, Thomas Edison, Leo Tolstoy, Henry David Thoreau, Mahatma Gandhi, and Clara Barton; all abstained from eating meat. Today's famous vegetarians include Chelsea Clinton, Brad Pitt, Madonna, and Beatle Paul McCartney.

The 1970s saw a resurgence in vegetarianism with the 1971 publication of

Frances Moore Lappé's *Diet for a Small Planet*. Lappé criticized the inefficiency of a diet based on animal foods, calling beef cattle "a protein factory in reserve" because cattle consume much more protein than they ever provide as meat. She raised the discussion to a global level by addressing the environmental effects of food production, like the destruction of rain forests and the politics of world hunger. She called for a large-scale move to a plant-based diet. Lappé wrote, "What we eat is within our control, yet the act ties us to the economic, political and ecological order of the whole planet. Even an apparently small change, consciously choosing a diet that is good for both our bodies and for the earth, can lead to a series of choices that transform our whole lives."

Public attention also turned to issues of animal cruelty. People for the Ethical Treatment of Animals (PETA) and others brought the stories and photographs of slaughterhouse conditions to the forefront. Formed in 1980, PETA encourages vegetarianism for humane reasons and works through a combination of advocacy, public relations, and advertising to expose the American people in sensational and graphic terms to what the organization calls the inhumanity of animal agriculture.

As is true of a diet that includes meat, variety is fundamental. A look at the U.S. Department of Agriculture's (USDA) Food Guide Pyramid lists meat, fish, and poultry as the primary sources of protein. In 1998, a vegetarian alternative to the USDA Food Guide Pyramid was unveiled at the Inter-

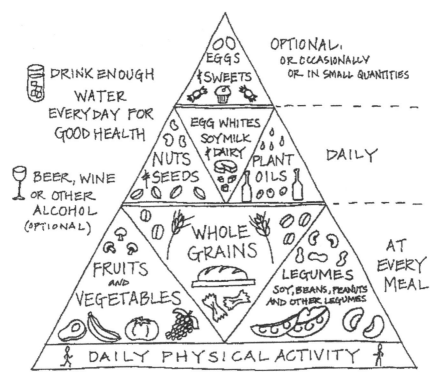

Figure 4 Vegetarian Diet Pyramid
Source: © 2000 Oldways Preservation & Exchange Trust. www.oldwayspt.org Used with permission.

national Conference on Vegetarian Diets. That alternative pyramid promotes protein from soy, legumes, dairy, nuts, and seeds, and emphasizes a wide base of foods to be eaten at every meal, including fruits and vegetables, whole grains, and legumes. The middle band of the pyramid, to be eaten from daily, includes nuts and seeds, egg whites, dairy and soy milk, and plant oils. The pyramid top shows optional foods or foods that should be eaten in small quantities, and includes eggs and sweets. The Vegetarian Diet Pyramid was developed by nutrition scientists and medical specialists from the Cornell-China-Oxford Project on Nutrition, Health and Environment; the Harvard School of Public Health; and the Oldways Preservation and Exchange Trust. Oldways is a Massachusetts-based nonprofit organization devoted to preserving food traditions and promoting healthy, environmentally sustainable, and multicultural foods. The Vegetarian Pyramid is the fourth in a series of Oldways pyramids that include diets from Asia, the Mediterranean, and Latin America. Oldways is not the only option either; the Nutrition Council of the Seventh-day Adventist Church, which advocates a vegetarian diet, also has its own vegetarian pyramid.

A vegetarian diet is not, by definition, either a healthy or a low-calorie eating plan.

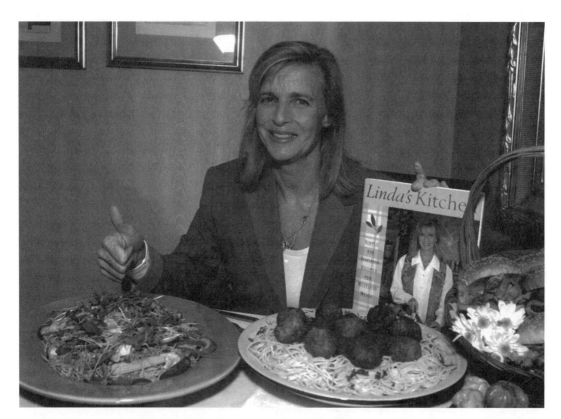

Linda McCartney poses with her cookbook and some of her favorite vegetarian dishes during an interview in New York on October 4, 1995. McCartney, wife of former Beatle Paul McCartney, built a food empire around her crusade for vegetarianism, including two cookbooks, a line of meatless frozen dinners, and a line of vegetarian dog food. Linda McCartney died in 1998 at age 56 of breast cancer. (AP/Wide World Photos)

Nutritionists say the biggest mistake new converts make is to fill up on fattening foods such as cheese, french fries, pizza, avocados, and nuts. They say the best diet is rich in fiber and complex carbohydrates and low in fat—consider apples, oranges, bananas, bagels, popcorn, pretzels, bean tacos or burritos, salads, frozen juice bars, smoothies, or rice cakes. Other good meal choices include non-cream soups and salads.

Misuse of vegetarian eating has also been associated with eating disorders like anorexia and bulimia. Teens who choose to be vegetarian should be doing it correctly and with the right motivation rather than trying to camouflage an eating disorder. A report in the *Archives of Pediatric Adolescent Medicine* in August 1997 looked at how some teens hid eating disorders behind the healthy façade of vegetarianism. The study reported that although vegetarian teens ate more fruits and vegetables than their meat-eating peers did, they were also twice as likely to diet frequently. The meatless teens were also four times as likely to diet intensively and eight times as likely to abuse laxatives. According to the study, this was the first population-based look at eating disorders and their connections to vegetarianism. The authors suggested that due to the increased social acceptance of vegetarian diets, teens who adopt a meatless diet should be evaluated carefully by their parents and health care professionals. Excessive dieting, binge eating, intentional vomiting, and laxative abuse are more obvious red-flag behaviors associated with anorexia and bulimia and teens may try to hide them by changing to a vegetarian diet. This is not to say that every teen who decides to go vegetarian is going to develop an eating disorder, but when it is pursued to extremes there is potential for serious problems.

Additional Reading

Atlas, Nava. *Vegetariana: A Rich Harvest of Wit, Lore and Recipes.* New York: Little Brown, 1984.

Bode, Janet. *Food Fight: A Guide to Eating Disorders for Pre-Teens and Their Parents.* New York: Simon and Schuster, 1997.

David, Marc. *Nourishing Wisdom: A New Understanding of Eating.* New York: Random House, 1994.

Harel, Zeev. "Adolescents and Calcium: What They Do and Do Not Know and How Much They Consume." *Journal of the American Medical Association,* 279, no. 21 (3 June 1998): 1678.

"How Many Teens Are Vegetarian? How Many Kids Don't Eat Meat?" *Vegetarian Journal,* xix, no. 6 (January/February 2001), www.vrg.org/journal/v2001jan/2001janteen.htm. Accessed 12 June 2003.

Katzen, Mollie. *Vegetable Heaven.* New York: Hyperion, 1997.

Krizmanic, Judy. *A Teen's Guide to Going Vegetarian.* New York: Viking and Puffin Books, 1994.

———. *The Teen's Vegetarian Cookbook.* New York: Viking and Puffin Books, 1999.

Lappé, Frances Moore. *Diet for a Small Planet* (20th Anniversary edition). New York: Ballantine Books, 1991.

Lemlin, Jeanne. *Quick Vegetarian Pleasures.* New York: HarperCollins, 1992.

Maradino, Cristin. "The Pyramids Go Veg: New Food Guide." *Vegetarian Times,* January 1998, 18.

Messina, Virginia, and Mark Messina. *The Vegetarian Way: Total Health for You and Your Family.* New York: Crown, 1996.

Neumark-Sztainer, Dianne, Mary Story, Michael D. Resnick, and Robert W. Blum. "Adolescent Vegetarians: A Behavioral Profile of a School-Based Population in Minnesota." *Archives of Pediatrics and Adolescent Medicine,* 151, no. 8 (August 1997): 833.

O'Connor, Amy. "8 Nutritional Myths: Debunking Accepted 'Truths' About Your Diet." *Vegetarian Times,* July 1997, 78.

Oldways Preservation & Exchange Trust. http://oldwayspt.org.

Newman, Judith. "Little Girls Who Won't Eat: The Alarming New Epidemic of Eating Disorders." *Redbook,* October 1997, 120.

Parr, Jan. *The Young Vegetarian's Companion.* New York: Franklin Watts, 1996.

Pierson, Stephanie. *Vegetables Rock!* New York: Bantam Books, 1999.

Reilly, Lee. "Bites of Passage: What You Need to Know When Your Teen Goes Vegetarian." *Vegetarian Times,* November 1997, 78.

Richmond, Akasha. *The Art of Tofu.* Torrance, Calif.: Morinaga Publications, 1997.

Robbins, John. *Diet for a New America.* Walpole, N.H.: Stillpoint Publishing, 1987.

Spencer, Colin. *The Heretic's Feast, A History of Vegetarianism.* London: The Fourth Estate, 1993.

Springer, Ilene. "Are You Ready to Go Vegetarian?" *Cosmopolitan,* October 1995, 130.

Stepaniak, Joanne. *The Vegan Sourcebook.* Los Angeles: Lowell House, 1998.

VanTine, Julia. "When Kids Say 'No More Meat!'" *Prevention,* November 1999, 52.

Vegetarian Times Vegetarian Beginner's Guide. New York: Macmillan, 1996.

Visser, Margaret. *Much Depends upon Dinner.* New York: Macmillan, 1988.

Vitamins

Vitamins are the natural components in food—different from proteins, carbohydrates, and fats—which help ensure normal metabolism. They are essential for good health and growth and when they are deficient or absent dramatic problems can develop. Vitamins fall into two categories, essential and nonessential. The essential vitamins are needed to sustain life and to maintain good health but the body must get them from outside sources. Nonessential vitamins are vital but the body can manufacture them on their own.

The word *vitamin* was derived from the term *vitamine*, Latin's *vita* for "life" and *amine* for "organic compound." The term was coined by biochemist Casimir Funk to describe an organic base, or amine, later found to be thiamine. In 1912, biochemists Sir F. G. Hopkins and Funk formulated the vitamin hypothesis of deficiency disease, meaning that certain diseases are caused by a dietary lack of specific vitamins. Dramatic examples of these diseases include scurvy from lack of vitamin C; pellagra from lack of niacin; and beriberi from lack of thiamine.

Vitamins are classified by their ability to be absorbed in fat or water. The water-soluble vitamins are the eight B vitamins and vitamin C. They must be eaten frequently because they cannot be stored, with the exception of some B vitamins. The fat-soluble vitamins—A, D, E, and K—are generally eaten along with fat-containing foods and can be stored in the body's fat, so they do not need to be eaten every day. Vitamin D is the only one manufactured by the body; all the others must come from the diet.

A well-balanced diet should satisfy the Recommended Dietary Allowance (RDA) of each vitamin. RDAs are guidelines first developed by the Food and Nutrition Board and the National Academy of Sciences–National Research Council based on the nutritional needs of an average healthy person. The U.S. government eventually adopted the National Research Council's RDAs. They are expressed in milligrams or international units (IU) and these recommendations differ for adults and children as well as for people who must follow special diets or women who are pregnant or lactating.

The vitamins include vitamin A; the eight vitamin B complex group of B^1, or thiamine; B^2, or riboflavin; B^3, or niacin; vitamin B^6, or pyridoxine; pantothenic acid; biotin; folic acid; and vitamin B^{12}, or cobalamin; vitamin C; vitamin D; vitamin E; and vitamin K.

Vitamin A is fat-soluble and comes from animal foods like liver, egg yolks, cream, or butter or from beta carotene that occurs in leafy green vegetables and in yellow fruits and vegetables. Vitamin A is important to skeletal growth as well as the health of the skin and mucous membranes. A deficiency of this vitamin can cause slowed skeletal growth, skin abnormalities, and susceptibility to serious infection. In very severe cases it can cause death.

Thiamine, B^1, is part of the vitamin B complex and plays an important role in the metabolism of carbohydrates. It also helps maintain appetite, normal intestinal function, and the health of the cardiovascular and nervous systems. Yeast, legumes, whole grains, thiamine-enriched cereal products, and nuts are all good sources of thiamine.

Riboflavin, also known as B^2, is needed for the body to effectively metabolize carbohydrates, fats, and respiratory proteins. Good sources of riboflavin include liver, milk, meat, dark-green vegetables, whole-grain and enriched cereals, and mushrooms. Deficiency can cause skin lesions and sensitivity to light.

Niacin, B^3, aids in the release of energy from nutrients. A deficiency of niacin causes pellagra, whose symptoms include a sunburnlike eruption that breaks out when skin is exposed to sunlight. Other symptoms are a red and swollen tongue, diarrhea, mental confusion, and depression. Large doses of niacin have been used to reduce levels of cholesterol in the blood but over long periods they can cause liver damage. Good sources of niacin are liver, poultry, meat, tuna and salmon, dried beans and peas, and nuts.

Pyridoxine, or vitamin B^6, is needed for the absorption and metabolism of amino acids, glucose, and fatty acids. It also plays a role in the formation of red blood cells. The best sources are liver and other organ meats, along with spinach, avocados, green beans, bananas, whole-grain cereal, and seeds.

Pantothenic acid, another B vitamin, plays a role in the metabolism of many substances, including fatty acids, steroids, and carbohydrates. The adrenal gland is an important site of pantothenic acid activity. Pantothenic acid is abundant in many foods, including liver, kidney, eggs, and dairy products, and there is no known problem with deficiency since is it also manufactured by intestinal bacteria.

Biotin, a B vitamin, also plays a role in the metabolism of carbohydrates, fats, and amino acids. It is synthesized by intestinal bacteria and is widespread in foods, especially egg yolk, tomatoes, yeast, kidney, and liver. There is no known deficiency in humans.

Folic acid, or vitamin B^9, comes from green leafy vegetables, fruits, dried beans, sunflower seeds, and wheat germ. It works to form body protein and hemoglobin, and deficiencies have been linked to neural tube defects, a type of birth defect that causes serious brain or neurological disorders such as spina bifida. Folic acid is lost in foods stored at room temperature and during cooking, so to increase access to this important vitamin the government has required enrichment of flours, cornmeal, rice, and pasta with folic acid since 1998. Unlike other water-soluble vitamins, folic acid is stored in the liver and does not need to be eaten daily.

Vitamin B^{12}, cobalamin, is the most complex of all known vitamins and is important in nervous system functioning. It comes only from animal sources—liver, kidneys, meat, fish, eggs and milk—and vegans or vegetarians, who eat few or no dairy products, are advised to take a supplement to ensure that they have adequate amounts. This vitamin is also necessary for folic acid to fulfill its role, and both are involved in the synthesis of proteins.

Vitamin C is perhaps the best known of the vitamins and is important in the formation and maintenance of collagen, a protein that help form bones and teeth. Vitamin C also enhances the absorption of iron from foods. Deficiency of this vitamin causes scurvy, whose symptoms include hemorrhages, loosening of teeth, and bone problems, especially in children. The use of large doses of vitamin C in treating common colds is the subject of continuing research.

Vitamin D is needed for healthy bones and for the retention of calcium and phosphorus in the body. Called the sunshine vitamin, it can be manufactured in the body with as little as a half-hour of sunlight. Rickets, from vitamin D deficiency, is usually caused by a lack of exposure to sunlight rather than a dietary deficiency. Symptoms include bowlegs, knock knees, and other bone deformities, or, in adults, softening of the bones. However, because this is a fat-soluble vitamin, it is stored in the body. To prevent deficiencies the government requires milk to be fortified with Vitamin D. On the other hand, excessive consumption can cause nausea, loss of appetite, and kidney damage. Good food sources of vitamin D include egg yolk, liver, tuna, and vitamin D–fortified milk or juice.

Vitamin E plays a role in forming red blood cells and muscle and other tissues. It is also a potent antioxidant, and studies show that it protects against arterial plaque buildup and cancer. It is found in vegetable oils, wheat germ, green leafy vegetables, and liver. Scientists believe it may have an anticoagulant effect on the blood, but that has not been substantiated although research is ongoing.

Vitamin K is necessary for the clotting of blood and its richest sources are alfalfa and fish livers. Other sources include leafy green vegetables, egg yolks, soybean oil, and liver. The bacterial synthesis of this vitamin usually provides enough for a healthy adult but those suffering from blood diseases can experience some deficiency.

Walking

Never underestimate the power of a good pair of sneakers. Walking is something nearly everyone can do—and it's one of the easiest, most convenient, and least expensive ways to begin an exercise regimen. On the Physical Activity Pyramid (see *exercise*), walking is listed as one of the "everyday activities." These first-level activities should total 30 minutes and should be repeated most days of the week. If you can't find one 30-minute interval, try finding two 15-minute opportunities to take a walk around the block, run an errand on foot instead of getting in the car, hop off the bus a stop or two before your usual one, or take the stairs instead of the elevator.

Set reasonable goals for yourself. Don't insist on walking 5 miles per day only to realize after two days that it's too much. Instead, say to yourself that you're going to "go for a walk" twice a day. As time goes on, either find a route that involves more hills or walk for longer stretches of time. Encourage a friend to walk with you. Time seems to go faster when you're enjoying conversation. And realize that even though it's "just" walking, it is exercising and it has cumulative benefits. Walking briskly can burn off about 100 calories per mile.

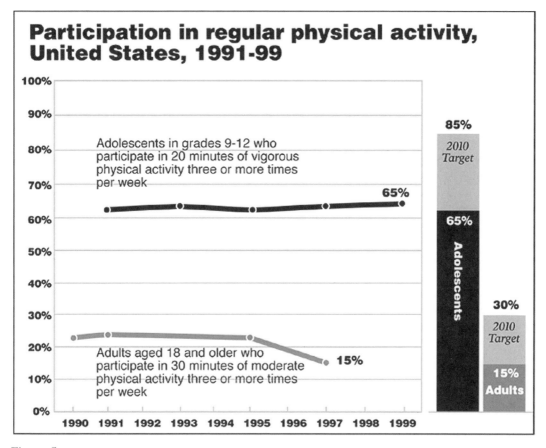

Participation in regular physical activity, United States, 1991-99

Adolescents in grades 9-12 who participate in 20 minutes of vigorous physical activity three or more times per week

65%

Adults aged 18 and older who participate in 30 minutes of moderate physical activity three or more times per week

15%

85%
2010 Target

65%
Adolescents

30%
2010 Target

15%
Adults

Figure 5 Participation in Regular Physical Activity, United States, 1991–99.

Weigh Down Diet

The Weigh Down Diet (1997) could literally be called an answer to author Gwen Shamblin's prayers. A registered dietitian with a master's degree in food and nutrition, Shamblin describes in the book how for many years she was "food focused," constantly struggling with her weight. Then she happened upon the simple concept that God can take away the desire to overeat and the Weigh Down Diet was born. The premise is simple; you don't have to starve yourself to lose weight. Overeating is a problem of the soul, and those who can put their spiritual life in order can, and will, lose weight.

The diet does not focus on the usual diet strategy of counting calories and makes very little mention of exercise. Still this 1997 best-seller has grown into a multimillion-dollar, Nashville-based corporation, called the Weigh Down Workshop, Inc. The diet now comes as part of a ten-week program that starts by teaching participants what hunger is. Instructors do not prescribe a specific menu nor do they encourage participants to cut out bad foods or empty calories from their lives. Instead, dieters focus on when they are physically hungry as opposed to when they are spiritually hungry.

In her book Shamblin gives a sample of her daily menu, but cautions participants to choose the foods they want in the amounts they select. Day 1 of her example includes a breakfast of a biscuit with butter and jelly and three slices of bacon. Lunch is a sandwich with white bread, ham, mayonnaise, a few potato chips, a small Snickers bar, and diet soda. Supper is lasagna, salad with blue-cheese dressing, a roll, lemon pie, and unsweetened tea. Her example also includes another slice of lemon pie as a late snack. She suggests that some food should remain on your plate at the end of each meal as a sign that you are only eating food you are really and truly hungry for.

Although fasting is not a goal in the diet, the program starts with an initial fast so dieters can feel hunger pangs, something they may not have felt in a long time. With Weigh Down, the use of fasting is seen as a way to gain more control over eating problems. Shamblin writes, "Fasting is all over the Old and the New Testaments as an offering to God. God would not be asking us to damage the body." But doctors say fasting poses health risks and is sometimes used by women to mask the signs of anorexia or bulimia. Although the book briefly cautions anorexics not to fast, Shamblin suggests that those with eating disorders work to "be obedient to hunger or emptiness by eating every time they sense emptiness." Critics question the program's use of fasting and lack of insight into its related risks.

While instructors spend the first few weeks teaching that participants should eat the way God intended, many skeptics point out that the diet offers no upfront nutritional information, leaving people with bad eating habits doomed to failure. In place of nutritional guidelines, people are told they can eat chocolate, biscuits and gravy, or any other food by listening to their own senses and letting God and their bodies dictate when, what, and how much they will eat. Opponents of Weigh Down call this approach shortsighted, charging that it ignores documented scientific principles such as the U.S. Department of Agriculture's (USDA) Dietary Guidelines for Americans.

An even more controversial aspect of the Weigh Down Diet is the clear message that fat is sin and God wants people to be thin. However, Shamblin makes no apologies for this approach, saying that if you crave a food, you should eat it, and God will help you stop when you are satisfied. But critics worry about the people who do not lose or who gain their weight back. Those people, theologians fear, might believe they are letting God down, they may question their faith, or even give up on God.

Although Weigh Down teaches people to trade an obsessive focus on food for an all-out focus on God, there are other Christian dieting programs that offer more nutritional direction and regimentation. Consider the program 3D—Diet, Discipline and Discipleship. 3D was founded in 1973 by Carol Showalter, a Presbyterian pastor's wife, who believes that Christians, meeting in small groups, can lose weight if they lead disciplined lives, a combination of disciplined eating and disciplined prayer. Another similar program, First Place, was founded in 1981 in Houston. Its national director, Carole Lewis, says this program supports a recognized food plan using food exchanges and the USDA Food Guide Pyramid.

Early Christian diet books have also enjoyed success long before the *Weigh Down Diet* was written. *Pray Your Weight Away* (1957), by Presbyterian minister Charlie Shedd, is believed to be the first overtly Christian diet book published for a mainstream audience. Shedd, pastor of the Memorial Drive Presbyterian Church of Houston, lost 100 pounds after which he wrote this best-seller explaining how to wage war against gluttony and overeating through prayer. Fifteen years later he wrote a second book, titled *The Fat in Your Head* (1972) based on his experiences as a board member of a psychiatric hospital. Other popular Christian diet book titles include *Help Lord, The Devil Wants Me Fat!* (1978), by Dr. C. S. Lovett, and *I Prayed Myself Slim* (1960) by Deborah Pierce.

See also:

anorexia nervosa; bulimia nervosa; Dietary Guidelines for Americans.

Additional Reading

Brown, Deneen. "Dieting Faithfully; Proponents of the Weigh Down Diet Turn to God for the Will to Resist Overeating." *Washington Post,* 11 April 2000, Z14.

Goodman, Ellen. "The Perils of Paunches and Pounds." *Washington Post,* 12 December 1977, A23.

Kennedy, John W., and Todd Starnes. "Gwen in the Balance." *Christianity Today,* 23 October 2000, 15.

Shamblin, Gwen. *The Weigh Down Diet.* New York: Doubleday, 1997.

Winner, Lauren F. "The Weigh & the Truth." *Christianity Today,* 4 September 2000, 50.

Weight Watchers

Weight Watchers is one of the best-known weight loss support organizations in the world. Sarah Ferguson, the Duchess of York, is the U.S. spokesperson for the international organization. Weight Watchers helps people lose weight at a moderate pace and keep it off with a program that offers a healthy food plan, exercise, and behavior modification in a group support environment.

The Weight Watchers concept was begun by Jean Nidetch in 1961—at the time, a 200-plus-pound New Yorker who met with friends to talk about effective weight loss and provide each other with moral support. With the support of other overweight friends, Nidetch lost 72 pounds and the organization was formally launched in 1963. Since then, the organization has enrolled millions of members worldwide. In 1978, Weight Watchers was purchased by H. J. Heinz and, twenty years later, it was purchased by Luxembourg's Artal Group. In November 2001, the company went public and listed on the New York Stock Exchange.

Weight Watchers offers the Points weight-loss system that includes the Daily Points Range. The Daily Points Range is assigned based on the amount of weight to lose. Rather than measure portion size or count calories, points are easier to track, and accomplishes much the same. Stay within the Daily Points Range and you'll lose weight. For example, a scoop of ice cream is 4 points; a bottle of beer is 3 points, a slice of pizza is 9 points, and a cup of grapes is 1 point. Weight Watchers members are encouraged to eat the daily allowance of food points and are told not to go below the Daily Points Range in an effort to speed up weight loss. People can, however, "earn" extra points by stepping up their physical activity level.

An adult who wants to lose at least 5 pounds can join Weight Watchers. Weight Watchers stresses that it does not market to teens. All members who join start with a preliminary goal to lose 10 percent of their body weight. For example, a person who weighs 200 pounds and has perhaps been struggling and yo-yo dieting for years to try to reach 150 pounds

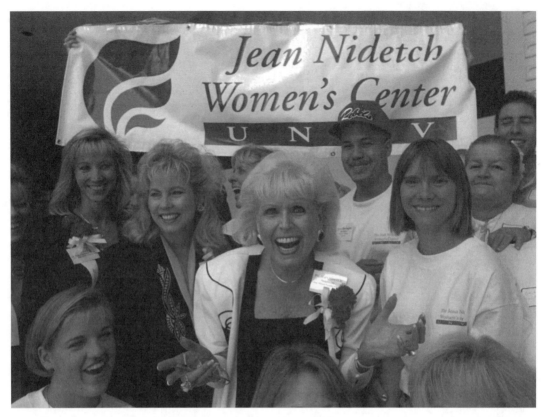

Dr. Jean Nidetch, founder of Weight Watchers International, center, interacts with a group of workers from the Jean Nidetch Women's Center during a Jobs Fair on the campus of the University of Nevada at Las Vegas, on September 9, 1995, in Las Vegas. (AP/Wide World Photos)

may quickly find herself or himself disappointed. With the 10 percent goal, the person would reach the first goal at 180 pounds—a weight loss of 20 pounds. That builds up confidence in ability to lose weight. Then he or she can set the next goal.

Weight Watchers is not a quick-fix diet scheme. On its Web site, www.weightwatchers.com, it states that the organization promotes a "healthy rate of weight loss—up to two pounds per week after the first three weeks."

Weight Watchers produces a bimonthly magazine and numerous cookbooks and inspirational books for those trying to lose weight and maintain that

weight loss. Weekly meetings are key to the concept of Weight Watchers. The Weight Watchers Web site states, "Preliminary scientific research shows that people who regularly attend Weight Watchers meetings lose more weight than people who try to lose weight on their own. Weight Watchers Leaders, who have all risen through the ranks as Weight Watchers meeting members and learned how to lose and successfully control their weight, lead meetings that follow a weekly curriculum. Their experience, techniques, and suggestions for solving problems can help you do what you're having trouble doing on your own: lose weight. Weight Watchers meeting members are also encouraged to share their weight-loss challenges and to celebrate their weight-loss victories at meetings...knowing that others are facing the same issues you're facing and hearing firsthand how they've solved or are working to solve similar problems can help keep you motivated and inspire you to stay the course."

For those who cannot join weekly meetings, Weight Watchers also offers on-line support through an Internet-based journal for tracking daily points, an online newsletter, and other support.

Weight Watchers generally receives good ratings from nutritionists because its emphasis is on moderate fat and balanced nutrients.

The Web site contains a FAQ section, success stories, and a search engine that allows a user to find the closest Weight Watchers meetings. Membership charges and special promotions are listed on the local group's contact information.

Additional Reading

Ferguson, Sarah, Duchess of York. *Dining With the Duchess: Making Everyday Meals A Special Occasion.* New York: Fireside, 1999.
———. *Win the Weight Game: Successful Strategies for Living Well.* New York: Simon and Schuster, 2000.
Ferguson, Sarah, ed. *Reinventing Yourself With the Duchess of York: Inspiring Stories and Strategies.* New York: Simon and Schuster, 2001.
Ferguson, Sarah, Duchess of York with Weight Watchers. *Energy Breakthrough: Jump-Start Your Weight Loss and Feel Great.* New York: Simon and Schuster, 2002.
Fletcher, Anne M. "Inside America's Hottest Diet Programs." *Prevention,* March 1990, 54.
Frascella, Larry. "An Exclusive Visit with Jean Nidetch." *Weight Watchers Magazine,* January 1988, 37.

Heshka, Stanley, James W. Anderson, Richard L. Atkinson, Frank L. Greenway, James O. Hill, Stephen D. Phinney, Ronette L. Kolotkin, Karen Miller-Kovach, and F. Xavier Pi-Sunyer. "Weight Loss With Self-help Compared With a Structured Commercial Program: A Randomized Trial." *Journal of the American Medical Association,* 289 (9 April 2003): 1792.
"Meet the Patrons of Prevention's Hall of Fame." *Prevention,* September 2000, 158.
Miller, Holly G. "Hips, Hips Away!" *Saturday Evening Post,* November 1988, 48.
Neal, Mollie. "Weight Watchers' Winning Marketing Strategy." *Direct Marketing,* August 1993, 24.
Nidetch, Jean. *Story of Weight Watchers.* New York: New American Library, 1979.
Tisdale, Sallie. "A Weight That Women Carry: The Compulsion to Diet in a Starved Culture." *Harper's Magazine,* March 1993, 49.
Weight Watchers International, editor. *Weight Watchers New Complete Cook Book.* New York: John Wiley & Sons, 1998.
———. *Weight Watchers Stop Stuffing Yourself: 7 Steps to Conquering Overweight.* New York: John Wiley & Sons, 1999.

Xenical

Xenical is a weight loss drug that was approved by the Food and Drug Administration (FDA) in May 1999. The drug works by blocking an enzyme needed to digest fat and prevents about 30 percent of ingested dietary fat from being absorbed by the body. That undigested fat accumulates in the intestines and is excreted in the stool. Side effects associated with Xenical include bloating, flatulence, oily stool, diarrhea, and fecal incontinence. Company officials say that maintaining a diet with no more than 30 percent of calories from fat can minimize these side effects.

Clinical trials also show that Xenical partially depletes fat-soluble vitamins A,

D, E, and K and beta carotene. Physicians advise patients taking the medication to also take a multivitamin. The drug is recommended only for patients considered clinically obese, with a BMI of 30 or higher, or those who suffer from other risk factors of obesity, including high blood pressure and diabetes. In a clinical study reported in the June 2001 edition of *Chemist & Druggist*, results showed more than 15,500 overweight men and women lost an average of 11 percent of body weight over a period of seven months while taking Xenical. The drug was taken in combination with a reduced-calorie diet.

Xenical differs from weight control medications that work on brain chemistry to control appetite, like Redux and fen-phen. The FDA withdrew both Redux and fen-phen from the market in 1997, citing concerns over reported cases of heart-valve abnormalities in users. Diet industry analysts consider Xenical a competitor of the obesity drug Meridia. Sales figures for Xenical's first full year in 2000 came to $225 million in U.S. retail sales. Sales in 2001 dropped to $157 million. Hoffmann–La Roche officials, makers of the medication, had originally predicted annual sales at $1 billion. The company attributed the slower-than-expected sales to the failure of physicians to treat obesity with drug therapy and to patients' difficulties securing insurance reimbursements for Xenical.

See also:

fen-phen; Meridia.

Additional Reading

Freeman, Miller. "Weight Loss Pill Offers Added Health Benefits," *Chemist & Druggist,* 9 June 2001, 10.

Gleick, Elizabeth. "Available from a Doctor Near You." *Time International,* 25 October 1999, 65.

Morehouse, Macon. "Girth Control: Despite Nasty Side Effects, Americans Are Tripping over Their Scales to Get the New Diet Drug Xenical. Is it Safe?" *People Weekly,* 7 June 1999, 113–14.

Wilhelm, Carolyn. "Growing the Market for Anti-Obesity Drugs," *Chemical Market Reporter,* 256, no. 20 (15 May 2000): 23.

Yo-Yo Dieting

Yo-yo dieting, also known as weight cycling, occurs when a person experiences cycles of weight loss and weight gain resembling the up and down of a yo-yo. The pattern begins with rapid weight loss normally associated with the use of fad diets or diet pills. However, once a goal weight is reached, dieters return to their original, poor eating habits. This causes the lost pounds to return, followed by extra weight gain. Each time yo-yo dieters lose weight through the use of pills, liquid diet drinks. or fads like a high-protein, high-fat, and low-carbohydrate diet, they lose mostly lean muscle and water but only a small amount of fat. However, when those pounds return, it is in the form of fat with very little muscle regained. The psychological effects of yo-yo dieting include depression and the erosion of confidence and self-esteem.

While research shows weight cycling may not benefit individuals who have only small amounts of weight to lose, doctors caution that severely obese individuals should not allow concerns about the hazards of weight cycling to deter them from efforts to control their body weight. Instead, individuals who undertake a weight loss program should consult a doctor first. They should also expect to make lifelong changes in their eating, behavior, and physical activity. The National Task Force on the Prevention and Treatment of Obesity said studies show that, for obese individuals, keeping off just 5 to 15 pounds permanently can have a positive impact on overall health.

The Zone

The Zone, published in 1995 by Barry Sears, is a one-man crusade against carbohydrates. The "Zone" is defined by its creator as a metabolic state in which the mind is relaxed and focused, and the body is strong and works at peak efficiency. As Sears explains, Zone is not some mystical place but instead relates to keeping hormones, such as insulin, within specified ranges. To reach the "Zone," dieters must eat a ratio of 40 percent carbohydrates, 30 percent proteins, and 30 percent fat per meal. In other words, eat the butter, not the bread. And stay away from the "danger" zone foods like pasta, bagels, rice, potatoes, bananas, carrots, apple juice, and ketchup.

Sears calls the Zone diet a moderate-carbohydrate, moderate-protein, and moderate-fat program. A typical day's Zone menu includes protein in a percentage considerably above what the U.S. Department of Agriculture (USDA) suggests. The recommended dietary allowance (RDA) for a young man between the ages of 15 and 24 years is from 58 to 59 grams of protein per day, although intake often reaches as high as 90 grams per day. The RDA for a young woman in that same age range is from 44

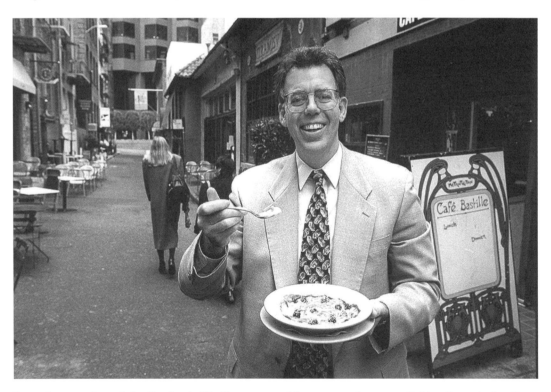

Barry Sears, author of the diet book *The Zone*, poses with a creamy dessert on Belden Street in San Francisco, a virtual restaurant alley. According to Sears, you can eat within the Zone at any restaurant and not deny yourself any foods as long as you balance carbohydrates with protein in the Zone formula of 40 percent carbohydrates, 30 percent fat, and 30 percent protein. (Knight Ridder/Tribune/NewsCom)

to 46 grams per day, but the average woman in this category often eats up to 65 grams of protein per day. Sears maintains that The Zone diet is not high in protein because a typical day's menu is not over 100 grams of protein a day, which he says does not exceed the newest protein guidelines set by the American Heart Association. Those guidelines urge adults to get less than 30 percent of total daily calories from fat and less than 10 percent from saturated fat. That recommendation means eating no more than 6 ounces (cooked) per day of lean meat, fish, or skinless poultry. The AHA also suggests that high-fiber plant foods and grains are an important part of a nutritionally balanced diet because they help lower cholesterol.

A Zone breakfast might include four scrambled egg whites with one ounce of low-fat cheese, a cup of strawberries, and a small cup of oatmeal. Lunch possibilities could be a chicken Caesar salad, two cups of vegetables, and a medium apple. Dinner might consist of six ounces of fish with slivered almonds, combined with four cups of vegetables such as broccoli, onions, mushrooms, bell peppers, and tomatoes, with fresh fruit for dessert. The Zone allows an average person, defined by the American Dietetic Association as a 154-pound active male, up to 1,500 calories per day. In contrast, the ADA suggests that same person eat a balanced diet of some 2,600 calories each day to maintain their current weight.

Sears claims a person in the "Zone" will experience permanent body-fat loss, optimal health, greater athletic performance, and improved mental productivity. Zoners will burn fat while they also fight heart disease, diabetes, premenstrual syndrome, chronic fatigue, depression, and cancer. The Zone literature suggests that when carbohydrate intake is controlled, the body burns fat faster and food cravings disappear. According to Sears, non-Zoners produce excess insulin from eating carbohydrates and this "excess" somehow creates food cravings, especially for more carbohydrates. The cycle of excess insulin production from complex carbohydrates like pasta, breads, and bagels, is kept in motion by the resulting lowered blood sugar levels that the cravings produce. Sears says his theory is supported by published clinical research.

Critics argue that people develop excess insulin, a condition called insulin resistance, from being overweight and sedentary. When insulin resistance takes place, a person's cells won't absorb glucose unless an abnormally large amount of insulin is on hand. Nutrition and health critics maintain that this is not a consequence of eating too many carbohydrates and they say medical research has not linked insulin levels to weight gain in healthy people. Critics also point to studies showing that eating fat in the form of steak, cheese, or bacon can contribute to a number of health problems from high cholesterol levels to the development of cardiovascular disease.

Although *The Zone* contradicts decades of nutritional wisdom, scientists agree with one aspect of this diet: the body does turn carbohydrates into glucose. In fact, eating anything—whether it's carbohydrates, protein, or fat—causes blood sugar levels to rise, which in turn stimulates insulin production. Critics say problems develop when a person loads up on protein and limits carbohydrates. Sears answers critics by saying The Zone cannot be considered a high-protein diet, since an individual who follows the program is eating more carbohydrates than protein. And The Zone doesn't forbid all carbohydrates; high-fiber fruits and vegetables are fine, but it discourages the more complex carbohydrates, which nutritionists say are important to a well-balanced diet.

In 2001 the American Heart Association issued a strong recommendation against what the association called high-protein weight loss programs, listing the Atkins Diet, The Zone, Protein Power, and Sugar Busters! The report in the AHA journal *Circulation* cited a lack of credible scientific evidence of long-term weight loss for these programs and the possibility of increased risk for those with diabetes and heart disease.

Dieters following plans that limit specific categories of foods, like carbohydrates, will initially see pounds melt off due to water loss and because of a lowered total calorie intake. Although carbohydrates are essential for fueling muscles and the brain, the body can't store a very large amount. So when dieters eat fewer carbohydrates than their body needs, the body reacts as though it were starving and releases the water that's stored, along with its small supply of carbohydrates. In addition, the ongoing glucose shortages will cause the body to start burning fats for fuel, releasing fatty acids called ketones into the bloodstream. Doctors say abnormally high ketone levels lead to ketosis, and ketosis sets the stage for gout or kidney disease in susceptible people. Sears says it is impossible to develop ketosis on The Zone diet because it has more carbohydrates than protein, but critics maintain that the amount of carbohydrates eaten on The Zone diet still falls below daily intake requirements for a healthy diet.

Throughout *The Zone*, Sears cites his own studies, case histories, and testimonials as proof that this diet works. Critics point out none of his studies have been published in peer-reviewed journals where experts evaluate the articles before being accepted for publication. Sears says that investigators, including those from Harvard Medical School, have reconfirmed his data in peer-reviewed research. Many critics sarcastically suggest the real "zone" is actually a money zone, since there are over 2 million copies of his best seller in print and it has been translated into fourteen languages. Sears followed *The Zone* with more titles: *Mastering the Zone,* which spent eleven weeks on the best-seller list; *The Anti-Aging Zone; The Soy Zone;* and *Zone Perfect Meals in Minutes.*

Although the Zone diet may provide short-term weight loss, its long-term effectiveness is still questionable. Skeptics include the American Heart Association, whose Nutrition Committee reported in 2001 that the initial, rapid weight loss often produced by high-protein diets is due mostly to a temporary fluid loss caused by eating fewer carbohydrates. The committee also noted that high-protein diets could compromise vitamin and mineral intake and cause heart, liver, and kidney abnormalities.

Representatives of the American Cancer Society (ACS) also had harsh words for what they called high-protein diets, which they charge can raise cholesterol levels, promote development of cardiovascular disease, and raise the risk of various cancers. In contrast, the ACS suggests a diet high in fruits and vegetables, low in fat, and lower in protein. Sears says his diet is in line with those recommendations because it is rich in fruits and vegetables. But the real answer to losing weight, according to nutritionists, is through hard work, changed eating habits, and increased exercise, a plan more commonly known as "eat less, exercise more."

See also:

Food Guide Pyramid; Dietary Guidelines for Americans; Sears, Barry; Sugar Busters!

Additional Reading

Kaufman, Frederick. "The Zone." *Harper's Magazine,* January 2000, 72.

Proulx, Lawrence G. "To Each His Zone: Best-Selling Book Promises Amazing Rewards from its Unorthodox Approach to Eating." *Washington Post,* 4 February 1997, Z16.

Ratnesar, Romesh. "Against the Grain: The Low-Carb Zone Diet Rises from Fad to Fixture." *Time,* 15 December 1997, 86.

Shaffer, Alyssa Lustigman. "The Great Nutrient Debate: Hollywood Loves 'the Zone' and Americans Love Their Pasta Bowls." *Weight Watchers Magazine,* March/April 1998, 39–42.

Squires, Sally. "Heart Association Skewers Atkins Diet; High Protein Plans Called Unproven, Risky." *Washington Post,* 9 October 2001, F01.

Appendix A

Timeline

1847

Physicians form the American Medical Association (AMA) with two goals: to draw up a code of moral ethics and to seek educational reform to raise the standards of medical training and establish uniform minimum requirements for medical degrees.

1850

The American Vegetarian Society is founded.

1863

William Banting writes what historians believe is the first diet book, *A Letter on Corpulence*. At his death in 1878 more than 58,000 copies of the book have been sold and "banting" is a popular term for dieting.

1879

Saccharin becomes the first sugar substitute. The discovery is the result of an accidental spill during research being done on food preservatives.

1894

The U.S. Department of Agriculture (USDA) develops the first food composition tables and dietary standards for Americans.

1906

Pure Food and Drug Act is enacted. This first federal food and drug law means manufacturers involved in interstate sales cannot make false statements on their product's label. However diet aids are exempt, since they not considered drugs and obesity is not considered a disease.

1907

Yale scientists announce the results of a series of experiments proving that the strict diet and thorough mastication of food, practiced by Horace Fletcher and known as Fletcherism, has been an effective aid in treating obesity, gout, and dyspepsia. Researchers say the studies also prove that nerves play an important part in digestion, agreeing with Fletcher that many emotions actually stop the flow of gastric juices. They agree with Fletcher's rule for eating: do not eat when you are mad or sad, only when you are glad.

1909

At a meeting of the Society of Internal Medicine in Paris, French doctor Marcel Labbé calls for an end to the medical treatment of obesity. He recommends that the best course of action is to reduce the intake of fats, bread, pastries, sweets, and salt and to exercise to lessen fat and increase muscular tissue.

1911

Dr. W. Wayne Babcock, a Philadelphia surgeon, announces the latest method of reducing stoutness, the surgical removal of abdominal fat. In his demonstration, he cut open the patient's abdomen, turned back the flesh, and removed superfluous fat. He cautions that great care must be taken to avoid severing any muscles. After the operation Dr. Babcock reports that the woman is twelve pounds lighter.

1917

The U.S. government releases dietary recommendations in a publication titled "How to Select Foods," and calls for five food groups: milk and meat; cereals; vegetables and fruits; fats and fat foods; and sugars and sugary foods.

1924

A scrub brush, slightly softer than a kitchen scrub brush, is introduced as a flesh reducer and weight-loss tool. For maximum results every part of the body is massaged four or five times a day. After rubbing, the dieter is told to take a cold shower. Promoters say dieters can expect a pound or so of "excess" fat to magically disappear each week.

Dr. Lulu Hunt Peters, a popular diet-book author, publishes the first diet book for children, *Diet for Children (and adults) and the Kalorie Kids* (New York, Dodd, Mead and Company).

1925

Pennsylvania officials with the Delaware County Tuberculosis Association declare that survey results show local high school girls are "starving themselves" in an effort to maintain stylish silhouette figures and are "dangerously underweight." Weight-loss methods range from starvation diets to eating pickles and ice cream instead of regular meals. The association secretary claims the girls start dieting when they reach fifteen years old, the flapper age.

1927

A noted British dietitian pronounces obesity the result of a state of mind. He suggests that the way to get thin is to adopt the correct attitude along with a correct diet and exercise.

1930

A slump in English potato sales is attributed to the "slim-figure craze" of English women. The Ulster Minister of Agriculture blames women who are no longer eating potatoes and announces that the government is searching for other markets.

1933

An overweight San Francisco physician dies from a violent fever generated by an overdose of the diet drug dinitrophenol, according to a report published in the *Lancet*. Dinitrophenol and the more powerful dinitro-ortho-cresol are both drugs that accelerate metabolism, and the report recommends that dieters seek medical guidance before taking either drug.

1934

Results of a scientifically supervised, 30-day diet of bananas and skim milk shows that three women participants were able to lose a total of 32 pounds. Dr. Herman N. Bundesen, the Chicago Health Commissioner, supervised the diet and recommends it to anyone with excess pounds.

1935

The New York State Hairdressers and Cosmetologists Association calls for government legislation to ban dieting by women. They say "public health protection" is needed to stop the starvation mania endangering the health of its members.

1938

Congress passes the Food, Drug, and Cosmetic Act, requiring that products must be proven safe before they reach the market. Diet aids are covered by the Act for the first time.

1939

The Metropolitan Life Insurance Company reports a trend toward "fashionable thinness" among American women. The company compared average weights among insured women from the years 1922–23 and 1932–34 and noted a general 3- to 5-pound decline in average weight for each height and at every age.

1941

The Food and Nutrition Board of the National Academy of Sciences announces the development of its recommended daily allowances, or RDAs.

1942

The American Medical Association (AMA) issues a public statement disapproving of amphetamines for the treatment of obesity because of problems of dependence.

The U.S. Department of Agriculture announces the "Basic Seven" food groups as part of its year-old recommended daily allowances. The seven food groups include green and yellow vegetables; oranges, tomatoes, and grapefruit; potatoes and other vegetables and fruit; milk and milk products; meat, poultry, fish, eggs, and dried peas and beans; bread, flour, and cereals; and butter and fortified margarine. The guide also suggests alternate choices in the event of wartime shortages.

1943

Overweight American women are compromising the nation's wartime food supply, according to the Metropolitan Life Insurance Company. Company officials release a new "ideal" weight table with three separate groups of women, those with slight, medium, and heavy builds. And company officials suggest wartime rationing of food can help with weight reduction programs.

1946

A U.S. Department of Agriculture bulletin advises overweight Americans to reduce their consumption of wheat and fats, pointing out that these are the foods most needed in Europe due to food rationing.

1947

A Cornell University doctor reports that nonglandular obesity in women should be regarded as a neurosis and must be treated with intensive psychotherapy.

1948

Milwaukee, Wisconsin, resident, Esther Manz, founds the organization Take Off Pounds Sensibly (TOPS), the first of the national dieting groups.

1950

The American Society of Bariatric Physicians begins as the National Obesity Society. After several name changes it becomes the ASBP with a shift in treatment of obesity away from glands toward appetite and exercise.

1952

Dietary experts with the U.S. Department of Health announce that New Yorkers lost 3.2 million pounds during a two-week heat wave. Director of the department's Bureau of Nutrition attributed the loss to the drop in appetite when temperatures soared. He calculated that 8 million New Yorkers ate 100 calories less each day, meaning an individual weekly loss of two-fifth of a pound during the early July record temperatures.

1954

A rounded plastic device to relieve hunger pangs is patented by the U.S. government. The device, invented by Dr. William S. Kroger of Evanston, Illinois, will abolish the hunger pangs that occur around mealtime, according to the doctor. He said pressing the device into the stomach just below the breastbone will produce a feeling of fullness. He blamed 98 percent of overweight on eating due to emotional tension. He believes his device will help in the national battle of the bulge.

1955

A patent is issued for a calorie counter, a small instrument to be carried in the pocket or handbag by dieters. The user records calories eaten during the day to gauge how much of a daily quota has been consumed. The patent is issued to Charles G. Hallowell of West Hartford, Connecticut.

1956

President Dwight D. Eisenhower establishes the President's Council on Physical Fitness to encourage American children to lead healthy, active, and physically fit lives. First named the President's Council on Youth Fitness by Eisenhower, the name was changed to the President's Council on Physical Fitness by President John F. Kennedy to reflect its expanded mandate to serve all Americans.

The American Medical Association's Council on Foods and Nutrition warns against the indiscriminate use of new low-protein diets, also known as "Rockefeller" or "fabulous formula" diets. Based on experimental diets developed at the Rockefeller Institute of Medical Research, both plans call for lowered protein intake. One diet, the fabulous formula, is a liquid combination of corn oil, evaporated milk, and dextrose. The Rockefeller diet calls for low-protein foods. The council pointed to serious hazards not made clear in any publicity for the diets.

The American Academy of Pediatrics, at its twenty-fifth and largest meeting, opens its session with a discussion of childhood obesity. The speakers caution American mothers who feed their babies on the "self-demand" regime that they may be overfeeding and subsequently setting their children up for a progression of problems with overweight.

The U.S. Department of Agriculture "Basic Seven" food groups are condensed to the "Basic Four" in a publication titled *Essentials of an Adequate Diet.*

1957

The modern Christian dieting industry begins when Charlie Shedd, a minister who lost 100 pounds, publishes *Pray Your Weight Away.*

1958

Congress passes the Food Additives Amendment to the Food, Drug, and Cosmetic Act, which requires premarket approval from the Food and Drug Administration (FDA) for food additives developed after 1958.

1960

Overeaters Anonymous, a dieting group similar in style to Alcoholics Anonymous, is founded.

1961

Weight Watchers is established.

The Food, Drug, and Cosmetic Act is revised to require that all new drugs and old drugs claiming new uses have to show that they are safe as well as effective.

1962

Findings released from the Hormone Research Laboratory of the University of California's Berkeley campus find the pituitary hormone ACTH has fat-dissolving activity and may greatly improve treatment of glandular obesity. Lab tests on rats and rabbits show a rapid breakdown of the solid form of fats into liquid fats that can be removed from the body by natural clearing mechanisms.

1963

The Federal Trade Commission (FTC) issues a complaint against the author and publisher of the former best-seller *Calories Don't Count.* The FTC charges that the book made false claims for the value of safflower oil in promoting improved health and weight loss. The commission files charges against Simon and Schuster, Inc., and the author, Dr. Herman Taller.

1964

The first time an advertising agency is indicted because of the ads it prepared for a client. A federal grand jury indicts a New York advertising agency on charges of writing fraudulent advertising copy for Regimen Tablets, a weight-loss pill.

1965

The first time an advertising agency is convicted for promoting the product of a client. A federal jury finds the advertising agency of Kastor Hilton Chesley Clifford & Atherton, Inc., guilty of promoting a fraudulent claim that Regimen tablets cause a substantial weight loss without dieting.

1967

The Oregon State Medical Examiner announces that six deaths have been linked to weight-reducing pills. Citing a two-year investigation into the pills by the State Crime Laboratory, he concludes that the pills depleted the dieters of potassium, leading to death. Although no brand name is released, the pills contained drugs that allegedly interacted to cause death, including amphetamines, Phenobarbital, digitalis, plain vegetable laxative, and a thiazide diuretic. The women who died ranged in age from 19 to 52.

1968

The Relaxacisor is promoted as a pleasant, effortless way to firm, tone, and tighten muscles without exercise. The handheld device delivers a mild electric shock to the skin, causing muscles to involuntarily contract. More than 400,000 Americans buy the machine before the FDA bans it as ineffective and dangerous.

1971

A group of New York doctors announce the first voluntary ban in the United States on prescribing amphetamines for use in treating obesity.

1972

The FDA announces a move to restrict unnecessary and potentially harmful use of diet pills and vitamins. The agency's action against diet pills is made public in testimony before a U.S. Senate subcommittee.

Dr. Robert Atkins publishes *Dr. Atkin's Diet Revolution*.

1973

The U.S. Senate Select Committee on Nutrition and Human Needs holds hearings devoted to people with "overnutrition," the estimated 30 percent of the U.S. population who are overweight. Dr. Robert Atkins appears before the committee to answer questions about the safety of his diet.

1974

The FDA announces that a drug produced from the urine of pregnant women must bear a label saying it is worthless for weight loss. The hormone human chorionic gonadotropin (HCG) has been used in antifat clinics around the country but the FDA declares that there is no evidence it is effective in treating obesity.

The U.S. Postal Service bans "Slimmer Shake" or "Joe Weider's Weight Loss Formula XR-7" from the mail on the grounds of false advertising. The product promises a 14-pound weight loss in 14 days but the company only provides a 12-day supply. The advertising also claims there is no need to restrict caloric intake but the product arrives with instructions to eat only the "slimmer shake" plus 1 quart of milk per day and no other food.

1975

A New York man pleads guilty to mail fraud and false advertising for "Slim-Tabs Slenderizing tablets," a concoction allegedly designed to slim a dieter down 48 pounds in eight weeks. The company received $1.1 million in orders within a six-month period and promised that if customers were dissatisfied they would receive a $25 U.S. Savings Bond.

1977

The Food and Drug Administration proposes a ban on the artificial sweetener saccharin after evidence links its use to bladder tumors in experimental animals. Weight-watching groups lobby in Washington, D.C., and force Congress to place a moratorium on the FDA ban.

1978

The Food and Drug Administration reverses its earlier order calling for warning labels on all liquid protein diets. The new regulation requires warning labels only on protein products that provide more than 50 percent of a person's calories if those products are promoted for weight loss or as a food supplement.

1979

Advertisements for an "electronic diet fork" explain that the eating utensil induces weight loss through behavior modification. The fork has lights in the handle: a green light tells dieters when to start eating; a red light tells them when to stop.

1980

Dr. Herman Tarnower, physician and author of the best-selling *Complete Scarsdale Medical Diet*, is shot and killed in the bedroom of his home. His longtime companion, Jean S. Harris, is tried and convicted of murder.

The first Dietary Guidelines for Americans are released by the USDA and the Department of Health and Human Services, to be revised every five years.

1981

The *Beverly Hills Diet* is published, based on the notion that undigested food, stuck in the body, causes weight gain. During the first ten days of the diet, only fruits are allowed. The book also claims two-hour rests are needed between different food types so those different enzymes will not interfere with digestion. The *Journal of the American Medical Association* publishes a scathing criticism of the diet.

1982

The Food and Drug Administration orders starch blockers off the market after it receives reports of adverse reactions, including thirty cases requiring hospitalization and one death. Makers of starch blockers claim that enzymes extracted from beans can block digestion of significant amounts of dietary starch, causing weight loss.

1983

The first liposuction surgery to reduce subcutaneous body fat is performed in the United States.

U.S. soft drink companies begin using NutraSweet artificial sweetener in diet beverages.

Popular singer Karen Carpenter's death brings national attention to the serious consequences of anorexia nervosa and bulimia nervosa.

1984

A National Institutes of Health panel calls obesity a major killer in the United States.

1985

The Center for Science in the Public Interest (CSPI) indicts fast-food chains for deep-frying with beef fat rather than with oils lower in saturated fats.

1986

The Food and Drug Administration allows only two drugs to be used in nonprescription diet aids, phenylpropanolamine (PPA), an appetite suppressant, and benzocaine with caffeine, which numbs the tongue to reduce the sense of taste.

The McDonalds Corporation announces that it will make a booklet available listing the ingredients of its fast foods following pressure from consumer groups to release that information.

Coca-Cola announces that it is replacing its ninety-nine-year-old formula with a sweeter-tasting formula. Consumer protests convince the company to reintroduce the old formula as Coca-Cola Classic.

1987

The FDA approves Lovastatin, a cholesterol-lowering drug.

1988

A report published in the *Journal of the American Medical Association* concludes that 80 percent of middle-aged American men run a sizable risk of dying prematurely from heart disease due to high cholesterol levels in their blood.

1989

The Food and Drug Administration *Consumer* magazine issues a report listing questionable and unsafe diet remedies, including skin patches, herbal capsules, grapefruit diet pills, and Chinese magic weight-loss earrings.

1990

The Nutrition Labeling and Education Act of 1990 takes effect.

1991

The U.S. government introduces its Food Guide Pyramid, which encourages the consumption of grains, vegetables, and fruits, and recommends fewer servings each day of dairy and meat foods along with fats and sweets.

1992

Researchers speaking before the annual meeting of the New York Society of Behavioral Medicine in New York announce a newly defined eating disorder more common than anorexia or bulimia, called "binge eating disorder," marked by frequent, uncontrolled eating episodes. Unlike people with bulimia, those with binge eating disorder do not try to lose or purge extra calories; they simply gain weight. Experts say commercial weight-loss programs only increase the problem.

1994

The death of gymnast Christy Henrich due to anorexia nervosa and bulimia nervosa focuses attention on eating disorders among female athletes, especially in sports like gymnastics where thinness is stressed.

1995

The National Center for Health Statistics reports that the proportion of American children who are overweight has more than doubled in the last three decades, following its most recent study from 1988–1991.

1996

The American Cancer Society releases guidelines recommending that people lower their cancer risk by eating very little meat and consuming a higher proportion of plant foods.

The Food and Drug Administration proposes new warning labels for over-the-counter diet pills containing phenylpropanolamine (PPA).

1997

The U.S. Surgeon General declares childhood obesity to be an epidemic in America.

The Food and Drug Administration withdraws Redux and fen-phen diet drugs from the market, citing concerns over reported cases of heart-valve abnormalities in users.

1998

The National Institutes of Health estimates that 97 million adult Americans are overweight or obese. The newly released figures also show that 300,000 unnecessary deaths a year can be attributed to the disease of obesity. Obesity is defined by the federal government as excessive mass when compared to height.

1999

The Food and Drug Administration approves the obesity drug Xenical (Orlistat), a lipase inhibitor that decreases absorption of dietary fat by 30 percent.

2000

The U.S. Department of Agriculture Food Guide Pyramid is revised to reflect changing nutritional information.

The USDA sponsors the Great Nutrition Debate, a discussion panel featuring popular diet-book authors as well as nutrition and weight-loss researchers.

The FDA issues a public health warning cautioning consumers against taking products containing phenylpropanolamine. The FDA also asks manufacturers to voluntarily replace it with alternative active ingredients.

2001

The Electronic Retailing Association, in collaboration with the Federal Trade Commission, is awarded one of the largest false advertising settlements in history—a $10 million judgment against Enforma Natural Products for best-selling pills called Exercise in a Bottle and Fat Trapper. Fat Trapper was advertised as being able to "trap up to 120 grams of fat per day." Infomercials told consumers they "could eat what you want and never, ever, ever have to diet again."

2002

The Internal Revenue Service recognizes obesity as a disease, clearing the way for taxpayers to claim weight-loss expenses as a medical deduction. To take the deduction, a person must participate in a weight-loss program for medical reasons. Only those who itemize and whose medical expenses total more than 7.5 percent of their adjusted gross income can take the deduction.

2003

Illinois becomes the first state to ban ephedra-based products.

Appendix B

Checklist for Evaluating Weight-Loss Products and Services

Use this checklist to gather and compare information from all weight-loss programs or services you're considering. Make several copies of the blank form so you can fill out one for each program. A provider's willingness to give you this information is an important factor in choosing a program. If you need help to evaluate the information you gather, talk with your primary health-care provider or a registered dietitian.

In this program, my daily caloric intake will be:

My daily caloric intake is determined by:

I will/will not be evaluated initially by program staff.

The evaluation will be made by (check all that apply):

___Physician   ___Nurse   ___Registered Dietitian   ___Other company-trained employee

My progress is supervised by (check all that apply):

___Physician   ___Nurse   ___Licensed Psychologist

___Registered Dietitian   ___Company-trained employee

I will/will not be evaluated by a physician during the course of my treatment.

During the first month, my progress will be monitored:

___Weekly   ___Biweekly   ___Monthly   ___Other

After the first month, my progress will be monitored:

___Weekly   ___Biweekly   ___Monthly   ___Other

My weight loss plan includes (check all that apply):

___Nutrition information about healthy eating

___At least 1,200 calories/day for women or 1,400 calories/day for men

___Suggested menus and recipes

___Keeping food diaries or other monitoring activities

___Portion control

___Liquid meal replacements

___Prepackaged meals

___Dietary supplements (vitamins, minerals, botanicals, herbals)

___Prescription weight-loss drugs

___Help with weight maintenance and lifestyle changes

___Surgery

My plan includes regular physical activity that is (check both if both apply):

Supervised (at the program site) ____times per week , ____minutes per session.

Unsupervised (on my own time) ____times per week, ____minutes per session.

The physical activity includes (check all that apply):

___Walking   ___Swimming   ___Stationary cycling

___Strength training   ___Aerobic dancing   ___Other

The weight-loss plan includes (check all that apply):

___Family counseling   ___Group support   ___Lifestyle modification advice

___Weight maintenance advice   ___Weight maintenance counseling

The staff explained the risks associated with this weight loss program. They are:

The staff explained the costs of this program. (Check all that apply and fill in the blanks.)

I will be charged a one-time entry fee of $_____.

I will be charged $_____ per visit.

Food replacements will cost about $_____ per month.

Prescription weight-loss drugs will cost about $_____ per month.

Vitamins and other dietary supplements will cost about $_____ per month.

Diagnostic tests are required and will cost about $_____ .

Other costs include _____ at $_____.

Total costs: $_____

The program gave me information about:

___The health risks of being overweight.

___The difficulty many people have maintaining weight loss.

___The health benefits of weight loss.

___How to improve my chances at maintaining my weight.

Other information to ask for:

Participants in this program have lost an average of _____ lbs. over _____ months/years.

Participants in this program have kept off _____% of their weight loss for year(s).

This information is based on the following (check one):

___All participants.

___Participants who completed the program.

___Other

Source: Partnership for Healthy Weight Management, "Weight Loss: Finding a Weight Loss Program that Works for You." Available online www.consumer. gov/weightloss/moreinfo.htm. Accessed 12 June 2003.

Appendix C

What's on the Web

American Anorexia/Bulimia Association, Inc. (AABA)

Address: 165 West 46th Street, Suite 1108, New York, NY 10036
Phone: 212-575-6200
Web address: www.aabainc.org
Web site: The AABA is a national nonprofit organization comprising health care professionals and others dedicated to the prevention and treatment of eating disorders. This site is geared toward the general public, with information, articles, and lists of risk factors for suffers as well as helplines, referral networks, public information, support groups, and prevention programs. Articles and information work to expose and change the idealization of thinness. This site provides information for all ages.

American Council on Science and Health (ACSH)

Address: 1995 Broadway, Second Floor, New York, NY 10023-5860
Phone: 212-362-7044 / Fax: 212-362-4919
Web address: www.acsh.org
Web site: The ACSH is a consumer education consortium made up of scientists, physicians, and policy advisors. The council tracks the accuracy of nutrition articles in the popular magazines and publishes its survey online. This site is geared for the general public and offers a useful, conservative interpretation of current health information, from product safety to food labeling to safety of "natural" products.

American Culinary Federation, Inc.

Address: 10 San Bartula Drive, St. Augustine, FL 32086
Phone: 904-824-4468 / 800-624-9458 / Fax: 904-825-4758
Web address: www.acfchefs.org
Web site: The ACF, founded in New York City in 1929, is a professional not-for-profit organization for chefs working to promote a professional

image of the American chef worldwide through education. The site includes a job bank, directories of accredited culinary programs, and apprenticeship programs plus information on receiving certification and a calendar of culinary events. The section titled "Chef and Child" provides a look at a culinary education program designed to teach nutrition and cooking to youngsters. The site also includes material appropriate for high school vocational educators.

American Diabetes Association (ADA)

Address: 1701 North Beauregard Street, Alexandria, VA 22311
Phone: 800-342-2383
Web address: www.diabetes.org
Web site: The ADA motto is to prevent and cure diabetes and to improve the lives of all people affected by diabetes. This easy-to-use Web site has information about the disease, risk factors, complications, and warning signs of diabetes. There are also sections on nutrition, exercise tips, and recipes, as well as general information. Users can request an information packet but the association cautions that representatives cannot make a diagnosis or recommend medical treatment. There are links to other Internet resources and to magazines and journals dealing with diabetes and related health issues.

American Dietetic Association (ADA)

Address: 216 West Jackson Boulevard, Chicago, IL 60606
Phone: 312-899-0040 / 800-366-1655
Web address: www.eatright.org
Web site: The number-one feature of this attractive and easy-to-use site is its ability to help people "Find a dietitian," plus a toll-free hotline for professional advice on improving your diet. Users can also link to many other nutrition-related sites. Informational categories include consumer education and public policy, dietetic practice groups, medical and health professionals, and dietetic associations. This fact-filled site includes a "Tip of the day," as well as in-depth monthly features. Users can find information on the USDA Food Guide Pyramid, fact sheets, and a nutrition reading list, along with a link to the ADA's journal and other highly rated nutrition books.

American Heart Association (AHA)

Address: 7272 Greenville Avenue, Dallas, TX 75231
Phone: 214-373-6300 / 800-242-8721
Web address: www.americanheart.org
Web site: This association Web site is colorful and user-friendly with an easy-to-use A to Z guide that provides clear, concise information

on heart disease and stroke-related illness. There are sections dealing with nutrition, exercise, and professional publications, and a news bureau. Users can link to a special site for women who want heart health information or link to an additional site titled "Living with Heart Failure," designed for caregivers and patients. Visitors can send a message to Congress about various biomedical issues and other health care initiatives.

American Institute for Cancer Research (AICR)

Address: 1759 R Street, NW, Washington, D.C. 20009
Phone: 202-328-7744 / 800-843-8114
Web address: www.aicr.org
Web site: This national cancer charity has created a Web site that offers information on food, nutrition, the prevention of cancer, news updates, critiques of fad diets and diet books, plus a helpful resource that answers common questions posed by newly diagnosed cancer patients and their families. It features recipes as well as a nutrition hotline and kids' newsletter. Users can also link to other cancer and nutrition sites.

American Medical Association (AMA)

Address: 515 North State Street, Chicago, IL 60610
Phone: 312-464-5000
Web address: www.ama-assn.org
Web site: While this site is clearly geared toward physicians, there are useful resources for the layperson, including a section on consumer health information. There is a members-only portion to this site with an AMA Staff Directory. Journals and the American Medical News are available, as well as *JAMA* (*Journal of the American Medical Association*) and its related links on HIV/AIDS, asthma, migraines, and women's health.

American Obesity Association (AOA)

Address: 1250 24th Street, NW, Suite 300, Washington, D.C. 20037
Phone: 800-986-2373 / 202-776-7711 / Fax: 202-776-7712
Web address: www.obesity.org
Web site: The focus of this site is information about obesity and its treatment, and includes helpful resources for understanding insurance issues as well as a body mass index. There are links to other sites like the American Heart Association. The AOA offers a health newsletter as well as a section called Hot Issues that covers topics like a patient's bill of rights.

American Society of Bariatric Physicians

Address: 5600 South Quebec Street, Suite 109A, Englewood, CO 80111
Phone: 303-770-2526 / Fax: 303-779-4834
Web address: www.asbp.org
Web site: While there is a members-only section on this Web site, there is also easy access for the general public to information about obesity and its related surgical treatments. Other features include medical updates, related links, and frequently asked questions, and the site offers assistance in finding a bariatric physician. Bariatrics is the medical treatment of obesity and its associated problems, and is currently one of the fastest-growing specialties in medicine.

Ask the Dietitian

Web address: http://www.dietitian.com
Web site: This site, developed by nutritionist Joanne Larsen, has a cool feature, the Healthy Body Calculator, found at http://www.dietitian.com/ibw/ibw.html. Have a tape measure handy and know your weight. This interactive tool creates a dietary recommendation as well as graphics to show where you fall in the ideal health and body mass index ranges.

Atkins Center for Complementary Medicine

Address: 152 East 55th Street, New York, NY 10022
Phone: 888-ATKINS-8 / 212-758-2110
Web address: atkinscenter.com
Web site: This site is the complete guide to finding and using any and all of the Dr. Atkins's New Diet Revolution diet products. There is information on the diet, success stories from dieters, recipes, and access to Atkins stores across the country.

Burger King Corporation

Address: 17777 Old Cutler Road, Miami, FL 33157-6347
Phone: 305-378-7011 / Fax: 305-379-7262
Web address: www.burgerking.com
Web site: This colorful site is filled with feel-good information about Burger King but also gets high marks for better-than-average nutritional information. Unlike sites that bury their numbers on fats and calories, Burger King provides an Interactive Nutritional Information Wizard, where users can select menu items, theoretically eat a reasonable amount of calories, and limit their fat intake if they choose. But advertising is still the most important part of this site, with entry to a Kids Club filled with toys, games, and a clubhouse, plus a What's Hot

section that highlights the latest toy giveaway. Franchise locations are listed as well as the company information.

Centers for Disease Control and Prevention (CDC)

Address: 1600 Clifton Road, NE, Atlanta, GA 30333
Phone: 404-639-3311 / 800-311-3435
Web address: www.cdc.gov
Web site: The CDC is an agency of the Department of Health and Human Services. The Web site is designed to answer a multitude of questions from the general public and Health Topics A–Z or Frequently Asked Questions are filled with updated documents for that purpose. Categories of Frequently Asked Questions range from Diabetes or E.coli to Hanta Virus and Listeriosis. The site includes access to data and statistics, and training and employment information, as well as links to other sites. Geared for the general public, it is a useful first stop for anyone with concerns about a medical condition. But keep in mind that the CDC strongly recommends against self-diagnosis or self-management without involvement of health care professionals.

Center for Food Safety

Address: 666 Pennsylvania Avenue, SE, Suite 302, Washington D.C., 20003
Phone: 202-547-9359 / Fax: 202-547-9429
Web address: www.centerforfoodsafety.org
Web site: The Center for Food Safety is a public interest and environmental advocacy organization addressing the impacts of the food production system on human health, animal welfare, and the environment. The site contains legislative alerts and information on food safety issues such as genetically modified organisms (bioengineered foods), irradiation, sludge, and methyl bromide. New is www.foodsafetynow.org—an interactive tool for the public to use in submitting food safety comments to government officials, agencies, and members of Congress.

Center for Science in the Public Interest (CSPI)

Address: 1875 Connecticut Avenue, NW, Suite 300, Washington, D.C. 20009
Phone: 202-332-9110 / Fax: 202-265-4954
Web address: www.cspinet.org
Web site: The CSPI is a nonprofit education and advocacy organization working to improve the safety and nutritional quality of food. CSPI promotes health education about nutrition and alcohol and also represents the public's interests in the legislative, regulatory, and judicial arenas. The site offers excellent links to both private and government nu-

trition sources as well as access to CSPI's *Nutrition Action Healthletter*. An interesting nutrition quiz and a document library add to the wealth of information on this site. Special reports, such as "Liquid Candy: How Soft Drinks Are Harming America's Health," spell out the facts on soft drinks and health.

Consumer Information Center (CIC)

Address: P.O. Box 100
Pueblo, CO 81002
Phone: 888-878-3256
Web address: www.pueblo.gsa.gov
Web site: The CIC is part of the General Services Administration (GSA), and has a large catalog of some 200 consumer publications currently in print. The Health and Food sections cover everything from fitness and medications to food safety, nutrition, and food preservatives. The site receives high marks for the access it provides consumers to highly accurate information. Order a free catalog by calling the toll-free number, 1-888-878-3256.

Council for Responsible Nutrition (CRN)

Address: 1875 Eye Street, NW, Suite 400, Washington, D.C. 20006-5409
Phone: 202-872-1488 / Fax: 202-872-9594
Web address: www.crnusa.org
Web site: The CRN is a trade association representing companies that make nutritional supplements. This site offers comprehensive links to many government sites that deal with nutrition, legislation, and regulation of dietary supplements. Other useful information includes the section on Scientific Affairs with current scientific articles on dietary supplements.

DietWatch

Web address: www.dietwatch.com
Web site: DietWatch began as DietWatch Diary, offering free software for anyone interested in healthy weight control. This virtual diet center does not support any specific diets, but does recommend sensible calorie levels based on realistic weight goals as well as individualized weight loss counseling available for a fee. The highlight of the site is still the "Diary" analysis tool that helps dieters track food intake. The database from which to select foods is outstanding and there is also room to log workouts as well as a section on diet-related news.

Drsears.com

Web address: www.drsears.com

Web site: Anyone looking for The Zone Technology Network and the Web site of the Zone diet by Dr. Barry Sears, need look no further. This Web site offers a chance to ask questions of Zone founder Sears, plus things like helpful hints, information, and an array of Zone tools and services. And make no mistake, this site is not affiliated in any way with the ZonePerfect Nutrition Company's Web page or with its products. To ensure that people make the connection, Dr. Sears offers an "Ask Dr. Sears" section along with a member center, recipes, tips for staying in the Zone, testimonials, a Physicians' Member Network to answer questions, health news updates, and, of course, access to Zone products.

Ethnic Grocer

Address: 1033 University Place #350, Evanston, IL 60201
Phone: 800-523-1961 / Fax: 847-475-7717
Web address: www.EthnicGrocer.com
Web site: This site makes ethnic cooking and eating as easy as possible for the average family. With choices like Chef Chat, Comfort Foods, and Select a Dish, users can choose by region or by meal parts like entrée, salad, dessert, soup. For each type of ethnic eating, like Japanese, Swedish, or Greek, you pick from a list of choices. Ingredient lists are provided as well as step-by-step directions. There is also a culinary world tour and history of each region's foods plus featured products. Visitors can also fill up grocery carts with specials like raspberry champagne vinegar, maple syrup, or grape leaves.

FitDay

Web address: www.fitday.com
Web site: This attractive and colorful site is based on an interactive and informative food diary to help users lose weight and meet fitness and nutritional goals. For those who like to keep track of numbers and chart activities, this is a great place to get a handle on eating habits and food intake. There is also accurate weight loss and healthful eating advice as well as information on the USDA Food Guide Pyramid.

Five-a-Day

Address: 5301 Limestone Road, Suite 101, Wilmington, DE 19808-1249
Phone: 302-235-ADAY / Fax: 302-235-5555
Web address: www.5aday.gov
Web site: This site was created by the National Cancer Institute and the Centers for Disease Control and Prevention. Users can find a health chart that rates health habits along with how-to ideas and recommended portion sizes. The site provides information on the basics of eating five or more servings of fruits and vegetables per day plus recipes

and tips on physical activity for optimum health. There is also a direct link to the USDA Dietary Guidelines for Americans.

Food Allergy Network

Address: 10400 Eaton Place, Suite 107, Fairfax, VA 22030-2209
Phone: 703-691-3179
Web address: www.foodallergy.org
Web site: This helpful site offers facts on food allergies with sections that answer common questions, dispel myths, and offer the latest research on food allergies. Users can also sign up for "Product Alerts," a free service via e-mail.

Food and Drug Administration (FDA)/U.S. Dept. of Health and Human Services

Address: 200 Independence Avenue, SW, Washington, D.C. 20201
Phone: 888-463-6332
Web address: www.fda.gov
Web site: This FDA site is user-friendly for a government site and includes information on a wide range of topics from cosmetics to articles on acne, sports, asthma, and eating disorders. There is a special section, titled "For Kids, Teens & Educators," that has a wealth of information in formats from crossword puzzles to a food safety word match and food safety quiz. There are also links to many nutrition sites and a useful resource list.

Food and Nutrition Board (FNB)/Institute of Medicine (IOM)

Address: Institute of Medicine, 2101 Constitution Avenue, NW, Washington, D.C. 20418
Phone: 202-334-1601 / Fax: 202-334-2419
Web address: www4.nas.edu/IOM/IOMHome.nsf
Web site: The FNB is part of the National Academy of Sciences (NAS). The NAS is a private, nonprofit corporation created by Congress and made up of biomedical scientists with expertise in nutrition and food science. The Board makes recommendations to improve food quality and to promote public health and prevent diet-related diseases. This Web site provides access to ongoing FNB studies and upcoming events, plus links to related food and nutrition sites and to the Institute of Medicine (IOM) and NAS. Not for the casual user, this site is difficult to navigate because information is presented in highly technical terms.

Food Finder/Olen Publishing, Inc.

Phone: 415-383-4280 / 800-424-6536
Web address:www.olen.com

Web site: This site is based on the book *Fast Food Facts* by the Minnesota Attorney General's Office. The site allows users to search by individual fast-food restaurants or by different fields like fat, cholesterol, or sodium. For example, you can find all fast-food restaurants that offer items with less than 10 grams of fat by putting 10 in the Maximum Fat field and leaving all other fields empty. A great way to compare and make better fast-food choices.

George Ohsawa Macrobiotic Foundation, Inc.

Address: P.O. Box 3998, Chico, CA 95927-3998
Phone: 800-232-2372 / 530-566-9765
Web address: www.gomf.macrobiotic.net
Web site: The George Ohsawa Macrobiotic Foundation, Inc., is a nonprofit organization dedicated to educating people about the teachings of George Ohsawa and the principles and practices of macrobiotics. The site is straightforward and easy to navigate. Users can find information about macrobiotics and Ohsawa's published works, along with access to its magazine, *Macrobiotics Today.* There is also information about the annual macrobiotic summer camp sponsored by the Foundation, held in the Sierra Nevada mountains. With resource connections and links to other health-related sites, this is a good starting point for anyone interested in learning more about a macrobiotic diet.

Good Karma Café

Web address: www.goodkarmacafe.com
Web site: A vegetarian-oriented site, Good Karma Café provides practical, how-to advice for new vegetarians. Users can also purchase books, locate restaurants, find recipes, or link to an eclectic variety of other Web sites. The recipe section also offers vegetarian versions of familiar foods. The Teen Veggie Forum offers information on how other teens cope with friends and family when they go vegetarian, and allows teens to chat with one another about getting healthy and exchange recipes.

Harvard Eating Disorders Center

Address: 356 Boylston Street, Boston, MA 02116
Phone: 617-236-7766 / 888-236-1188 / Fax: 617-236-2068
Web address: www.hedc.org
Web site: This national nonprofit organization is dedicated to research and education about eating disorders and their treatment. The site includes excellent resources; a question-and-answer section titled "Do I Have a Problem?" along with lots of facts about eating disorders. There is also a list of events and programs, and referrals for help and support for anyone dealing with an eating disorder.

Healthfinder/U.S. Department of Health and Human Services

Address: 200 Independence Avenue, SW, Washington, D.C. 20201
Phone: 202-619-0257 / 877-696-6775
Web address: www.healthfinder.gov
Web site: The Department of Health and Human Services' site covers every thing from current topics like breastfeeding and folic acid to nutrition information from federal and state agencies. There is also a list of online medical journals, a database of toll-free numbers, a medical dictionary, a library locator, and information about support and self-help groups. There is a search engine for subject searches or for browsing by topics. This site is easy to navigate and is filled with understandable and useful information.

Health Mall

Address: 2051 Springdale Road, Cherry Hill, NJ 08003
Phone: 800-204-1902
Web address: www.healthmall.com
Web site: With a database of some 4,800 health food stores, Health Mall calls itself the most comprehensive source for information concerning health, nutrition, and alternative medicine. The site has a handy Health Food Store Directory, and a way to check for drug interactions between prescription drugs and vitamins. There is a database of chiropractors and a page of health-related links, plus more alternative features like a directory of herbal remedies and a naturopath search or a list of massage therapists. The section on symptoms and remedies is heavily visited. The monthly newsletter contains an alternative medicine update, which focuses on nutrition and herbal remedies.

Healthy People 2010

Web address: http://www.health.gov/healthypeople/default.htm
Web site: This site details the goals of the Healthy People 2010 initiative of the U.S. Department of Health and Human Services. It contains progress reports and reviews, links to community Healthy People initiatives, and information on how Americans' health compares with that of people in other countries. The 10 Leading Health Indicators, for which there are updated statistics, are physical activity; overweight and obesity; tobacco use; substance abuse; responsible sexual behavior; mental health; injury and violence; environmental quality; immunization; and access to health care.

iEmily

Address: 136 West Street, Suite 201, Northampton, MA, 01060
Phone: 413-587-0244

Web address: www.iemily.com
Web site: This unique site was created for an underserved population—teenage girls. Look for solid and sensible nutrition information in the "Healthy Eating" section plus articles that explain topics like organic foods, eating disorders, and strategies for fitness. The section on the fact and fiction of fad diets offers honest evaluations of current best-selling weight-loss plans, and the site encourages girls to give up on diets and eat for health. Teens can also find information on vegetarianism, ethnic cuisine, sport-specific nutrition, and how to develop a basic healthy, active, and realistic lifestyle. The attractive site continues to change and grow, like the audience it serves.

Images of Health—The Nutrition Link

Address: Department of Family Medicine, East Carolina University, Greenville, NC 27858
Phone: 252-816-5459
Web address: www.preventivenutrition.com
Web site: Sponsored by the East Carolina University School of Medicine, this site was originally designed as a tutorial for students in the medical program. Each section links to assessment tools for use in clinical settings where students learn to teach patients the relationship between disease and diet. The four areas of information on the site are the U.S. Dietary Guidelines, the Natural History of Cancer, physician interventions research, and case studies.

International Food Information Council (IFIC)

Address: 1100 Connecticut Avenue, NW, Suite 430, Washington, D.C. 20036
Phone: 202-296-6540 / 202-296-6547
Web address: http://ificinfo.health.org
Web site: The IFIC collects and disseminates scientific information on food safety and nutritional health to nutritional professionals and educators, plus government officials, journalists, and consumers. The IFIC was founded in 1985 and is a nonprofit organization. Information for educators is included, along with sections on general nutrition facts, current nutrition developments, and additional resources. A lengthy glossary, plus the variety of food safety and nutritional information, makes this site better than average.

Mayo Health Oasis/Mayo Foundation for Medical Education and Research

Address: 200 First Street, SW, Rochester, MN 55905
Phone: 507-266-4057

Web address: www.mayohealth.org

Web site: Presented by the famous Mayo Health Clinic, this site is rated among the best by the Tufts University Nutrition Navigator. The format is user-friendly and offers information on anything from past articles concerning nutritional topics to a virtual cookbook where readers send recipes to be "made over" into a healthier version. Ask the Mayo Dietitian is in a question-and-answer format, and there are quizzes and tests, some interactive, so users can test their nutrition knowledge.

McDonalds Corporation

Address: 1 McDonalds Plaza, Oak Brook, IL 60523-1928

Phone: 630-623-3000

Web address: www.McDonalds.com

Web site: An attractive and easy-to-use site; business comes first as it features all the promotional products McDonalds has to offer consumers. However, there is good nutritional information to be had if you click on menu choices like Nutrition Facts and Nutrient Card. Consumers can find the breakdown on all McDonalds food products as well as fat grams and calories of each. The information gives interested consumers the opportunity for informed menu selections, something that chains like Mrs. Fields Cookies and Cinnabon lack.

McDougall On-Line Wellness Center

Address: P. O. Box 14039, Santa Rosa, CA 95402

Phone: 800-570-1654 / 707-576-1654 / Fax: 707-576-3313

Web address: www.drmcdougall.com

Web site: The Wellness Center and Web site were founded by Dr. John McDougall who has written several books about the effects of nutrition on disease as well as diet books based on low-fat, starch-based foods. This easy-to-use site offers access to McDougall products and books, as well as recipes, information on the California-based health center, and articles dealing with nutrition and disease.

Meals for You (My Menus)/Point of Choice

Address: P.O. Box 2309, Fairfield, IA 52556

Phone: 515-472-3434 / 800-446-3687

Web address: www.MealsForYou.com

Web site: Welcome to a Web site that is free, fast, and easy-to-use, where it's possible to find thousands of recipes by type, ingredients, or nutrient content. This site is sponsored by My Menus/Point of Choice, a small independent company founded in 1991. Users can search by categories of menus for diabetics, vegetarians, and dieters. The site offers menu plans, complete with nutrient analysis and a shopping list, which can be organized based on the floor plans of participating stores. Meals for You/Point of Choice has tested in-store interactive recipe centers in several U.S. grocery store chains.

National Academy of Sciences (Institute of Medicine/Food Nutrition Board)

Address: 2101 Constitution Avenue, NW, Washington, D.C. 20418
Phone: 202-334-2587
Web address: www4.nas.edu
Web site: The NAS is a private, nonprofit corporation made up of biomedical scientists with expertise in nutrition, food science, food safety, and other areas. They provide independent advice on scientific issues to government. The site sections include news, current projects, publications, reports, books, articles, and a subject index for searching. This site offers important information but is difficult for the casual browser to navigate.

National Association of Anorexia Nervosa and Associated Disorders (ANAD)

Address: P.O. Box 7, Highland Park, IL 60035
Phone: (Hotline) 847-831-3438 / Fax: 847-433-4632
Web address: www.anad.org
Web site: The ANAD was founded in 1976 and is among the oldest national nonprofit organizations helping eating disorder victims and their families. The site offers access to free hotline counseling, an international network of support groups for sufferers and their families, and referrals to health care professionals. There are sections on insurance discrimination and legislative news. The association also provides educational speakers, programs, and presentations for schools, colleges, public health agencies, and community groups. There is an online form to request information or to volunteer.

National Center for Health Statistics (NCHS)

Address: 6525 Belcrest Road, Hyattsville, MD 20782-2003
Phone: 301-458-4636
Web address: www.cdc.gov/nchs
Web site: This center is affiliated with the Centers for Disease Control and Prevention (CDC), under the U.S. Department of Health and Human Services. Health Topics A–Z is a list of disease and health subjects found on the CDC Web site. Those are divided by categories from teens to environmental health and women's health. This site links to vital records for the entire United States and also links to the U.S. State Department.

National Coalition for Promoting Physical Activity (NCPPA)

Address: 1010 Massachusetts Avenue, Suite 350, Washington D.C. 20001
Phone: 202-454-7521 / Fax: 202-454-7598
Web address: www.ncppa.org
Web site: The NCPPA is a national network of public, private, and industry organizations working to improve access and knowledge of physical activity through physical fitness, sports, education, and worksite health promotion. Founded by the American College of Sports Medicine, the American Heart Association, and the American Alliance for Health, Physical Education, Recreation and Dance, it now includes over 150 organizations working to promote fitness on the local, state, and national levels. The site contains a wealth of information and includes a direct link to the Healthy People 2010 site as well as a list of state coalitions and a national calendar of events.

National Council Against Health Fraud

Address: 119 Foster Street, Building R, Second Floor, Peabody, MA 01960
Phone: 978-532-9383 / Fax: 978-532-9450
Web address: www.ncahf.org
Web site: The NCAHF is a nonprofit voluntary health agency focused on health fraud, misinformation, and quackery as public health problems. This straightforward format is user-friendly and contains hundreds of articles to educate consumers and health professionals about fraud and quackery. The site also supports sound consumer health laws and will assist with legal actions against fraudulent products or product claims.

National Institutes of Health (NIH)

Address: Building 1, Room B156, 1 Center Drive, MSC 0122, Bethesda, MD 20892-0148
Phone: 301-496-4000
Web address: www.nih.gov
Web site: This government site offers a very comprehensive list of hotline resources on any imaginable health problem from A to Z. There are sections about the NIH, news and events, scientific resources from journals to research labs, and health information in the form of publications as well as access to resources like MEDLINEplus. Information is also provided in Spanish. The NIH is part of the U.S. Department of Health and Human Services.

Nutrition on the Web—For Teens/ThinkQuest

Address: 200 Business Park Drive, Armonk, NY 10504
Phone: 914-273-1700
Web address: http://library.thinkquest.org
Web site: The ThinkQuest site was developed by students and is written especially for the third- to twelfth-grade audience. Informative sections include Exercises, Myths, Case Files, Teen Health, and Recipes, among others, and interactive areas allow users to take a Nutri-Quiz, to ask fellow users questions, to find the number of calories in common foods, and to log in to the diet planner for healthy meal planning. There is also access to a chatroom and users can choose from several languages with which to view the Web site.

New York Online Access to Health (NOAH)

Web address: www.noah.cuny.edu/wellness.nutrition/nutrition.html
Web site: NOAH is a consumer health Web site of quality filtered materials in English or Spanish. The volunteer staff receives the information from medical librarians working in academic, special, hospital, and public libraries throughout New York. Page editors organize and arrange the full-text consumer information, which is available through an effective keyword search.

Oldways Preservation and Exchange Trust

Address: 25 First Street, Cambridge, MA 02141
Phone: 617-621-3000 / Fax: 617-621-1230
Web address: www.oldwayspt.org
Web site: This is a nonprofit education organization that promotes healthy eating based on the "old ways," or traditional cuisines from around the world. They have created four food pyramids: Asian, Latin, Mediterranean, and Vegetarian. The Oldways site also offers educational programs, nutritional news, and a bookstore. Users can browse an assortment of health issues by searching Oldways' archive of articles.

Overeaters Anonymous (OA)

Address: P.O. Box 44020, Rio Rancho, NM 87174-4020
Phone: 505-891-2665 / Fax: 505-891-4320
Web address: www.overeatersanonymous.org
Web site: With a focus on recovery, the Overeaters Anonymous site provides information about the organization, from finding a meeting to ordering from an online catalog of literature and specialty items. OA makes no claims for weight loss; instead it works to help members overcome their problem with compulsive overeating. Fashioned after the

12-step program of Alcoholics Anonymous, OA addresses the physical, emotional, and spiritual aspects of recovery. Members are encouraged to seek professional help with every aspect of their recovery. The Web site is not fancy but is packed with information.

Physicians Committee for Responsible Medicine (PCRM)

Address: 5100 Wisconsin Avenue, NW, Suite 400, Washington, D.C. 20016
Phone: 202-686-2210
Web address: www.pcrm.org
Web site: PCRM promotes preventive medicine and a nutrition program, the New Four Food Groups that includes a nutrition curriculum for schools. It supports research into diabetes, cancer, and other health care issues, and has also developed a program for healthful eating for businesses, hospitals, and schools, called the Gold Plan. A keyword search can locate topics like restaurant reviews and physician referrals, and there are special resources available for medical students and educators. Dr. Neal Barnard founded PCRM in 1985 to promote preventive medicine through the use of diet and exercise.

President's Council on Food Safety

Address: 200 Independence Avenue, SW, Washington, D.C. 20201
Phone: 888-SAFEFOOD
Web address: www.foodsafety.gov
Web site: The President's Council on Food Safety was established in August 1998 to coordinate the nation's food safety policy and resources. This site is a gateway to government food safety information and is jointly sponsored by the Department of Commerce, the Environmental Protection Agency, the U.S. Department of Health and Human Services, and the U.S. Department of Agriculture and is maintained by the FDA's Center for Food Safety and Applied Nutrition. Sections include Consumer Advice; Kids, Teens and Educators; Report Illnesses; and Product Complaints. There is also quick access to current government publications on safety topics and links to federal and state government agencies.

President's Council on Physical Fitness and Sports

Address: Department W, 200 Independence Avenue, SW, Room 738H, Washington, D.C. 20201
Phone: 202-690-9000 / Fax: 202-690-5211
Web address: www.fitness.gov

Web site: This government site, part of the U.S. Department of Health and Human Services, has information about the history of the Council as well as links to other federal agencies and health organizations. There are exercise and nutrition tips aimed at youngsters and information about health and exercise plus a resource link for coaches, teachers, and fitness professionals. This site links to a huge index of government health publications and gives information about the Presidential Sports Award.

Preventive Medicine Research Institute (PMRI)

See WebMDHealth.

Pritikin Longevity Center

Address: 19735 Turnberry Way, Aventura, FL 33180
Phone: 800-327-4914 / 305-935-7131 / Fax: 305-935-7111
Web address: www.pritikin.com
Web site: The Pritikin Longevity Center was originally founded by Nathan Pritikin and is now run by his son, Robert. The Web site explains the Pritikin approach in great detail, offers products and services, answers requests for information, and has updates on current nutritional information. Pritikin products have been carried in local grocery stores for years and range from pasta, cereal, and salad dressings to soups and beverages.

Quackwatch

Web address: www.quackwatch.com
Web site: Quackwatch is a nonprofit corporation designed to combat health-related frauds, fads, and faulty products. Founded by Dr. Stephen Barrett in 1969 as the Lehigh Valley Committee Against Health Fraud, it assumed its current name following the launching of its Web site in 1997. This no-frills site provides access to health-related articles. Quackwatch has also sponsored research projects to look at dubious advertising and questionable methods used by advertisers as well as several other projects. The site launched NutriWatch, www.nutriwatch.org, in 2000 as a monitor of sensible nutrition and any quackery associated with diet, nutrition, or diet products.

Shape Up America

Address: 6707 Democracy Boulevard, Suite 306, Bethesda, MD 20817
Web address: www.shapeup.org
Web site: Shape Up America is a national initiative to promote healthy weight and nutrition, and increased physical activity across America.

Made up of a large coalition of industry, physical fitness, medical, health, and nutritional experts, Shape Up America works to promote the importance of a healthy weight; works to education people about ways to achieve appropriate body weight; and cooperates with other organizations to advance a healthy lifestyle. The site offers a support center for practical tips on weight loss, an interactive weight-loss program, a cyber kitchen, and a center to determine your body mass index (BMI).

Snack Food Association

Address: 1711 King Street, Suite 1, Alexandria, VA 22314
Phone: 703-836-4500 / 800-628-1334
Web address: http://www.sfa.org
Web site: Ever thought of snacking across America? This site provides regional recipes using every possible snack food from chocolate-covered potato chips to spicy Santa Fe trail mix. The association was founded in 1937 and continues to grow just as the industry it supports does. Users can find information on the state of the snack food industry and on consumer snacking behavior, plus an interesting timeline and a history of snack foods. If you wanted to know who invented the potato chip, the information is easily available.

Society for Nutrition Education (SNE)

Address: 9202 North Meridian Street, Suite 200, Indianapolis, IN 46260
Phone: 317-571-5618 / 800-235-6690 / Fax: 317-571-5603
Web address:www.sne.org
Web site: The Society for Nutrition Education is an international community of professionals involved in nutrition education and health promotion. While the Web site is geared for nutrition educators, it provides access to the society's official publication, the *Journal of Nutrition Education and Behavior* (JNEB), a great resource on the history of and up-to-date developments in nutrition education.

Taco Bell/Trigon Global Restaurants

Address: 17901 Von Karman Avenue, Irvine, CA 92614
Phone: 949-863-4500
Web address: http://www.tacobell.com
Web site: This fast-food restaurant site offers easy-to-find nutritional information plus the usual company information about franchise locations, employment information, and even an online gift shop. Though not as interactive as the McDonalds site, this is still a colorful and informative tool. Also links to Kentucky Fried Chicken (KFC) and Pizza Hut, both under the Trigon corporate umbrella.

Teenage Research Unlimited (TRU)

Address: 707 Skokie Boulevard, Suite 450, Northbrook, IL 60062
Phone: 847-564-3440
Web address: www.teenresearch.com
Web site: Teenage Research Unlimited was founded in 1982 and calls itself the first marketing-research firm to specialize exclusively in the teenage market. From this site users can subscribe to a syndicated teen study, along with news releases and descriptions of the firm's marketing strategy and biographies of company officials. Although much of the information must be purchased, the news released includes current facts useful to teens and educators.

Take Off Pounds Sensibly (TOPS)

Web address: www.TOPS.org
Web site: The oldest of the weight loss self-help groups, TOPS offers a chapter locator plus an easy-to-access schedule of events and speakers for across the country. TOPS provides information generated by its own in-house health-care professionals. Users can click on to the TOPS store or look at TOPS 10, encouraging words that provide positive, helpful suggestions for TOPS members.

U.S. Department of Agriculture (USDA)

Address: 14th and Independence Avenues, SW, Washington, D.C. 20250
Phone: 202-720-2791
Web address: www.usda.gov / www.usda.gov/cnpp
Web site: The USDA site has a wealth of government information, starting with a message from the Secretary, and including a history of American agriculture. One cool feature is the interactive Healthy Eating Index. Plug in what you've eaten in recent days and the site produces a score on how healthy your overall diet is. There is also access to the Code of Federal Regulations for agriculture, animals, and forests, and a link to the USDA Fraud Hotline. The site also links to the USDA Center for Nutrition Policy and Promotion. That site offers professionals who work on nutrition and hunger issues access to USDA documents but it is not for the casual browser. The documents include a healthy eating index and resources for nutrition educators.

USDA Food and Nutrition Information Center

Address: 10301 Baltimore Avenue, Beltsville, MD 20705-2351
Phone: 301-504-5719
Web address: www.nal.usda.gov/fnic

Web site: Sponsored by the USDA National Agricultural Library, this site connects users to the resources of the National Agricultural Library, which contains educational materials, research briefs, and food-composition data. This site is geared toward professionals looking for technical information. However, there is some information aimed at consumers.

U.S. Department of Health and Human Services (HHS)

Address: 200 Independence Avenue, SW, Washington, D.C. 20201
Phone: 202-619-0257 / 877-696-6775
Web address: www.hhs.gov
Web site: The Department of Health and Human Services is the U.S. government's principal agency overseeing all aspects of American health, with more than 300 programs on everything from food and drug safety to Medicare and Medicaid. The site links to other HHS agencies and sponsored sites, such as News and Public Affairs, What's New, and a calendar of events and health observances. It also links to YouthInfo, a Web site developed to provide the latest information about America's adolescents. That site contains a profile of youth, resources for parents, and speeches on topics of interest to youth. The department also sponsors and links to Healthy People 2010 as a way to promote physical activity across the nation.

University of Missouri Food and Nutrition

Address: 225 University Hall, Columbia, MO 65211
Phone: 573-882-2428
Web address: http://outreach.missouri.edu/hes/food.htm
Web site: Sponsored by the University of Missouri in partnership with Columbia Extension Service, this site is designed to help consumers of all ages improve their health by selecting nutritious foods. Consumer tip sheets and the Food and Nutrition Resource Newsletters are consumer-friendly, easy to search, and answer questions from the latest diet and sports supplements to food safety and educational resources. A Resource Network Hotline links to different categories of companies, organizations, and Web sites. Educators will find information divided by grade level with activities and links. A nice addition is a health days calendar.

Vegetarian Pages

Web address: www.veg.org/veg
Web site: This online guide for vegetarians and vegans is a vast collection of information geared toward anyone interested in becoming a vegetarian or anyone who wants to quit eating a lot of meat. Sections

range from Frequently Asked Questions to the Mega Index of Everything Vegetarian, plus recipes, nutrition, a list of famous vegetarians, and contacts with many organizations.

Vegetarian Resource Group (VRG)

Address: P.O. Box 1343, Baltimore, MD 21203
Phone: 410-366-VEGE
Web address: www.veg.org
Web site: The VRG is a nonprofit organization that works to educate the public on vegetarian and related issues such as health, ecology, world hunger, and nutrition. Financial support comes largely from membership, contributions, and book sales. The site provides news, recipes, and a huge list of nutrition and related links. There is a lengthy section on vegetarian nutrition, geared for anyone interested in meatless eating. Although developed for students and consumers, health care professionals may find useful information as well.

Vegetarian Society of the UK

Address: Parkdale, Dunham Road, Altrincham, Cheshire, WA144QG, United Kingdom
Phone: 0161-925-2000
Web address: www.vegsoc.org
Web site: For new vegetarians this resource offers a glimpse into the lifestyle of the British vegetarian. The site is geared to student users, who can find anything from tips on stumbling blocks to being vegetarian to a section for matching up with a vegetarian pen pal.

Wake Forest University—Baptist Medical Center

Address: School of Medicine, Medical Center Boulevard, Winston-Salem, NC 27157
Phone: 336-716-2011
Web address: www.bgsm.edu/nutrition
Web site: Run by Wake Forest University's Bowman Gray School of Medicine and its Center for Research on Human Nutrition and Chronic Disease Prevention, this site gives a nutritional breakdown of common foods, including fast food, and offers quizzes on diet and fitness. The school's research center devised this site to promote preventive health care. It also offers a calorie calculator to estimate calories, fat, cholesterol, and sodium levels in a variety of common foods and beverages. Unsure that you're eating a balanced diet? Take the "How's Your Diet?" quiz. Eating habits are compared to the U.S. Dietary Guidelines put out by the USDA.

WebMDHealth

Address: 669 River Drive, Center 2, Elmwood Park, NJ 07407
Phone: 877-GO-WEBMD
Web address: my.webmd.com
Web site: This site features an enormous amount of medical information, from nutrition to pregnancy, sports fitness to news on drugs and herbs. The site is affiliated with Dr. Dean Ornish, founder of the Preventive Medicine Research Institute in Sausalito, California. Special features include My HealthRecord, where users can list all important personal health information, from current medications to allergies, doctors, and health plan information. "Ask Our Experts" provides answers to general questions and users can also ask Dr. Ornish questions. The site reminds users that it is not a substitute for seeing a doctor or other health care professional, and it provides links to other health related web pages.

Weight-Control Information Network

Address: 1 Win Way, Bethesda, MD 20896-3665
Phone: 202-828-1025 / 877-946-4627 / Fax: 202-828-1028
Web address: www.niddk.nih.gov/health/nutrit/win.htm
Web site: This site is sponsored by the National Institute of Diabetes and Digestive and Kidney Diseases (NIDDK), part of the National Institutes of Health. The site offers information for health professionals as well as consumers on weight control, obesity, and nutritional disorders. With access to thousands of articles, books, and educational materials, this site is very helpful for consumers as well as professionals. It also features *WIN Notes,* a quarterly newsletter published by NIDDK.

Weight Watchers

Phone: 800-651-6000
Web address: www.weightwatchers.com
Web site: Like the other diet program Web pages, this site features everything from Frequently Asked Questions to information about the program and its new points system to tips from spokesperson Sarah Ferguson, the Duchess of York. There are recipes and weight-loss articles plus access to Weight Watchers' products and a history of the organization. The presentation is tasteful and the site is user-friendly.

Yale Center for Eating and Weight Disorders

Address: Yale University Department of Psychology, P.O. Box 208205, New Haven, CT 06520-8205
Phone: 203-432-4610
Web address: www.yale.edu/ycewd

Web site: This no-nonsense Web site is clear and concise. The home page includes a short introduction to the center, including its services, fees, and location. There is a brief description of various eating disorders but the obvious purpose of the site is to connect anyone who has a suspected eating disorder with appropriate treatment.

ZonePerfect: The Official Zone Diet Web site

Phone: 800-390-6690
Web address: www.zoneperfect.com
Web site: Another commercial diet program site, this one is designed for anyone who wants to enter the Zone—the Zone Diet, that is. The site offers easy access to support staff and every opportunity to purchase different Zone products. There are also recipes, success stories, and a look at a free newsletter. For those not yet in the Zone, there is an easy-to-use store locator to make ordering Zone foods for home delivery as simple as a mouse click.

Appendix D

Myths and Facts About Weight Loss

Myth: *Fad diets work for permanent weight loss.*

Fact: Fad diets are not the best ways to lose weight and keep it off. These eating plans often promise to help you lose a lot of weight quickly, or tell you to cut certain foods out of your diet to lose weight. Although you may lose weight at first while on these kinds of diets, they can be unhealthy because they often keep you from getting all the nutrients that your body needs. Fad diets may seriously limit or prohibit certain types of food, so most people quickly get tired of them and regain the lost weight.

Research suggests that losing 1/2 to 2 pounds a week by eating better and exercising more is the best way to lose weight and keep it off. By improving your eating and exercise habits, you will develop a healthier lifestyle and control your weight. You will also reduce your chances of developing heart disease, high blood pressure, and diabetes.

Myth: *Skipping meals is a good way to lose weight.*

Fact: Your body needs a certain amount of calories and nutrients each day in order to work properly. If you skip meals during the day, you will be more likely to make up for those missing calories by snacking or eating more at the next meal. Studies show that people who skip breakfast tend to be heavier than those who eat a nutritious breakfast. A healthier way to lose weight is to eat many small meals throughout the day that include a variety of nutritious, low-fat, and low-calorie foods.

Myth: *"I can lose weight while eating anything I want."*

Fact: This statement is not always true. It is possible to eat any kind of food you want and lose weight. But you still need to limit the number of calories that you eat every day, usually by eating smaller amounts of food. When trying to lose weight, you can eat your favorite foods—as long as you pay attention to the total amount of food that you eat. You need to use more calories than you eat to lose weight.

Myth: *Eating after 8 P.M. causes weight gain.*

Fact: It doesn't matter what time of day you eat—it's how much you eat during the whole day and how much exercise you get that make you gain or lose weight. No matter when you eat your meals, your body will store extra calories as fat. If you want to have a snack before bedtime, make sure that you first think about how many calories you have already eaten that day.

Try not to snack while doing other things, like watching television, playing video games, or using the computer. If you eat meals and snacks in the kitchen or dining room, you are less likely to be distracted and more likely to be aware of what and how much you are eating. (If you want to snack while watching TV, take a small amount of food with you, like a handful of pretzels or a couple of cookies—not the whole bag.)

Myth: *Certain foods, like grapefruit, celery, or cabbage soup, can burn fat and make you lose weight.*

Fact: No foods can burn fat. Some foods with caffeine may speed up your metabolism (the way your body uses energy, or calories) for a short time, but they do not cause weight loss. The best way to lose weight is to cut back on the number of calories you eat and be more physically active.

Myth: *Natural or herbal weight-loss products are safe and effective.*

Fact: A product that claims to be "natural" or "herbal" is not necessarily safe. These products are not usually tested scientifically to prove that they are safe or that they work.

Some herbal or other natural products may be unsafe to use with other drugs or may hurt people with certain medical conditions. Check with your doctor or other qualified health professional before using any herbal or natural weight-loss product.

Myth: *Nuts are fattening and you shouldn't eat them if you want to lose weight.*

Fact: Although high in calories and fat, most (but not all) types of nuts have low amounts of saturated fat. Saturated fat is the kind of fat that can lead to high blood cholesterol levels and increase the risk of heart disease.

Nuts are a good source of protein and fiber, and they do not have any cholesterol. In small amounts, nuts can be part of a healthy weight-loss program.

Myth: Eating red meat is bad for your health and will make it harder to lose weight.

Fact: Red meat, pork, chicken, and fish contain some saturated fat and cholesterol. But they also have nutrients that are important for good health, like protein, iron, and zinc.

Eating lean meat (meat without a lot of visible fat) in small amounts can be part of a healthy weight-loss plan. A serving size is 2 to 3 ounces of cooked meat, which is about the size of a deck of cards. Choose cuts of meat that are lower in fat, such as beef eye of the round, top round, or pork tenderloin, and trim any extra fat before cooking. The "select" grade of meat is lower in fat than "choice" and "prime" grades.

Myth: Fresh fruits and vegetables are more nutritious than frozen or canned.

Fact: Most fruits and vegetables (produce) are naturally low in fat and calories. Frozen and canned fruits and vegetables can be just as nutritious as fresh. Frozen or canned produce is often packaged right after it has been picked, which helps keep most of its nutrients. Fresh produce can sometimes lose nutrients after being exposed to light or air.

Myth: Starches are fattening and should be limited when trying to lose weight.

Fact: Potatoes, rice, pasta, bread, beans, and some vegetables (like squash, yams, sweet potatoes, turnips, beets, and carrots) are rich in complex carbohydrates (also called starch). Starch is an important source of energy for your body.

Foods high in starch can be low in fat and calories. They become high in fat and calories when you eat them in large amounts, or if they are made with rich sauces, oils, or other high-fat toppings like butter, sour cream, or mayonnaise. Try to avoid high-fat toppings and choose starchy foods that are high in fiber, like whole grains, beans, and peas.

The Dietary Guidelines for Americans recommend 6 to 11 servings a day from the bread, cereal, rice, and pasta group, even when trying to lose weight. A serving size can be 1 slice of bread, 1 ounce of ready-to-eat cereal, or 1/2 cup of pasta, rice, or cooked cereal.

Myth: Fast foods are always an unhealthy choice and you should not eat them when dieting.

Fact: Fast foods can be part of a healthy weight-loss program with a little bit of know-how. Choose salads and grilled foods instead of fried foods, which are high in fat and calories. Use high-fat, high-calorie toppings, like full-fat mayonnaise and salad dressings, only in small amounts.

Eating fried fast food (like french fries) or other high-fat foods like chocolate once in a while as a special treat is fine—but try to split an order with a friend or order a small portion. In small amounts, these foods can still be part of a healthy eating plan.

Myth: Fish has no fat or cholesterol.

Fact: Although all fish has some fat and cholesterol, most fish is lower in saturated fat and cholesterol than beef, pork, chicken, and turkey. Fish is a good source of protein. Types of fish that are higher in fat (like salmon, mackerel, sardines, herring, and anchovies) are rich in omega-3 fatty acids. These fatty acids are being studied because they may be linked to a lower risk for heart disease. Grilled, baked, or broiled fish (instead of fried) can be part of a healthy weight-loss plan.

Myth: High-protein/low-carbohydrate diets are a healthy way to lose weight.

Fact: A high-protein/low-carbohydrate diet provides most of your calories each day from protein foods (like meat, eggs, and cheese) and few calories from carbohydrate foods (like breads, pasta, potatoes, fruits, and vegetables). People on these diets often get bored because they crave the plant-based foods they are not allowed to have or can have only in very small amounts. These diets often lack key nutrients found in carbohydrate foods.

Many of these diets allow a lot of food high in fat, like bacon and cheese. High-fat diets can raise blood cholesterol levels, which increases a person's risk for heart disease and certain cancers.

High-protein/low-carbohydrate diets may cause rapid weight loss—but most of it is water weight and lean muscle mass—not fat. You lose water because your kidneys try to get rid of the excess waste products of protein and fat, called ketones, that your body produces.

This is not a healthy way to lose weight! It overworks your kidneys, and can cause dehydration, headaches, and bad breath. It can also make you feel nauseous, tired, weak, and dizzy. A buildup of ketones in your blood (called ketosis) can cause your body to produce high levels of uric acid, which is a risk factor for gout (a painful swelling of the joints) and kidney stones. Ketosis can be very risky for pregnant women and people with diabetes.

By following a reduced-calorie diet that is well-balanced between carbohydrates, proteins, and fats, you will still lose weight—without hurting your body. You will also be more likely to keep the weight off.

Myth: Dairy products are fattening and unhealthy.

Fact: Dairy products have many nutrients your body needs. They have calcium to help children develop strong bones and to keep adult bones strong and healthy. They also have vitamin D to help your body use calcium, and protein to build muscles and to help organs work properly.

Low-fat and nonfat dairy products are as nutritious as whole-milk dairy products, but they are lower in fat and calories. Choose low-fat or nonfat milk, cheese, yogurt (frozen or regular), and reduced-fat ice cream.

For people who can't digest lactose (a type of sugar found in milk and other dairy products), lactose-free dairy products can be used. These are also good sources of protein and calcium. If you are sensitive to some dairy foods, you may still be able to eat others, like yogurt, hard cheese, evaporated skim milk, and buttermilk. Other good sources of calcium are dark, leafy vegetables (like spinach), calcium-fortified juice, bread, soy products (like tofu), and canned fish with soft bones (like salmon).

Many people are worried about eating butter and margarine. Eating a lot of foods high in saturated fat (like butter) has been linked to high blood cholesterol levels and a greater risk of heart disease. Some research suggests that high amounts of trans fat can also cause high blood cholesterol levels. Trans fat is found in margarine, and in crackers, cookies, and other snack foods made with hydrogenated vegetable shortening or oil. Trans fat is formed when vegetable oil is hardened to become margarine or shortening, a process called "hydrogenation." More research is needed to find out how trans fat affects the risk of heart disease. Foods high in fat, like butter and margarine, should be used in small amounts.

Myth: *Low-fat or no fat means no calories.*

Fact: Remember that most fruits and vegetables are naturally low in fat and calories. Other low-fat or nonfat foods may still have a lot of calories. Often these foods will have extra sugar, flour, or starch thickeners to make them taste better. These ingredients can add calories, which can lead to weight gain.

A low-fat or nonfat food is usually lower in calories than the same size portion of the full-fat product. The number of calories depends on the amount of carbohydrate, protein, and fat in the food. Carbohydrate and protein have about 4 calories per gram, and fat has more than twice that amount (9 calories per gram).

Myth: *"Going vegetarian" means you are sure to lose weight and be healthier.*

Fact: Vegetarian diets can be healthy because they are often lower in saturated fat and cholesterol and higher in fiber. Choosing a vegetarian diet with a low fat content can be helpful for weight loss. But vegetarians—like nonvegetarians—can also make poor food choices, like eating large amounts of junk (nutritionally empty) foods. Candy, chips, and other high-fat, vegetarian foods should be eaten in small amounts.

Vegetarian diets need to be as carefully planned as nonvegetarian diets to make sure they are nutritious. Vegetarian diets can provide the recommended daily amount of all the key nutrients if you choose foods carefully. Plants, especially fruits and vegetables, are the main source of nutrients in vegetarian diets. Some types of vegetarian diets (like those that include eggs and dairy foods) contain animal sources, while another type (the vegan diet) incorporates no animal foods. Nutrients normally found in animal products that are not always found in a vegetarian diet are iron, calcium, vitamin D, vitamin B^{12}, and zinc. Here are some foods that have these nutrients:

- Iron: cashews, tomato juice, rice, tofu, lentils, and garbanzo beans (chick peas).

- Calcium: dairy products, fortified soymilk, fortified orange juice, tofu, kale, and broccoli.

- Vitamin D: fortified milk and soymilk, and fortified cereals (or a small amount of sunlight).

- Vitamin B^{12}: eggs, dairy products, and fortified soy milk, cereals, tempeh, and miso. (Tempeh and miso are foods made from soybeans. They are low in calories and fat, and high in protein.)

- Zinc: whole grains (especially the germ and bran of the grain), eggs, dairy products, nuts, tofu, leafy vegetables (lettuce, spinach, cabbage), and root vegetables (onions, potatoes, carrots, celery, radishes).

Vegetarians must eat a variety of plant foods over the course of a day to get enough protein. Those plant foods that have the most protein are lentils, tofu, nuts, seeds, tempeh, miso, and peas.

Claims That Raise a Caution Flag

http://www.ftc.gov/bcp/conline/pubs/alerts/paunch.html

Paunch Lines: Weight Loss Claims Are No Joke For Dieters

Are you one of the estimated 50 million Americans who will go on a diet this year? If so, you may be tempted by advertisements for products promising easy, quick ways to lose weight. You should know that, when it comes to losing weight, gimmicks usually don't deliver on their promises.

While some dieters succeed in taking off weight, perhaps as few as 5 percent manage to keep it off in the long run. Most experts agree that the best way to lose weight is to eat fewer calories and burn more energy by increasing physical activity. Experts suggest aiming for a goal loss of about a pound a week. This usually means cutting about 500 calories a day from your diet, eating healthy, low-fat foods, finding a regular exercise activity you enjoy, and sticking to it.

When it comes to evaluating claims for weight loss products, the Federal Trade Commission recommends a healthy portion of skepticism. Before you spend money on products or programs that promise fast or easy weight loss, weigh the claims and consider these tips:

- *"Lose 30 Pounds in Just 30 Days."* As a rule, the faster you lose weight, the more likely you are to gain it back. Also, fast weight loss could harm your health. Unless your doctor advises it, don't look for programs that promise quick weight loss.
- *"Lose All the Weight You Can For Just $39.99."* Some weight loss programs have hidden costs. For example, some don't advertise the fact that you must buy their prepackaged meals that cost more than the program fees. Before you sign up for any weight loss program, ask for a rundown of all the costs. Get them in writing.
- *"Lose Weight While You Sleep."* Claims for diet products and programs that promise weight loss without effort are phony.
- *"Lose Weight and Keep It Off for Good."* Be suspicious about products promising long-term or permanent weight loss. To lose weight and keep it off, you must change how you eat and how much you exercise.
- *"John Doe Lost 84 Pounds in Six Weeks."* Don't be misled by someone else's weight loss claims. Even if the claims are true, someone else's success may have little relation to your own chances of success.
- *"Scientific Breakthrough . . . Medical Miracle."* There are no miracle weight loss products. To lose weight, you have to reduce your intake of calories and increase your physical activity. Be skeptical about exaggerated claims.

Source: The Weight Control Information Network of the National Institute of Diabetes & Digestive & Kidney Diseases of the National Institutes of Health, posted December 2000. URL: http://www.niddk.nih.gov/health/nutrit/pubs/myths/index.htm.

The Smart Snacker's Guide to Substitutions

INSTEAD OF...	TRY...	TO SAVE...	
		Calories	Fat (gm)
CRUNCHIES			
Potato chips, regular 17–22 (1 oz.)	Pretzels, low-salt 6 (1 oz.)	60	11
Potato chips, light 17–20 (1 oz.)	Raw vegetables 1/2 cup	130	12
	Potato chips, baked 28–30 (1 oz.)	50	7
Popcorn, microwave reg. 2 cups	Popcorn, air-popped 2 cups	100	7
	Popcorn, microwave light 2 cups	80	5
Doritos tortilla chips 15–16 (1 oz.)	Tortilla chips, baked 22–26 (1 oz.)	30	6
Nachos made from tortilla chips with melted cheese 8 pieces	Baked tortilla wedges with salsa 8 pieces	40	7
Cheese crackers with peanut butter 3 "sandwiches" (0.7 oz.)	Ry Krisp crackers 2 triple crackers (1/2 oz.)	55	6
Ritz Bits crackers 22 (1/2 oz.)	Breadsticks, fat-free 2 (1/2 oz.)	25	4
Wheat Thins crackers 8 (1/2 oz.)	Premium fat-free crackers 5 (1/2 oz.)	20	3
SWEETS			
Snickers candy bar 2-oz bar	Cocoa, from mix, regular 6-oz cup	170	13
Oreo cookies 3 (1 1/2 oz.)	Fig or apple bar; nonfat 2 (1 1/2 oz.)	30	4
Chocolate chip cookies 2 (1 oz.)	Fat-free oatmeal raisin cookie 1 large	20	4
Chips Ahoy cookies with chocolate chunks 2 (1 oz.)	Ginger Snaps 3 (1/2 oz.)	140	9
Granola bar 1 (.8–1 oz.) squares 1/2 cup (1 oz.)	Frosted bite-size shredded wheat	30	6
Fun fruit or fruit roll-ups and wrinkles 1 pouch or 2 rolls	Fresh fruit 1 piece	40	1
	Dried fruit (raisins, apricots) 1/4 cup	20	1
Pop-tarts 1 pastry	Bagel—half with 2 tsp jelly	130	6
Double raspberry mocha	"Skinny" latte sprinkled with cinnamon (espresso and skim milk)	225	7

INSTEAD OF...	TRY...	TO SAVE...	
FROZEN SNACKS		**Calories**	**Fat (gm)**
Ice cream, regular 1 cup	Frozen yogurt, nonfat or lowfat ice cream 1 cup	90	11
Ice cream, premium 1 cup	Fruit sorbet 1 cup	150	24
Fudgesicle 1 bar (1.75 oz.)		280	24
SMOOTH SNACKS			
Yogurt, regular with fruit 1 cup	Yogurt, lowfat with fruit preserves	20	3
	Yogurt, plain nonfat with 1/2 cup fresh strawberries 1 cup	100	5
Dip, regular commercial 2 Tbsp.	Dip, from plain lowfat or nonfat yogurt with dab of light mayonnaise	25	2
	Dip from nonfat cottage cheese 2 Tbsp	30	5
MINI-MEALS			
Pizza, pepperoni 1 slice (5.25–5.5 oz)	English muffin or bagel pizza, low-fat cheese 1 piece (4.25 oz.)	25	4
Pizza, French bread, pepperoni 1 piece (5.25–5.5 oz.)	English muffin (see above)	245	15
Sandwich, w/3 oz. bologna, 1 oz. regular cheese, 2 tsp. regular mayo, lettuce, tomato	Sandwich, with 1 oz. turkey 1 oz. Lowfat cheese, 1 tsp mustard	320	36
Fast-food deluxe burger	Fast-food grilled chicken sandwich plain	260	26
Hamburger (80% lean) 4 oz.	Veggie burger	240	20
Fast-food French fries, large	Baked potato with 1 Tbsp. lowfat sour cream with fresh chives	260	28
Mashed potatoes 1 cup, with gravy	Baked potato (see above)	30	10
Regular hot dog (beef and pork)	Fat-free beef frank	109	13
BEVERAGES			
Soda, regular 8 oz.	Club soda or seltzer with lime 8 oz.	120	0
Blended juice drinks, regular 8 oz.	Club soda with 2 oz. juice	140	0
Wine cooler 8 oz.	Raspberry or peach ice tea, with 1 tsp. sugar, lemon	140	0
Beer 12 oz.	Tomato or V-8 juice 8 oz.	100	0
2% milk 8 oz.	nonfat (skim) milk 8 oz.	35	5

Source: American Institute for Cancer Research, *Sneak Health Into Your Snacks.* Washington, D.C.: American Institute for Cancer Research, December 1998, pp. 10–15.

Appendix F

Recommended Dietary Intakes for Young People

1989 RECOMMENDED DIETARY ALLOWANCES (RDA)

	MALES			FEMALES		
	11–14	15–18	19–24	11–14	15–18	19–24
Energy (calories)	2500	3000	2900	2200	2200	2200
Protein	45	59	58	46	44	46
Vitamin A	1000	1000	1000	800	800	800
Vitamin E	10	10	10	8	8	8
Vitamin K	45	65	70	45	55	60
Vitamin C	50	60	60	50	60	60
Thiamin (mg)	1.3	1.5	1.5	1.1	1.1	1.1
Riboflavin (mg)	1.5	1.8	1.7	1.3	1.3	1.3
Niacin (mg)	17	20	19	15	15	15
Vitamin B6 (mg)	1.7	2.0	2.0	1.4	1.5	1.6
Folate	150	200	200	150	180	180
Vitamin B12	2.0	2.0	2.0	2.0	2.0	2.0
Iron	12	12	10	15	15	15
Zinc	15	15	15	12	12	12
Iodine	150	150	150	150	150	150
Selenium	40	50	70	45	50	55

In April 2000, a panel of the National Academy of Sciences recommended increasing the RDA of vitamin E to 15 milligrams of alpha-tocopherol, increasing the vitamin C RDA to 75 milligrams per day and increasing the selenium recommendation to 55 micrograms per day.

Dietary Reference Intakes in 1997 for adolescents and young adults for vitamin D were 5 micrograms per day. Calcium recommendations were 1,300 milligrams daily until age 19, when the recommendation dropped to 1,000. Phosphorous recommendations were 1,250 milligrams until age 18, then 700. Magnesium requirements were slightly higher for men and pregnant women. Males aged 14 to 18 should have 410 milligrams; females in that age range should have 360 milligrams. The requirement for young adult males decreased to 400 and for young females it decreased to 310.

Sample Menus
at Various Calorie Levels

FIVE DAYS' MENUS AT 1,600 CALORIES

BREAKFAST

DAY 1

Orange juice	3/4 c
Oatmeal	1/2 c
White toast	1 slice
Margarine	1 tsp
Jelly	1 tsp
Skim milk	1/2 c

DAY 2

Grapefruit juice	3/4 c
*Breakfast pita	1 sandwich
Skim milk	1 c

DAY 3

Grapefruit	1/2
Ready-to-eat cereal flakes	1 oz
Toasted English muffin with raisins	1/2
Jelly	1 tsp
Skim milk	1/2 c

DAY 4

Fresh sliced strawberries	1/2 c
Whole-grain cereal flakes	1 oz
Toasted plain bagel	1/2
Cream cheese	1/2 Tbsp
2% fat milk	1 c

DAY 5

Cantaloupe	1/4 melon
*Whole-wheat pancakes	2
*Blueberry sauce	1/4 c
Skim milk	1

LUNCH

DAY 1

*Split pea soup	1 c
*Quick tuna and sprouts sandwich	1
Mixed green salad	1 c
Reduced-calorie Italian dressing	1 Tbsp
*Chocolate mint pie	1 serving

DAY 2

*Turkey pasta salad	1–1/4 c
Tomato wedges on lettuce leaf	1 serving
Hard roll	1
Margarine	1 tsp
Skim milk	1 c

DAY 3

*Taco salad greens	1 c
Chili	3/4 c
Sherbet	1/2 c

DAY 4

Broiled chicken fillet sandwich	1
Mayonnaise	1 pkt
*Confetti coleslaw	1/2 c
2% fat milk	1 c

DAY 5

*Chili-stuffed baked potato	1
*Spinach-orange salad	1 c
Wheat crackers	6

DINNER

DAY 1

*Savory sirloin	3 oz
*Corn and zucchini combo	1/2 c
Tomato and lettuce salad	1 serv
Reduced-calorie French dressing	1 Tbsp
Whole-wheat roll	1
Margarine	1 tsp
*Yogurt-strawberry parfait	1 c

DAY 2

*Creole fish fillet	3 oz
Small new potatoes with skin	2
Cooked green peas	1/2 c
w/margarine	1 tsp
*Whole-wheat cornmeal muffin	1
Margarine	1 tsp
*Peach crisp	1/2 c

DAY 3

*Pork & vegetable stir-fry	1 c
Rice	3/4 c
Cooked broccoli	1/2 c
White roll	1
Minted pineapple chunks	1/2 c

DAY 4

*Lentil stroganoff mixture	1–1/2 c
noodles	3/4 c
Cooked whole green beans	1/2 c
Tomato and cucumber salad	1 serv.
Reduced-calorie vinaigrette dressing	1 Tbsp
Honeydew	1/8 melon

DAY 5

*Apricot-glazed chicken	3 oz
*Rice-pasta pilaf	3/4 c
Tossed salad	1 c
Reduced-calorie Italian dressing	1 Tbsp
Hard roll	1
Vanilla ice milk	1/2 c

SNACKS

DAY 1

Graham crackers	3 squares
Skim milk	1 c

DAY 2

Bagel	1 medium
Margarine	1 tsp
Jelly	1 tsp

DAY 3

Wheat crackers	6
Skim milk	1 c

DAY 4

Roast beef sandwich	1/2

DAY 5

Fig bar	1
Skim milk	3/4 c

FIVE DAYS' MENUS AT 2,200 CALORIES

BREAKFAST

DAY 1

Orange juice	3/4 c
Oatmeal	1/2 c
White toast	2 slices
Margarine	2 tsp
Jelly	1 tsp
2% fat milk	1/2 c

DAY 2

Grapefruit juice	3/4 c
*Breakfast pita	1 sandwich
2% fat milk	1 c

DAY 3

Grapefruit	1/2
Banana	1 medium
Ready-to-eat cereal flakes	1 oz
Toasted English muffin with raisins	1
Margarine	2 tsp
Skim milk	1/2 c

DAY 4

Fresh sliced strawberries	1/2 c
Whole-grain cereal flakes	1 oz
Toasted plain bagel	1 medium
Cream cheese	1 Tbsp
2% fat milk	1 c

DAY 5

Cantaloupe	1/4 melon
Turkey patty	1–1/2 oz
*Whole-wheat pancakes	2
*Blueberry sauce	1/4 c
Margarine	1 tsp
Skim milk	1 c

LUNCH

DAY 1

*Split pea soup	1 c
*Quick tuna and sprouts sandwich	1
Mixed green salad	1 c
Reduced-calorie Italian dressing	1 Tbsp
*Chocolate mint pie	1 serving

DAY 2

*Turkey pasta salad	1–1/4 c
Tomato wedges on lettuce leaf	1 serv.
Hard rolls	2
Margarine	2 tsp
Oatmeal cookies	4
2% fat milk	1 c

DAY 3

*Taco salad greens	1 c
Chili	3/4 c
Ginger snaps	2

DAY 4

Broiled chicken fillet sandwich	1
Mayonnaise	1 pkt
*Confetti coleslaw	1/2 c
Fresh orange	1
2% fat milk	1 c

DAY 5

*Chili-stuffed baked potato	1
Lowfat, low-sodium cheddar cheese	3 Tbsp
*Spinach-orange salad	1 c
Wheat crackers	6
Skim milk	1 c

DINNER

DAY 1

*Savory sirloin	3 oz
*Corn and zucchini combo	3/4 c
Tomato and lettuce salad	1 serv
French dressing	1 Tbsp
Whole-wheat rolls	2
Margarine	1 tsp
*Yogurt-strawberry parfait	1 c

DAY 2

*Creole fish fillet	4 oz
Small new potatoes with skin	2
Cooked green peas	1/2 c
with margarine	1 tsp
Whole-wheat cornmeal muffins	2
Margarine	2 tsp
*Peach crisp	1/2 c

DAY 3

*Pork and vegetable stir-fry mixture	1 c
Rice	3/4 c
Cooked broccoli	1/2 c
White rolls	2
Margarine	2 tsp
Minted pineapple chunks	1/2 c

DAY 4

*Lentil stroganoff mixture	1–1/2 c
noodles	3/4 c
Cooked whole green beans	1/2 c
with margarine	1 tsp
Tomato and cucumber salad	1 serv.
Reduced-calorie vinaigrette dressing	1 Tbsp
Pumpernickel roll	1
Margarine	1 tsp
Honeydew	1/8 melon

DAY 5

*Apricot-glazed chicken	3 oz
*Rice-pasta pilaf	3/4 c
Tossed salad	1 c
Reduced-calorie Italian dressing	1 Tbsp
Hard rolls	2
Margarine	2 tsp
Vanilla ice milk	1/2 c

SNACKS

DAY 1

Graham crackers	6 squares
2% fat milk	1 c
Peanut butter	2 Tbsp
Fresh peach	1
Carrot sticks	7–8 medium

DAY 2

Bagel	1 medium
Margarine	2 tsp
Fresh pear	1

DAY 3

Wheat crackers	6
Cheddar cheese	1–1/2 oz
Turkey sandwich	1/2
No-salt-added tomato juice	3/4 c

DAY 4

No-salt-added vegetable juice	3/4 c
Roast beef sandwich	1
2% fat milk	1 c

DAY 5

Soft pretzel	1 large
Fresh apple	1/2

FIVE DAYS' MENUS AT 2,800 CALORIES

BREAKFAST

DAY 1

Orange juice	3/4 c
Oatmeal	1/2 c
White toast	2 slices
Margarine	2 tsp
Jelly	2 tsp
2% fat milk	1/2 c

DAY 2

Grapefruit juice	3/4 c
*Breakfast pita	1 sandwich
Bran muffin	1 large
Margarine	1 tsp
2% fat milk	1 c

DAY 3

Grapefruit	1/2
Banana	1 medium
Ready-to-eat cereal flakes	1 oz
Toasted English muffin with raisins	1
Margarine	2 tsp
Skim milk	1 c

DAY 4

Fresh sliced strawberries	1/2 c
Hard cooked egg	1
Whole-grain cereal flakes	1 oz
Toasted plain bagel	1 medium
Cream cheese	2 tbsp
2% fat milk	1 c

DAY 5

Cantaloupe	1/4 melon
*Turkey patty	1/2 oz
*Whole-wheat pancakes	3
*Blueberry sauce	6 tbsp
Margarine	2 tsp
2% fat milk	1 c

LUNCH

DAY 1

*Split pea soup	1 c
*Quick tuna and sprouts sandwich	1
Mixed green salad	1 c
Italian dressing	1 Tbsp
*Chocolate mint pie	1 serving
2% fat milk	1 c

DAY 2

*Turkey pasta salad	1–1/4 c
Tomato wedges on lettuce leaf	1 serv.
Hard rolls	2
Margarine	2 tsp
Tangerine	1
Oatmeal cookies	6
2% fat milk	1 c

DAY 3

*Taco salad greens	1 c
Chili	3/4 c
Sherbet	1/2 c
Ginger snaps	3
Skim milk	1 c

DAY 4

Broiled chicken fillet sandwich	1
Mayonnaise	1 pkt
*Confetti coleslaw	1/2 c
Fresh orange	1
*Lemon pound cake	1 slice
2% fat milk	1 c

DAY 5

*Chili-stuffed baked potato	1
Lowfat, low-sodium cheddar cheese	3 Tbsp
*Spinach-orange salad	1 c
Fresh grapes	12
Wheat crackers	6
Fig bars	2
2% fat milk	1 c

DINNER

DAY 1

*Savory sirloin	4 oz
*Corn and zucchini combo	1 c
Tomato and lettuce salad	1 serv.
Reduced-calorie French dressing	1 Tbsp
Whole-wheat rolls	2
Margarine	1 tsp
*Yogurt-strawberry parfait	1 c

DAY 2

*Creole fish fillets	4 oz
Small new potatoes with skin	2
Cooked green peas	3/4 c
with margarine	1 tsp
*Whole-wheat cornmeal muffins	2
Margarine	2 tsp
*Peach crisp	1/2 c

DAY 3

*Pork and vegetable stir-fry mixture	1 c
rice	3/4 c
Cooked broccoli	1 c
White rolls	2
Margarine	2 tsp
Minted pineapple chunks	1/2 c

DAY 4

*Lentil stroganoff mixture	1–1/2 c
noodles	3/4 c
Cooked whole green beans	1 c
with margarine	1 tsp
Tomato and cucumber salad	1 serv.
Reduced-calorie vinaigrette dressing	1 Tbsp
Pumpernickel rolls	2
Margarine	2 tsp
Honeydew	1/4 melon

DAY 5

*Apricot-glazed chicken	3 oz
*Rice-pasta pilaf	3/4 c

Steamed zucchini	1/2 c
Tossed salad	1 c
Italian dressing	1 Tbsp
Hard rolls	2
Margarine	2 tsp
Vanilla ice milk	1/2 c

SNACKS

DAY 1

Graham crackers	6 squares
Peanut butter-banana sandwich	1
Fresh peach	1
Nonfat fruit-flavored yogurt	8 oz
Carrot sticks	7–8 medium

DAY 2

Bagel	1 medium
Margarine	2 tsp
Jelly	2 tsp
Fresh pear	1
Low-fat fruit-flavored yogurt	1/2 c
Unsalted roasted peanuts (1/2 oz)	2–1/2 tbsp

DAY 3

Wheat crackers	6
Orange juice	3/4 c
Cheddar cheese	1–1/2 oz
Turkey sandwich	1
Raw vegetables	6 pcs
Spinach dip	2 Tbsp

DAY 4

No-salt-added vegetable juice	3/4 c
Roast beef sandwich	1
2% fat milk	1 c
Lemonade	1 c

DAY 5

Fresh apple	1/2
Soft pretzel	1 large
Lemonade	1 c
2% fat milk	1 c

Recipes for Five Days' Menus

Recipes appear in same order as five days' menus above.

Breakfast Menu Recipes

Breakfast Pita
   4 servings, 1 pita each
   PER SERVING:

Calories	170
Total fat	6 grams
Saturated fat	2 grams
Cholesterol	108 milligrams
Sodium	400 milligrams

Margarine, 2 teaspoons
Mushroom pieces, drained, 4-ounce can
Onion, chopped, 1/4 cup
Green pepper, chopped, 1/4 cup
Eggs, 2 large
Egg whites, 2 large
Lowfat cottage cheese, 1/4 cup
Pepper, 1/8 teaspoon
Lowfat cheddar cheese, shredded, 1/4 cup
Whole-wheat pita rounds, 4-inch, 4

1. Melt margarine in nonstick frying pan. Add mushrooms, onion, and green pepper; cook until onion and green pepper are tender, stirring often.

2. Combine eggs, egg whites, cottage cheese, and pepper; mix well. Pour over mushroom mixture.

3. Cook over medium heat, stirring frequently, until eggs are firm but still moist. Stir in cheddar cheese.

4. Using a sharp knife, split edge of pita open about 3 inches to make a pocket. Spoon 1/4 of mixture, about 1/2 cup, into each pita. Serve immediately.

EACH SERVING PROVIDES:
Meat alternate equal to 1/2 ounce from meat group
1 serving from bread group
1/4 serving from vegetable group

Turkey Patties
4 servings, 1 patty each
PER SERVING:

Calories   125
Total fat   6 grams
Saturated fat   2 grams
Cholesterol   46 milligrams
Sodium   200 milligrams

Ground turkey, 8 ounces (1/2 pound)
Ground sage, 1/2 to 3/4 teaspoon
Marjoram leaves, 1/4 teaspoon
Pepper, 1/4 teaspoon
Salt, 1/8 teaspoon
Vegetable oil, 1/2 teaspoon

1. Mix all ingredients, except oil, thoroughly.

2. Shape into 4 patties about 3 inches in diameter.

3. Heat oil in nonstick frying pan.

4. Cook patties in hot frying pan about 4 minutes, turning once to brown other side.

EACH SERVING PROVIDES:
1–1/2 ounces from meat group

Whole-Wheat Pancakes
4 servings, 2 4-inch pancakes each
PER SERVING:

Calories   170
Total fat   4 grams
Saturated fat   1 gram
Cholesterol   54 milligrams
Sodium   230 milligrams

Whole-wheat flour, 1 cup
Brown sugar, packed, 2 teaspoons
Baking powder, 1–1/2 teaspoons
Salt, 1/8 teaspoon
Egg, 1
Skim milk, 1 cup
Vegetable oil, 2 teaspoons

1. Preheat griddle.

2. Mix dry ingredients.

3. Beat egg, milk, and oil together.

4. Add milk mixture to dry ingredients; stir until dry ingredients are barely moistened. Batter will be lumpy.

5. For each pancake, pour 1/4 cup of batter onto hot griddle.

6. Cook until surface is covered with bubbles, then turn. Cook other side until lightly browned.

EACH SERVING PROVIDES:
2 servings from bread group

Blueberry Sauce
4 servings, 1/4 cup each
PER SERVING:

Calories	35
Total fat	Trace
Saturated fat	Trace
Cholesterol	0
Sodium	1 milligram

Cornstarch, 1 tablespoon
Sugar, 1 tablespoon
Water, 2/3 cup
Frozen blueberries, unsweetened, 2/3 cup
Lemon juice, 2 teaspoons

1. Mix cornstarch and sugar in a small saucepan.

2. Add water and stir until smooth. Add blueberries.

3. Bring to boil over medium heat, stirring constantly. Cook until thickened.

4. Remove from heat. Stir in lemon juice.

5. Serve warm over whole-wheat pancakes.

EACH SERVING PROVIDES:
1/3 serving from fruit group

Lunch Menu Recipes

Split Pea Soup
6 servings, 1 cup each
PER SERVING:

Calories	220
Total fat	2 grams
Saturated fat	1 gram
Cholesterol	5 milligrams
Sodium	190 milligrams

Boneless smoked pork chop, 1 small (about 3 ounces)
Dry green split peas, 1–1/2 cups
Onion, chopped, 1/2 cup
Carrot, shredded, 1/2 cup
Pepper, 1/8 teaspoon
Water, 2–1/2 cups
Low-sodium chicken broth, 3–1/2 cups

1. Cut fat from smoked pork chop; discard. Chop or dice meat.

2. Mix all ingredients in a large saucepan. Bring to a boil, cover, reduce heat, and simmer 1–1/2 hours. Stir occasionally.

EACH SERVING PROVIDES:
Meat alternate equal to 1–1/4 ounces from meat group
1/2 serving from vegetable group

Quick Tuna and Sprouts Sandwich
4 servings, 1 sandwich each
PER SERVING:

Calories	200
Total fat	4 grams
Saturated fat	1 gram
Cholesterol	10 milligrams
Sodium	320 milligrams

Mayonnaise-type salad dressing, 2 tablespoons
Celery seed, 1/4 teaspoon
Onion powder, 1/4 teaspoon
No-salt-added water-pack tuna, 1 can undrained (6–1/2 ounces)
Alfalfa sprouts, 1/2 cup
Whole-wheat hamburger rolls, 4

1. Mix salad dressing and seasonings in a bowl. Add tuna and sprouts; mix well.

2. Use 1/4 of filling per sandwich.

EACH SERVING PROVIDES:
1–1/2 ounces from meat group
2 servings from bread group

Chocolate Mint Pie
   8-inch pie, 8 servings
   PER SERVING:

Calories	175
Total fat	6 grams
Saturated fat	1 gram
Cholesterol	1 milligram
Sodium	175 milligrams

Graham Cracker Crust:
Graham crackers, crushed, 1–1/4 cups
Margarine, softened, 3 tablespoons
Filling:
Unflavored gelatin, 1 envelope (about 1 tablespoon)
Cold water, 1/4 cup
Sugar, 1/2 cup
Cocoa, 1/4 cup
Cornstarch, 2 tablespoons
Skim milk, 2 cups
Peppermint extract, 4 drops

To Make Crust

1. Mix graham cracker crumbs and margarine thoroughly. Reserve 1/4 cup of crumb mixture for top of pie.

2. Press remaining crumb mixture into 8-inch pie pan so the bottom and sides are completely covered.

To Make Filling

1. Soften gelatin in cold water.

2. Mix sugar, cocoa, and cornstarch in saucepan. Add milk. Cook, stirring constantly, until thickened.

3. Stir softened gelatin into hot mixture and cool 20 minutes, stirring occasionally. Stir in extract. Cool an additional 20 minutes.

4. Pour filling into crust.

5. Sprinkle reserved crumb mixture over top of filling.

6. Chill until set. Keep in refrigerator until served.

EACH SERVING PROVIDES:
1/4 serving from milk group
1/2 serving from bread group

Turkey Pasta Salad
4 servings, 1–1/4 cups each
PER SERVING:
Calories   265
Total fat   6 grams
Saturated fat   1 gram
Cholesterol   47 milligrams
Sodium   225 milligrams

Elbow macaroni, uncooked, 1 cup
Dried chives, 1–1/2 teaspoons
Salad dressing, mayonnaise-type, light, 1/4 cup
Cooked turkey, diced, 1–2/3 cups
Seedless red grapes, halved, 1 cup
Celery, thinly sliced, 1/3 cup
Salad greens, 4 leaves

1. Cook macaroni according to package directions. Drain.

2. Stir chives into salad dressing.

3. Mix macaroni, turkey, grapes, and celery together lightly.

4. Stir in salad dressing.

5. Chill well. Serve on salad greens.

EACH SERVING PROVIDES:
2 ounces from meat group
1 serving from bread group
1/2 serving from fruit group

Taco Salad
4 servings, 1 cup greens,
3/4 cup chili each
PER SERVING:

Calories	455
Total fat	19 grams
Saturated fat	6 grams
Cholesterol	43 milligrams
Sodium	545 milligrams

Lean ground beef, 1/2 pound
Kidney beans, undrained, 15–1/2-ounce can
No-salt-added tomato purée, 1 cup
Chili powder, 1–1/2 tablespoons
Instant minced onion, 1 tablespoon
Iceberg lettuce, torn, 2 cups
Spinach leaves, torn, 2 cups
Lowfat, low-sodium cheddar cheese, 3/4 cup shredded (3 ounces)
Unsalted tortilla chips, 40 chips (about 2–1/2 ounces)

1. Cook beef in hot frying pan until lightly browned. Drain off fat.

2. Add beans, tomato purée, chili powder, and onion.

3. Bring to a boil, reduce heat, cover, and simmer 10 minutes. Stir as needed.

4. Place 1/2 cup of lettuce and 1/2 cup of spinach in a salad dish. Top with 3/4 cup chili and 1/4 of the cheese. Place 10 chips around each salad.

EACH SERVING PROVIDES:
Meat and meat alternate equal to 2–1/2 ounces from meat group
3/4 serving from bread group
1/2 serving from milk group
1–1/2 servings from vegetable group

Confetti Coleslaw
4 servings, about 1/2 cup each
PER SERVING:
Calories   35
Total fat   Trace
Saturated fat   Trace
Cholesterol   0
Sodium   10 milligrams
Green cabbage, finely chopped, 2 cups
Green pepper, finely chopped, 1/4 cup
Red pepper, finely chopped, 1/4 cup
Onion, finely chopped, 1 tablespoon
Vinegar, 2 tablespoons
Water, 1 tablespoon
Sugar, 1–1/2 tablespoons
Celery seed, 1/8 teaspoon
Pepper, 1/8 teaspoon

1. Mix vegetables together lightly.

2. Mix remaining ingredients together for dressing.

3. Stir dressing into vegetables. Chill well.

NOTE: This salad keeps well in the refrigerator for one or two days. Green peppers may be used in place of red peppers. Add color by adding a small amount of shredded carrots.

EACH SERVING PROVIDES:
1 serving from vegetable group

Lemon Pound Cake
18 servings, 1 slice, about 1/2-inch thick
PER SLICE:
Calories   195
Total fat   8 grams
Saturated fat   2 grams
Cholesterol   48 milligrams
Sodium   120 milligrams

Margarine, softened, 2/3 cup
Sugar, 1–1/3 cups
Eggs, 4
Vanilla, 1 teaspoon

Flour, 2 cups
Baking powder, 1/4 teaspoon
Baking soda, 1/4 teaspoon
Lowfat lemon yogurt, 2/3 cup
Lemon juice, 3 tablespoons
Lemon peel, grated, 1 teaspoon

1. Preheat oven 325° F. Grease and flour 9″ × 5″ loaf pan.

2. Cream margarine in large mixing bowl. Gradually add sugar; beat until light and fluffy.

3. Add eggs one at a time, beating well after each addition. Add vanilla.

4. Mix dry ingredients.

5. Mix yogurt, lemon juice, and lemon peel.

6. Add dry ingredients and lemon mixture alternately to egg mixture, mixing until dry ingredients are just moistened.

7. Pour batter into pan.

8. Bake 1–1/4 hours until lightly browned.

9. Cool 10 minutes in pan on a rack before removing from pan.

EACH SERVING PROVIDES:
3/4 serving from bread group

Chili-Stuffed Baked Potato
Variation for Taco Salad
PER SERVING:

Calories	395
Total fat	9 grams
Saturated fat	3 grams
Cholesterol	38 milligrams
Sodium	460 milligrams

1. Omit lettuce, spinach, cheese, and tortilla chips from salad recipe. Prepare chili mixture as directed in the *Taco Salad* recipe.

2. Wash and bake 4 medium baking potatoes (in oven or microwave). Cut a slit in top of each potato. Top potatoes with chili, using about 3/4 cup for each. Shredded cheddar cheese may be added as a garnish.

EACH SERVING PROVIDES:
Meat and meat alternate equal to 2–1/2 ounces from meat group
1–1/2 servings from vegetable group

Spinach-Orange Salad
4 servings, about 1 cup each
PER SERVING:

Calories	110
Total fat	7 grams
Saturated fat	1 gram
Cholesterol	0
Sodium	25 milligrams

Spinach, torn into pieces, 4 cups
Orange, sectioned, 2 medium
Fresh mushrooms, sliced, 2/3 cup
Red onion, sliced, 1/2 cup
Vegetable oil, 2 tablespoons
Vinegar, 2 tablespoons
Orange juice (from sectioning of orange), 1/4 cup
Ground ginger, 1/2 teaspoon
Pepper, 1/4 teaspoon

1. Place spinach in bowl. Add orange sections, mushrooms, and onion. Toss lightly to mix.

2. Mix oil, vinegar, orange juice, ginger, and pepper well. Pour over spinach mixture. Toss to mix.

3. Chill.

EACH SERVING PROVIDES:
1–1/2 servings from vegetable group
1/2 serving from fruit group

Dinner Menu Recipes

Savory Sirloin

4 servings, about 3 ounces meat each
PER SERVING:

Calories	130
Total fat	5 grams
Saturated fat	2 grams
Cholesterol	52 milligrams
Sodium	155 milligrams

Boneless sirloin steak, lean, 1 pound
Garlic, minced, 1 clove
Rosemary, crushed, 1/4 teaspoon
Thyme leaves, 1/4 teaspoon
Margarine, 1 teaspoon
Plain lowfat yogurt, 1 tablespoon
Prepared mustard, 1 tablespoon
Worcestershire sauce, 1 tablespoon
Parsley, chopped, 1 tablespoon

1. Trim fat from meat.

2. Combine garlic and spices. Sprinkle over meat.

3. Melt margarine in a nonstick frying pan. Add meat and cook over medium heat 6 minutes on each side, or to desired doneness.

4. Place meat on serving platter and keep warm.

5. Combine yogurt, mustard, and Worcestershire sauce in a small microwave-safe bowl. Cover and microwave on high power for 1 minute. Spread mixture over warm meat.

6. Garnish with parsley.

7. To serve, slice meat on a diagonal into thin slices.

Note: Sauce may also be heated in a small saucepan over low heat. Stir constantly until warm.

EACH SERVING PROVIDES:
3 ounces from meat group

Corn and Zucchini Combo
4 servings, about 1/2 cup each
PER SERVING:

Calories	75
Total fat	2 grams
Saturated fat	Trace
Cholesterol	0
Sodium	15 milligrams

Margarine, 1 teaspoon
Onion, diced, 1/2 cup
Zucchini squash, sliced 1/8-inch thick 1–1/2 cups
Frozen whole kernel corn 1–1/2 cups
Basil leaves, 1/4 teaspoon
Oregano leaves, 1/8 teaspoon
Pepper, 1/8 teaspoon

1. Melt margarine in frying pan over low heat.

2. Add onion; cook 2 minutes.

3. Add zucchini, cover and cook 5 minutes. Stir occasionally.

4. Add corn and seasonings. Cover and cook over low heat 5 minutes or until corn is done. Stir as needed.

EACH SERVING PROVIDES:
1 serving from vegetable group

Yogurt-Strawberry Parfait
4 servings, 1/2 cup frozen yogurt and 1/2 cup fruit each
PER SERVING:

Calories	130
Total fat	2 grams
Saturated fat	1 gram
Cholesterol	5 milligrams
Sodium	60 milligrams

Frozen lowfat vanilla yogurt, 1 pint
Strawberries, sliced 2 cups
Mint leaves (optional), 8

1. Layer yogurt and berries in parfait glass.

2. Garnish with mint leaves and serve.

Note: For variety, use other berries or sliced fresh fruit in season.

EACH SERVING PROVIDES:
1/2 serving from milk group
1 serving from fruit group

Creole Fish Fillets
4 servings, 3 ounces fish and 1/2 cup sauce each
PER SERVING:

Calories	130
Total fat	1 gram
Saturated fat	Trace
Cholesterol	49 milligrams
Sodium	155 milligrams

No-salt-added tomatoes, cut up, 16-ounce can
Celery, chopped, 1/2 cup
Onion, chopped, 1/2 cup
Green pepper, chopped, 1/4 cup
Garlic, minced, 1 clove
Bay leaf, 1
Thyme leaves, 1/2 teaspoon
Red pepper flakes, 1/4 teaspoon
Salt, 1/8 teaspoon
Fresh cod fillets, 1 pound

1. Preheat oven to 400° F.

2. Combine all ingredients, except fillets, in a saucepan. Bring to a boil. Cover; reduce heat, and simmer 25 minutes, stirring occasionally. Remove bay leaf.

3. Place fillets in a baking dish. Bake, uncovered, for 15 minutes or until fish flakes easily when tested with a fork.

4. Pour sauce over fish and serve.

EACH SERVING PROVIDES:
3 ounces from meat group
1 serving from vegetable group

Whole-Wheat Cornmeal Muffins
8 Muffins
PER MUFFIN:

Calories	130
Total fat	4 grams
Saturated fat	1 gram
Cholesterol	27 milligrams
Sodium	130 milligrams

Yellow degerminated cornmeal, 2/3 cup
Whole-wheat flour, 2/3 cup
Sugar, 1 tablespoon
Baking powder, 2 teaspoons
Salt, 1/8 teaspoon
Skim milk, 2/3 cup
Egg, beaten, 1
Vegetable oil, 2 tablespoons

1. Preheat oven to 400° F.

2. Grease 8 muffin tins or use paper liners.

3. Mix dry ingredients thoroughly.

4. Mix milk, egg, and oil. Add to dry ingredients. Stir until dry ingredients are barely moistened. Batter will be lumpy.

5. Fill muffin tins 2/3 full.

6. Bake until lightly browned, about 20 minutes.

EACH SERVING PROVIDES:
2 servings from bread group

Pork and Vegetable Stir-fry

4 servings, 1 cup meat mixture,
1/4 cup sauce and 3/4 cup rice each

PER SERVING:

Calories	370
Total fat	9 grams
Saturated fat	3 grams
Cholesterol	69 milligrams
Sodium	240 milligrams

Boneless pork loin, lean, 1 pound
Tarragon leaves, 1/2 teaspoon
Pepper, 1/4 teaspoon
Garlic powder, 1/4 teaspoon
Salt, 1/4 teaspoon
Cornstarch, 2 teaspoons
Water, 1 cup
Lemon juice, 1/4 cup
Carrots, sliced, 1 cup
Fresh mushrooms, sliced, 1 cup
Celery, sliced, 1 cup
Onions, chopped, 1/2 cup
Rice, cooked, 3 cups

1. Partially freeze meat. Trim fat and slice meat across the grain into 1/4-inch thick slices.

2. Combine seasonings. Sprinkle mixture over meat.

3. Combine cornstarch, water, and lemon juice. Set aside.

4. Heat nonstick frying pan. Add meat and stir-fry until brown, about 5 minutes. Drain meat, remove to another container, and cover to keep warm.

5. In same frying pan, stir-fry carrots 5 minutes or until tender-crisp. Add remaining vegetables and stir-fry 2 minutes. Add meat and cornstarch mixture. Bring to a boil. Cook, stirring constantly, until thickened.

6. Serve over rice.

EACH SERVING PROVIDES:
3 ounces from meat group
1 serving from vegetable group
1–1/2 servings from bread group

Lentil Stroganoff

4 servings, 1–1/2 cups stroganoff and 3/4 cup noodles each

PER SERVING:

Calories   520
Total fat   5 grams
Saturated fat   1 gram
Cholesterol   48 milligrams
Sodium   340 milligrams

Lentils, dry, 1–1/2 cups
Water, 4–1/2 cups
Salt, 1/4 teaspoon
Vegetable oil, 1 teaspoon
Fresh mushrooms, sliced, 1–1/2 cups
Red or green pepper, cut in strips, 1 cup
Onion, chopped, 1/2 cup
Flour, 3 tablespoons
Dry mustard, 2 teaspoons
Black pepper, 1/4 teaspoon
Plain lowfat yogurt, 8-ounce container
Egg noodles, cooked, 3 cups
Green onion, sliced, 2 tablespoons

1. Combine lentils, water, and salt in a large saucepan. Bring to a boil; cover, reduce heat, and cook until lentils are tender, about 30 minutes. Drain; set lentils aside and keep warm. Save liquid; add water to make 1–1/2 cups.

2. Heat oil in a large frying pan. Add mushrooms, peppers, and onion. Cook until vegetables are just tender.

3. Mix flour and seasonings. Stir evenly into vegetable mixture. Add saved liquid, stirring constantly. Cook over medium heat until mixture is smooth and thickened.

4. Add lentils; mix well. Heat to serving temperature.

5. Just before serving, stir in yogurt.

6. Cook noodles according to package directions.

7. Serve stroganoff over noodles. Garnish with green onion slices.

EACH SERVING PROVIDES:
Meat alternate equal to 2 ounces from meat group
1–1/2 servings from bread group
1–1/4 servings from vegetable group
1/4 serving from milk group

Apricot-Glazed Chicken
4 servings, about 3 ounces chicken each
PER SERVING:
Calories   210
Total fat   2 grams
Saturated fat   Trace
Cholesterol   68 milligrams
Sodium   155 milligrams

Lemon juice, 2 tablespoons
Garlic, minced, 1 clove
Pepper, 1/4 teaspoon
Boneless skinless chicken breast halves, 4
Orange juice, 3/4 cup
Dried apricots, 12 halves
Vinegar, 1 tablespoon
Brown sugar, packed, 1 teaspoon
Prepared mustard, 1 teaspoon
Ground ginger, 1/4 teaspoon
Salt, 1/8 teaspoon
Raisins, 1/4 cup

1. Preheat oven to 400° F.

2. Combine lemon juice, garlic, and pepper. Brush chicken with the mixture.

3. Arrange chicken on a rack in a baking dish. Cover and bake 45 minutes.

4. Combine orange juice and apricots in a small saucepan. Simmer, uncovered for 10 minutes until apricots are tender. Stir in vinegar, sugar, mustard, ginger, and salt. Simmer 2 minutes longer. Remove from heat and pour into blender jar. Purée apricots about 15 seconds. Add raisins.

5. Spread half of the glaze on one side of the chicken; bake 3 minutes longer. Turn chicken and spread with remaining glaze. Return to oven for 3 more minutes or until chicken is tender.

EACH SERVING PROVIDES:
3 ounces from meat group
1/2 serving from fruit group

Rice-Pasta Pilaf
4 servings, about 3/4 cup each
PER SERVING:

Calories	205
Total fat	5 grams
Saturated fat	1 gram
Cholesterol	0
Sodium	225 milligrams

Brown rice, uncooked, 1/2 cup
Chicken broth, unsalted, 2–1/4 cups
Thin spaghetti, broken into 1/2 to 1-inch pieces, 1/2 cup
Margarine, 1 tablespoon
Green onions, chopped, 3 tablespoons
Green pepper, chopped, 3 tablespoons
Fresh mushrooms, chopped, 3 tablespoons
Garlic, minced, 1 small clove
Savory, 3/4 teaspoon
Salt, 1/4 teaspoon
Pepper, 1/8 teaspoon

1. Cook rice in 1–3/4 cups of the broth in a covered saucepan until almost tender, about 35 minutes.

2. Cook spaghetti in margarine in heavy pan over low heat until golden brown, about 2 minutes. Stir frequently; watch carefully.

3. Add browned spaghetti, vegetables, remaining 1/2 cup of chicken broth, and seasonings to rice.

4. Bring to boil, reduce heat, cover, and cook over medium heat until liquid is absorbed, about 10 minutes.

5. Remove from heat; let stand 2 minutes.

EACH SERVING PROVIDES:
1–1/2 servings from bread group
1/4 serving from vegetable group

Peach Crisp
10 servings, about 1/2 cup each
PER SERVING:

Calories   155
Total fat   4 grams
Saturated fat   1 gram
Cholesterol   0
Sodium   40 milligrams

Frozen, unsweetened peaches, 2 16-ounce bags
Cornstarch, 2 tablespoons
Lemon juice, 2 teaspoons
Flour, 1/2 cup
Sugar, 1/2 cup
Ground cinnamon, 1/2 teaspoon
Ground cloves, 1/4 teaspoon
Margarine, softened, 3 tablespoons
Quick rolled oats, 1/2 cup

1. Preheat oven to 375° F.

2. Place peaches in an 8″ × 8″ baking dish. Add cornstarch; toss to mix evenly.

3. Sprinkle lemon juice over peaches.

4. Mix flour, sugar, and spices.

5. Stir margarine into oats; add flour mixture. Mix until crumbly.

6. Sprinkle crumb mixture evenly over peaches.

7. Bake 45 minutes or until peaches are tender and top is lightly browned.

EACH SERVING PROVIDES:
3/4 serving from fruit group
1/2 serving from bread group

Source: Anne Shaw, Lois Fulton, Carole Davis, and Myrtle Hogbin, *Using the Food Guide Pyramid: A Resource for Nutrition Educators.* Washington, D.C., U.S. Department of Agriculture, Food, Nutrition, and Consumer Services, Center For Nutrition Policy and Promotion, pp. 86–88, 58–82.

Index

About the Authors

MARJOLIJN BIJLEFELD is a freelance writer and editor. She is the author of *The Gun Control Debate: A Documentary History* (Greenwood, 1997), *Teen Guide to Personal Financial Management* (Greenwood, 2000), and *Food and You: A Guide to Healthy Habits for Teens* (Greenwood, 2001).

SHARON K. ZOUMBARIS is a professional librarian, freelance writer, and storyteller. She is author of *Teen Guide to Personal Financial Management* (Greenwood, 2000) and *Food and You: A Guide to Healthy Habits for Teens* (Greenwood, 2001).